Rethinking Rhinoplasty and Facial Surgery

Howard D. Stupak

Rethinking Rhinoplasty and Facial Surgery

A Structural Anatomic Re-Analysis of the Face and Nose and Their Role in Aesthetics, Airway, and Sleep

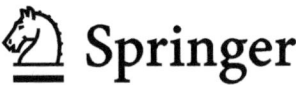 Springer

Howard D. Stupak
Otolaryngology/Head and Neck Surgery
Albert Einstein College of Medicine
Bronx, NY
USA

ISBN 978-3-030-44673-4   ISBN 978-3-030-44674-1   (eBook)
https://doi.org/10.1007/978-3-030-44674-1

This Springer imprint is published by the registered company Springer Nature Switzerland AG
The registered company address is: Gewerbestrasse 11, 6330 Cham, Switzerland

This book is dedicated to my mentor and fellowship director, Calvin M. Johnson, Jr., who helped foster the career of many prominent surgeons in our field. While he may or may not agree with many of the concepts in this book, without the framework of structural/anatomic understanding, surgical and diagnostic skills, and approach to patients that he taught me, I would hardly have even able to "rethink" anything. I am deeply indebted to his generosity in sharing his thoughts so openly.

I am also extremely grateful to the many other teachers and mentors who have helped shape my career and thoughts – especially to my public school teachers in the Caldwell school system for their patience in developing a late-bloomer, in particular gym teacher and coach Ed Gibbons, who encouraged competitiveness in sports and self-confidence. I thank my professors at Emory University and the Albert Einstein College of Medicine for a fun, wonderful, and broad education and for the introduction to many aspects of biology and medicine. I warmly thank my mentors from

Otolaryngology/Head and Neck Surgery residency at the University of California, San Francisco, especially Andrew Murr, Andrew Goldberg, and David Eisele, for making sure I became a competent and professional physician. I thank Marc Singer and Corey Maas for introducing me to the world of surgical innovation and to Facial Plastic and Reconstructive Surgery.

I would like to thank Marvin Fried, John Bent, Richard Smith, and the faculty and residents of the Otolaryngology Department at Montefiore/Einstein where I am very fortunate to be part of for permitting me to teach and practice with my own style. I also thank my colleagues at Jacobi Medical Center for such great support, from the chair of Surgery, John McNelis, to my fellow surgeons and patients, from whom I have learned so much over the years and for their tremendous effort in the Covid crisis. I also cannot overstate how happy I have been to work with the Jacobi Otolaryngology physician assistants, residents and staff over the years, who have always been so supportive: Nicole Santopietro, Katrina Falkovitch, Diana Kariyev, and Dila Kilaja. I thank Alan Cohen and Joanne Salerno and all of my patients for their tremendous and long-running support of my private practice in Westport.

Of course, I must thank my parents, Susan and Elliot, and brothers, Daniel and Jeffrey, for fostering an amazing family environment of creativity and fun and lifelong learning. Most importantly, this book is for Allison, Grant, Asher, and Harper – you are my true inspiration and love!

Preface/Summary

Disciplines involving the understanding of structure, like rhinoplasty, facial surgery, and otolaryngology, have achieved great strides by incorporating statistical evidence-based medicine in the twentieth century, moving from an anecdotal art form to a science-based series of algorithms. Despite these advances, a focus on specific therapeutic "maneuvers" and whether these tactics result in improvement has resulted in a general disregard for the probing into the structural origins of the physical causation of disorders. With an inquiry into the origins of these causative forces, disorders can be reversed or prevented much more efficiently and naturally than the statistically driven accumulated maneuvers that fuel our treatment algorithms.

Communication and education about topics like rhinoplasty today are largely dispensed by an oligarchy of the conventional, who, in the interest of standardization, control our academies with very fixed educational and research messaging. This is generally the reason why techniques, current knowledge, and results in this field have been largely frozen in time since the late twentieth century supported by mostly uninteresting confirmatory data.

In this environment, only few are willing to challenge the rigid standards, facing an uphill battle with substantial review board, hospital/institutional, legal, and publication obstacles.

With a little bit of reconsideration, one can see how wonderfully simple the external nose is and how it interacts with the underlying facial skeleton and soft tissue. Even more simply, surgical treatments can directly address the root cause of the problem, and not simply consist of a series of steps that fix only downstream manifestations of the problem.

This book is literally the opposite of the standard *comprehensive* rhinoplasty or facial surgery text, perhaps serving as a complement to these books. It questions everything we do and accepts nothing as granted. The stepwise tactic-style surgery that consists of additive (e.g., grafts or sutures) or subtractive (e.g., cartilage removal or scoring/turbinate reduction) that is the norm in surgery is the result of overly linear thinking. A multidimensional view of these problems, fostered by understanding the root cause of nasal and facial structural deficiencies, can help us design better plans, more focused on logic-based framework adjustments in three-dimensional space, which have the potential to create more efficient, aesthetic, and realistic results. This book is meant to actually be read in order, unlike most texts, and is designed to be engaging, not all-encompassing, with each chapter building on the next. It focuses on basic cause and effect using logic and reason, illustrated with the simplest diagrams designed to illustrate specific concepts, one at a time, like "chalk-talk." This is in contrast to the more technical, professionally illustrated guides that focus on optimizing maneuver-based surgery via photos or diagrams of graft or suture placement.

Here, the reader is not forced to swallow the rigid algorithms hoisted upon them by the experts, but is encouraged to reach their own deeper conclusions about the nature of facial and airway problems.

Bronx, NY, USA   Howard D. Stupak

Acknowledgement/Conflict of Interest Statement

This book is not intended to serve as a guide to the steps of surgical procedures and does not give specific medical advice for any disorder. Instead, this book is intended to help individuals reason in a more logical fashion than the conventionally accepted wisdom about anatomy and function of the human facial skeleton and airway. Many of the concepts in this book are just that – concepts. Many of these concepts will stand the test of time, and others will require further evolution. I personally use these concepts in their current form in my practice to assist in medical decisions, but many of these would be considered off-label treatments if devices were involved and can differ from the current "standard of care." I always recommend clearly understanding and explaining the "standard-of-care" treatments to patients before even discussing "off-label" alternatives to ensure maximal transparency. Finally, I do have a conflict of interest in owning intellectual property related to a nasal valve device discussed in Chap. 6, the Alar™ device, licensed to Medtronic ENT. The discussion of this device was purposely limited in this manuscript. I attempt to briefly discuss it as objectively as possible. But, of course, this does not remove all traces of bias, so use caution when interpreting this perspective. I also have applied for intellectual property related to mandible fracture repair devices, including a variation on the vertical plate described in Chap. 10, but this has not been commercialized.

Contents

Part I
Toward an Understanding
of Structure/Function Interaction

Chapter 1
The Problem We Face: The "Compartmentalized" Conventional View of Facial/Nasal Anatomy

Beyond Spreader Grafts: Do We Ask "Why?" Enough?

> When you develop your opinions on the basis of weak evidence, you will have difficulty interpreting subsequent information that contradicts these opinions, even if this new information is obviously more accurate.—Nassim Nicholas Taleb (from The Black Swan, with permission)

Deep, creative curiosity about the "why?" of our surgeries is never encouraged. Rounding as a surgical team, as logistics are discussed, everyone is quietly annoyed with the junior student or resident who insists that while yes, they understand that the algorithm recommends surgery as the next step, they want to know *why*? In other words, they want to engage reason and the language of causality. They do not just want to hear what the next step in the protocol is. Eventually, this apprentice, seeing the annoyance of his or her superiors will stop asking, and later, may even stop wondering about deeper reasoning as they advance into practice and embrace the routine of step-wise standards of care. We feel justified in disregarding these questions, as Judea Pearl says in his recent book on causality, that questions requiring imagination can appear unscientific [1].

On the whole, the surgical research establishment also tends to avoid straying too far in to deep reasoning questions, preferring primarily to reinforce and confirm the treatment standards, or expand treatment indications. Statistics are used to show that one maneuver is superior to another, and the field evolves slowly, preferring one treatment for a period, usually evolving into higher-tech alternatives over time, as devices improve. But beyond the occasional look at optimizing indications or the inflammatory cascade in wound healing, the algorithm itself is not questioned.

The overly conservative leadership, citing "safety," remains overly reliant on the simple recipe-like format of step-wise procedures and upon rote replication of adages taught to them by mentors. While this is not necessarily a problem minute to minute and case to case, possibly even providing a degree of stability and safety in preventing disasters, over the long-term, inability to see beyond the cookbook

© Springer Nature Switzerland AG 2020
H. D. Stupak, *Rethinking Rhinoplasty and Facial Surgery*,
https://doi.org/10.1007/978-3-030-44674-1_1

mentality of the "standard of care" can hinder us from evolving and providing real value to patients beyond very limited basics. The knowledge of these experts, despite extensive clinical experience may actually be expertise in a very rigid and flawed paradigm of understanding due to a significant lack of variability of approach.

Perhaps you, like me, have experienced some *frustration* in following practice guidelines that do not seem to match reason, particularly when following a seemingly disparate series of steps outlined in a procedural or algorithmic manual. Following the prescribed steps, we are led to believe that the series of steps we perform will yield a positive outcome, perhaps an esthetic or functional breathing outcome in the case of rhinoplasty. But, as in the case of the disappointed artist who expected a masterpiece to result from following a set of instructions, the results are limited and do not correlate with the degree of precision to which the steps were followed.

For example, in rhinoplasty, most conventional textbooks contend that placement of a "spreader graft," first described by Sheen in 1984 [2], will result in improved airway function and symmetry. However, it only takes a short exercise in logic and structure, as well as some thoughtful experience to see that a graft placed between the medial border or the upper lateral cartilage, and the dorsal septum will be a *space-occupying* object that impinges on the caliber of the airway and cannot possibly improve airflow even though it will make the nasal bridge wider. It can be mathematically proven as well: If the height of the septum and base of the sill were 1 cm, for example, and a spreader graft was placed that widened the airway apex (dorsal) by 3 mm (septal cartilage is 2 mm thick, but let us be generous) (Fig. 1.1) and had a depth of 3 mm, it would have a cross-sectional area of 45.5 mm², using the formula for area of a trapezoid: Area = (base1 + base2) × height/2. Without the spreader graft, the cross-sectional area of the pre-operative airway is *larger*, at 50 mm², using the formula for area of a triangle: A = (base × height)/2. Further,

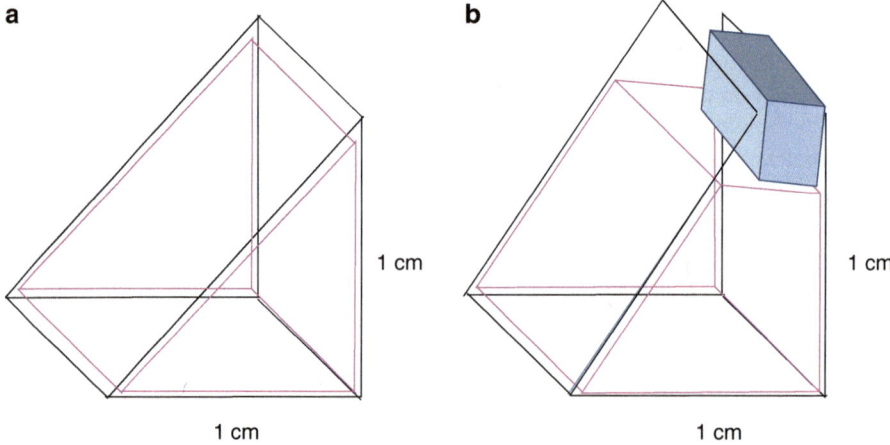

a   **b**

                                          1 cm   1 cm

          1 cm   1 cm

Fig. 1.1 Schematic of right "internal nasal valve." (**a**) Shows base or septal height of 1 cm, width at bony sill of 1 cm, and the diagonal component is upper lateral cartilage. (**b**) Shows the same height and width, but has a spreader graft between upper lateral cartilage and septum

while the cross-sectional area is made smaller, the entire premise of the spreader graft targeting the internal nasal valve is marginal, as only enlarging the nostril or vestibule *relative* to the nasal cavity is useful in increasing laminar flow, as we will discuss in future chapters. The two outcomes most reported in the literature that measure the outcomes from spreader grafts, internal nasal valve angle (abnormal is less than 15°), and Nasal Obstruction Severity Outcome (NOSE) scores are severely flawed in that the first is simply a reflection of the viewed mucosal angle that has no bearing on airflow, and as you can see in Fig. 1.1 actually represents a foreshortening of the airway at the level of graft placement. And the latter, while very popular and validated is not a measure of airflow at all but of *patient perception*. And while the illusion of patient satisfaction is an important concept in empathy, basing research upon solely subjective patient opinion as our "gold standard" surrogate of nasal airflow is a very big problem indeed [3]. Perception by individuals who have experienced only one nose in their lifetime (and thus have nothing to compare it to) is too variable to adequately correlate in a linear fashion with physical functions like flow. Much more about this is discussed later in the book.

At the end of the day, we need to strive toward measuring actual function and to predictably and systematically being able to create sound aesthetic and functional structure without an overly complex system that makes little practical sense. Most of the frustration and difficulty I experienced earlier in my practice was not related to executing or following steps in a procedure, but in achieving inconsistent results in functional and aesthetic outcomes. Was I not executing the plan as accurately as I was led to believe when attending conferences, or was I doing too much or too little? Were the patients just difficult, or did I not explain things very well in advance? The results were like a roller coaster, sometimes people were thrilled, other times, even with what results seemed OK, they were depressed. Patients breathed better but mostly only a little and inconsistently. Patients looked better, but also an inconsistent amount. Crooked noses were made a little less crooked, sometimes not by much, and always just camouflaged to look less crooked. I also felt limited by the procedures we had available. The sub-mucous-resection septoplasty that I learned as a resident that simply was the removal of a small patch of posterior septal cartilage and bone (with forbidden manipulation of the L-strut beyond preservation) was a far cry from the complex open rhinoplasty functional and aesthetic procedure that I learned from my fellowship director. But, in the patient who fell between these two procedural extremes, perhaps with moderate nasal obstruction and mild aesthetic issues, which was the correct procedure to choose? Choose over-operation or under-operation. Was there truly no middle ground? How could two procedures that addressed similar problems be so divergent, and why didn't the concepts make more sense? Did we have any idea of what the root physical and natural causes of the aesthetic and functional deformity was, or were we most interested in just following the accepted standard model of how these procedures are taught by the leaders of the rhinoplasty field?

Failure, I started to note was everywhere, but we do not even have the language terminology to discuss *incompletely achieving our goals*, but only terminology to discuss severe *complications* and malpractice. I also found that there was and is no shortage of revision rhinoplasty patients (despite a "conventional wisdom" revision rate of about 10%). Also, one could not help but notice how many nasal obstruction patients, many over- or under-treated, had undergone many procedures, but apparently not one that actually helped, and were called "refractory" by their surgeon. Even the "top" surgeons, the lecturers at the meetings had patients grumbling about them and seemed unable to find a procedure that was consistently beneficial.

The problem extended well beyond just rhinoplasty specialists. The same patients were seeing providers in different specialties for essentially the same problem (unbeknownst to themselves), but each specialist essentially would give an entirely different treatment plan, with usually very rigid parameters and totally different explanations. This dissociation of knowledge known as "compartmentalization." This condition is where specialists of one discipline are not aware of the knowledge of other disciplines and focus upon a problem from a uni-dimensional perspective, not even aware that other perspectives exist, and certainly unable to see causality of disorder, only treatment options. This is particularly a problem in the experienced and sometimes senior experts, who, believing that they were taught the only solution to a problem, only are capable of imagining slight variations as innovation in their field. One example is someone who fashions themselves as forward thinking because they have sampled multiple different energy devices in order to perform inferior turbinate reduction, without ever considering beyond "allergy" why the turbinates grew larger in the first place.

Classic compartmentalization occurs when different specialists treat the same problem but from vastly different perspectives, most failing to see the big picture, or doing a root cause analysis (Fig. 1.2). To me, this stems from algorithm or list-type

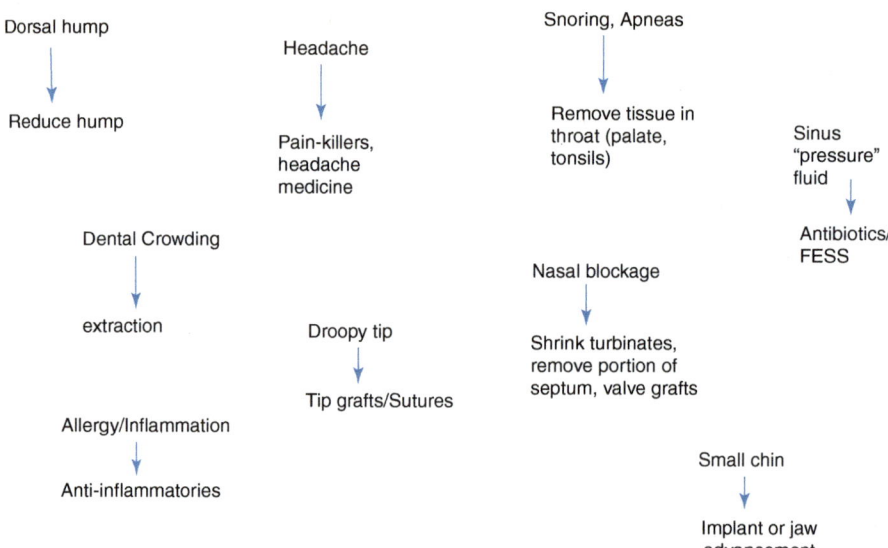

Fig. 1.2 Causal diagram of compartmentalized symptoms and the "appropriate" treatment without bigger picture thinking

(indications versus contra-indications) thinking and learning that we subject our trainees to. Once we hear a chief complaint, we launch into our compartmentalized targeted history and physical, perform the diagnostic tests, and eventually come up with the recommended therapeutic procedure or medication. Whether or not our therapy was successful is only an afterthought, and typically failure just triggers another step in the algorithm (i.e., refractory diagnosis and treatment).

While we tend to focus on hospital marketing materials on inter-specialty collaboration and access, in reality collaboration tends to mean referrals to colleagues in another specialty. And while this also seems harmless, it can make the tunnel-vision that specialists have even more complete. The tendency to rely on "expert" clinical consensus, like that on nasal valve compromise [4] can be equally limiting, with the opinions of the experts just serving to reinforce the conservative status quo, where no insight in to actual disease root cause or best treatment can be discerned.

In a clinical example, many patients can present to a practice with chief complaints that typically would require a specialist to follow a classic algorithm. For example, a patient with pain over the midface could present to many specialists and be sent on a vastly different diagnostic and treatment algorithm depending on who they are sent to by their primary doctor, by the internet, or even by a billboard. A sinus specialist would no doubt perform endoscopy and possibly order a CT (computed tomography) scan to evaluate and treat sinusitis. A dental specialist might consider dental caries and dry mouth, while an oral surgeon might evaluate the patient for wisdom tooth impaction and plan removal, and an orthodontist may focus upon crowding and occlusion irregularities. An otolaryngologist may be most interested in the deviated septum, large turbinates, and long uvula and soft palate that the patient has and will evaluate with fiberoptic endoscopy. The plastic surgeon may be most interested in discussing the patient's dorsal hump and weak chin. The headache specialist will rule-out various organic causes of headaches before prescribing medication and the internist diagnoses chronic fatigue syndrome and depression. In reality, the tunnel-blindness and two-dimensional thinking exhibited by all of the specialists in this sample (but based on reality) case, fail to even consider why the patient has such a slew of symptoms or even why this patient needs to see so many specialists. As we will discuss in future chapters, the patient's underlying problem is limited facial structural growth, not within the disease spectrum of a syndromic facial growth disorder, but part of the general weakening and shrinking of the facial bone structure of the general human population. This is possibly due to "gracilization" of *Homo sapiens* as taught by anthropologists occurring as technology and sedentariness take the place of heavy activity that had been required once to survive. This subtle limitation in facial growth causes aesthetic limitations, a predictable pattern of nasal deformity and predisposes to mouth-breathing, all of which we will discuss in future chapters. This mouth-breathing phenomenon predisposes the individual to a broad spectrum of worsening sleep apnea, headaches, depression, dry mouth, and is associated with dental crowding and decay due to insufficient mandibular space and dry mucosal barriers.

So, how did we get this so wrong, especially in the age of technology and evidence-based medicine (EBM)? The answer may lie in how we are trained to consider problems. From the moment we begin clinical training we are taught that the "Chief Complaint" is the essence and primary goal of the visit to the doctor. While noble sounding, patient-centric, in many ways, it is focusing on this chief complaint that may be the cause of inefficient thinking. The chief complaint will trigger a clinical algorithm that determines which specialist will be seen, and in this multifactorial example, will be determined by the problem that the patient decides to communicate first, regardless of its relationship to root cause. Instead, while less socially inviting, we perhaps should focus on a root cause analysis (RCA) of the patient's spectrum of problems, and anatomic deficiencies. RCA has been used successfully in medicine as an analysis of major errors and accident prevention [5]. In contrast, I am not suggesting a post-care RCA, but that we reconsider how we approach problems, and consider a RCA for every patient as they enter care. One way is to strategically rethink patient visits themselves, and even how to analyze our care and treatment decisions from another perspective.

For example, imagine that five clones, all with a similar disorder like the one described above visited five different specialists. While all five clones have the same disorder, they all present to the five specialists with five different chief complaints. Perhaps one is focused upon the "sinus" pain, another on the fatigue, another on the dental crowding, and yet another on nasal discharge, and the final one on an aesthetic deformity. Five different chief complaints to five specialists, all will follow different algorithms to treat the patient five different ways, all inadvertently chosen by the patient. In reality, there is possibly a best solution, or perhaps multiple long-term solutions, but we are not equipped, due to narrow thinking, specialty compartmentalization and current business practices and fee structuring to handle this adequately.

From a surgical perspective, even the way we call our techniques "procedures" narrows our perspective causing us to focus upon the series of steps involved instead of a logical approach to strategy, risk-benefit analysis, and the actual physical forces involved in causing the disease. In rhinoplasty, for example we are taught that only the delicate placement of grafts and sutures, as dictated by the experts are paramount to a successful result. We are repeatedly taught this at meetings by panels of these experts, in residency, in textbooks, and even in peer-reviewed articles. But, evidence-based medicine (EBM) and "expertise" should protect us from incorrect conclusions, right? The answer is complicated: Of course, analyzing clinical data does provide real evidence of association or efficacy, but it does NOT explain cause and effect, and never makes sure we are asking the right questions! If we do not ask the correct question, we cannot find the correct answers.

So, while we can analyze various maneuvers in rhinoplasty with outcome measures, the data will never give us an understanding of how the nose really develops, becomes pathologic, or requires treatment without *reason*. "Reason" is the missing ingredient for too long in our fields. As Judea Pearl reminds us in his book, even extensive mining of data will not reveal answers if we do not know what we are looking for [1].

Rhinoplasty surgery, with so many variables and steps involved in its modern form, is almost impossible to scientifically evaluate without confusion by confounding data. However, it only takes occasional deeper thought, if one has the interest in questioning the well-established dogma that we accept during our training indoctrination to realize that there are many inconsistencies in what is generally taught. For example, only a limited understanding of the forces of nature or the physical world will dictate that the placement of objects like sutures for example beyond their role in reinforcement, cannot possibly result in permanent changes to spring-like cartilaginous structures, and provide almost zero therapeutic value in any surgery beyond as an agent for scarification (despite what appears frequently in lectures, meetings, and textbooks). Along the same line of thinking, grafts cannot make existing cartilage stronger, but can only replace absent cartilage, as the existing cartilage, despite suturing, without adequate release will revert to its original position, as any spring-like structure in nature (think of the bent sapling). Only the principles of approach, release, reposition, and reinforcement (see Chap. 7) will permit lasting change in any surgical procedure.

Because of this, one cannot help but question how over half of a century of expertise in multiple fields could have a created a well-intentioned, but incomplete framework of understanding of how to consider facial surgery and its interaction with structure and the airway.

By creating and then replicating a framework of "rules" of medical treatment and procedures, many based on untestable adages, the experts of the past few generations have failed to notice that the educational system now fails to match the unbendable dictates of nature. Unfortunately, the hierarchical and rigid system of medical education (blindly replicate your mentors techniques and principles, as they once did for their mentor), as embodied in the "see one, do one, teach one" mentality has only served to prevent deviation from this pathway. Further, because specialists are financially rewarded for performing existing procedures by insurance codes and financial structures, and not for questioning paradigms, there are few who even begin to seriously question the existing model, as there is no incentive to. This reliance on a series of rules of management that does not mirror nature is called the Ludic Fallacy by Nicholas Taleb [5]. This essentially is a set of instructions, as for a board-game or sport, but that does not actually match the real-world environment. Taleb uses the example of the chess-master who assumes through his knowledge of strategy that he/she will be a great military general as well, only to find during battle/reality that they are excellent only at playing chess.

As we discussed earlier, this is only enforced more by compartmentalization, or failure to see beyond the narrow borders of our own specialty, and has also created a sort of myopia, or failure to understand the big picture *of the actual cause* and not just the manifestations of disease (e.g., an Otolaryngologist who fails to see the dental/facial structure root cause of a sleep disorder because he/she has never trained on, or paid attention to anything related to jaw structures, and instead focuses only on the internal pharyngeal aspect of sleep via a fiberoptic scope). This is literally, a form of "tunnel-vision" that encourages some of these providers to think the endoscope will provide all of the answers, while in reality it completely fails to identify the invisible forces that are the root cause as we will discuss in future chapters.

In many ways, I believe that it is this dissociation of the hierarchical set of rules from actual reality and the laws of nature that is subconsciously responsible for what is increasingly called "physician burnout" in increasingly self-aware physicians who may not have the words to describe their condition.

So, What Is the Solution?

Never ask the doctor what you should do. Ask him what he would do if he were in your place. You would be surprised at the difference.—Nassim Nicholas Taleb, Antifragile: Things That Gain from Disorder, 2018 [6] (with permission)

A workable analogy for our problem was provided in the book *Topgun: An American Story* (2019) by Dan Pedersen [7], a cofounder of the program of the same name that was the inspiration for the film starring Tom Cruise. In this book, Pedersen describes how the once great US naval fighter aviation program that had achieved tremendous rates of success over their enemies during World War II and Korea had slipped into mediocrity against their enemies in the sky during the 1960s Vietnam conflict largely due to disconnect from the leadership in Washington. After a "manifesto" for improvement was written by a junior officer on ways to radically rethink dogfight strategy and tactics, the Topgun program was established and run by these young radicals to disseminate the information to the fleet. After this *knowledge* (this was not a change in high-tech weapons systems) became widespread throughout the Navy, the success rates during the later Vietnam conflict returned to that of the prior generations, and the program remains today, supporting this success.

In the same way, we must take a critical eye to even our beloved EBM, peer review process, and even our rigid residency training paradigms to recognize that the root of our problems today may be our system itself, and how it is self-reinforcing. Instead of the forlorn hope that data will give us causal answers, we must use logic and intuition combined with data to understand cause and effect [1].

All of the concepts discussed above will be expanded further in this book, but we will also begin to discuss how we can acknowledge that reason has a place in surgery *every day*. As you can see, our purpose in this text is not, like usual to provide a comprehensive view of existing EBM to confirm the use of conventional maneuvers in rhinoplasty, or simply show how subtle nuances in technique ("how I do it") or how high-tech improvements like the DaVinci "robot" can help your practice. If you read further, you will see how with we can completely rethink the paradigms of the "how" and "why" of structural disorders of the nose and facial skeleton in humans. Further, we will discuss why reframing the origins of this process will help us plan better, more efficient treatment, including preventative strategies for function, aesthetics, and overall health.

This book is not about a single way to do more thoughtful nasal airway and aesthetic treatment planning, but about *why* we need to look at problems from multiple perspectives, and *not* just one.

References

1. Pearl J. The book of why: the new science of causality. London: Penguin; 2019.
2. Sheen JH. Spreader graft: a method of reconstructing the roof of the middle nasal vault following rhinoplasty. Plast Reconstr Surg. 1984;73(2):230–9.
3. Teymoortash A, Fasunla JA, Sazgar AA. The value of spreader grafts in rhinoplasty: a critical review. Eur Arch Otorhinolaryngol. 2012;269(5):1411–6.
4. Rhee JS, Weaver EM, Park SS, Baker SR, Hilger PA, Kriet JD, Murakami C, Senior BA, Rosenfeld RM, DiVittorio D. Clinical consensus statement: diagnosis and management of nasal valve compromise. Otolaryngol Head Neck Surg. 2010;143(1):48–59.
5. Wu AW, Lipshutz AK, Pronovost PJ. Effectiveness and efficiency of root cause analysis in medicine. JAMA. 2008;299(6):685–7.
6. Taleb NN. Antifragile: Things that gain from disorder. New York: Penguin Random House; 2014.
7. Pedersen D. Topgun. An American story. New York: Hachette; 2019.

Chapter 2
The Invisible Forces in Our Nasal Airway: Air Flow and Cavity Negative Pressure

Nasal Obstruction Versus Nasal Underuse: Are the Turbinates the Problem or the Solution?

The problem with experts is that they do not know what they do not know (with permission).—Nassim Nicholas Taleb, The Black Swan: The Impact of the Highly Improbable

Imagine for a moment that we have just arrived in our world from a faraway planet or time where of course the laws of nature and physics are the same, but all of our technology and cultural norms are different. As we begin to explore this foreign world, one of the first places we chance upon is a massive airplane hangar housing a jumbo jet that is being serviced for an unknown mechanical problem. With wonder, we gaze at the tremendous beast before us, and we search our memory for a similar type of object, finding nothing. We try to consider what such an object is used for, but we cannot come up with a reasonable function.

So, we use the diagnostic equipment we have to find a purpose of the machine. A magnifying type device reveals little but that the device's skin is of a strong substance that appears to be weather resistant, with few sharp edges. We guide an endoscope into the bulging protrusions along the body of the object, which reveals large blade-like objects arranged around an axle in a circular fashion. And of course we notice the platform-like extensions on either side of the object. We apply a primitive X-ray type device to these platforms and only find more beams and much hollow useless space. The large wheels and robust tires suggest that the device is used for ground transportation, perhaps like a bus.

When we observe the jet, nonoperational in its hangar, despite the opportunity to investigate, we fail to understand the full context of this structure and the huge advantage of seeing this structure in action. The tools we used to further study our device, seemingly high-technology served us poorly to identify its purpose, and in reality may have further misled our thinking. Only viewing the jet plane in flight would reveal its secrets, or considering alternative paradigms of understanding.

When we evaluate the human facial skeleton inside with an endoscope, speculum, or headlight, or from externally with an imaging device, we experience similar tunnel vision to the observer in the above scenario. When we see enlarged turbinates for example, in a patient with a nasal complaint we automatically assume that this

© Springer Nature Switzerland AG 2020
H. D. Stupak, *Rethinking Rhinoplasty and Facial Surgery*,
https://doi.org/10.1007/978-3-030-44674-1_2

enlargement is the *origin* of the problem, because this is what we *see*, and the framework of our education has reinforced this belief, as has our business model of providing the shrinking turbinate solution. Typically, we do not consider the alternative possibility that the enlargement could be compensatory or secondary to restricted or absent airflow. Due to our extensive training in the conventional model of turbinate enlargement, its origins based on cause and effect models that predate evidence-based medicine (EBM), we experience confirmation bias and follow established norms. Further, just as magnification offered little help to our observation of the jumbo jet to discern function, the histologic analysis of enlarged turbinates suggests a general picture of inflammation, possibly related to an allergy/infectious etiology. Thus, misguided by our endoscopes and biopsies, we generally believe in an inflammatory→turbinate enlargement→nasal obstruction cascade. Using this flawed framework, we focus our research efforts and pharmaceutical efforts on disrupting the inflammatory cascade, from complex biotechnology research to simple nasal steroid nasal spray. Further, we focus our surgical efforts on reducing the size of these turbinates or removing parts using a whole variety of energy and technologic devices. These devices include lasers, radiofrequency devices, electrocautery devices, and micro-debriders, each technology encouraged by their respective device makers as superior to its predecessors. In reality, it is hard to discern which treatment is better, despite EBM, as our entire understanding of the turbinate paradigm may be flawed. To complete our metaphor, just as the uninitiated observer of the jumbo jet may have considered the large hanging jet turbines to be obtrusive, non-aerodynamic vestiges and could consider removing them for efficiency, we routinely partially remove or damage turbinates in patients without really understanding their purpose or why they enlarge in the first place.

Our confirmation bias is due to an over-reliance on a hypothesis, or set of rules that are accepted nearly universally and almost never questioned. This may be also a result of the medical education process, where trainees are tested, evaluated, and rewarded for their abilities to emulate and reiterate texts, lectures, and "standard-of-care" algorithms. Even the way complications, research, and malpractice law is discussed, practising physicians are always judged relative to the existing set of "treatment rules" and standards, with almost no value given to creativity or rethinking paradigms. Even this short discussion on this topic will tempt many readers to pronounce that we are promoting danger by even suggesting that standards should be reconsidered. On the contrary, we are not suggesting giving license to suggest daily improvisation by practitioners to find or try new treatments, but to thoughtfully, using reason, feedback, and evidence re-evaluate deeply held notions, particularly when possibly destructive to tissue from time to time. Despite certain surgeries being considered as well-established "standards of care," it is my opinion that the burden of evidence should be placed upon the invasive option, not the option of doing less or observation. In other words, as we re-evaluate our treatments critically, the null hypothesis should assume that observation (doing nothing) is equivalent to surgery, until the surgery is proven worthwhile.

As early as a 1932 article, the Royal Society [1] suggested that reduction of the turbinate should enter the "limbo of forgotten industries" after an analysis of the face and airway. Several European clinical studies agreed when published that inferior turbinate enlargement was simply a compensation to septal obstruction, and was not part of the obstruction itself, and "does not add to the relief of nasal obstruction beyond that attained by septal surgery" [2, 3].

A recent study demonstrated that the turbinates of allergy sufferers was no different than that of non-allergic individuals [4].

A German study in 2006 more accurately explained the phenomenon using the only reliable way to evaluate cause and effect: a physiologic model. They found that "on the opposite side of the deviation, the enlargement of the stream channel did not generally lead to a reduction in flow resistance, but rather to a 'dead space', where only a slow-circling eddy was observed. This eddy causes an increase in turbulence. In vivo turbinate hypertrophy occurs to fill this dead-space, thereby reducing turbulent flow without a significant increase in resistance. In cases of moderate septal deviation, compensatory mechanisms of the turbinates can lead to a normalization of nasal airflow and surgical therapy would not be indicated" [5].

The findings of these authors made great strides in understanding the true function of the turbinates as playing a role in reducing nasal "dead space," thus improving the flow of the column of air that reaches the pharynx. Already this is an improvement over the over-simplified concept that more space created in the nasal cavity (turbinate reduction/excision) will improve airflow, as suggested by the majority of studies in the literature that enthusiastically justify turbinate surgery via various means. In reality, these procedures can worsen airflow by increasing physiologic dead-space and creating turbulent circular airflow patterns. One could speculate that this concept and not "airflow sensation" could be partially responsible for the disease entity known as "empty nose syndrome," and why septal perforation patients, despite massive amounts of space in the nasal cavity complain of obstruction.

However, these studies are incomplete in that they only explain the appearance of enlarged turbinates on the contralateral side of septal deviation as a compensatory mechanism to fill overly cavernous dead-space. So, what about all of the patients that have no substantial septal deviation or symmetric turbinates? Surely this must demonstrate that this concept is flawed, or at best limited?

In reality, these earlier studies describing inferior turbinate enlargement as a compensatory process to septal deviation serves as the basis for the understanding the expanded concept of why inferior turbinate enlargement is much more common in patients without septal deviation or other physically obstructive nasal findings. The answer lies in a pervasive physical entity we refer to as "Nasal Underuse."

The Key to Understanding Nasal Pathology: Nasal Obstruction Versus Nasal Underuse

The understanding of this single concept may be the most important in planning successful treatment of nasal and airway problems and avoiding more failure. Essentially, the easily understandable concept of "nasal underuse" is just another

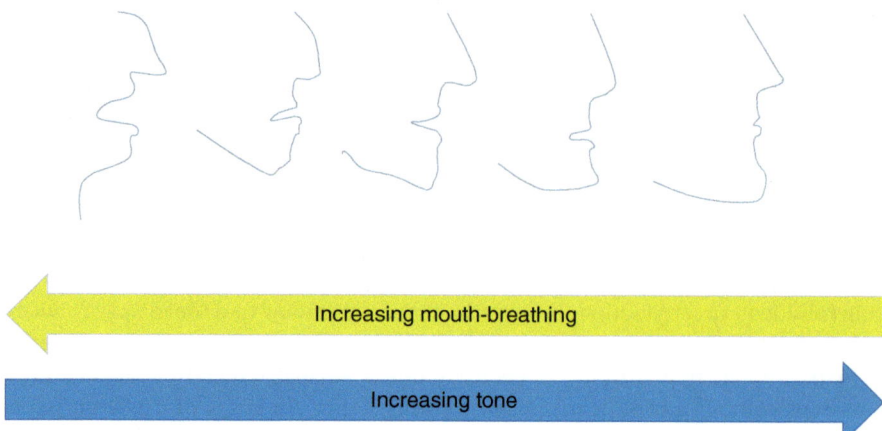

Fig. 2.1 Nocturnal mouth-breathing is inversely proportional to tone, with yellow arrow displaying increasing mouth-breathing while blue arrow indicates increasing tone

variation of the above described mucosal tissue and turbinate enlargement that is compensatory to states of low nasal airflow in *both* chambers of the nasal passage due to various degrees of … *mouth-breathing*. Thus, instead of how nasal "dead-space" and turbulent eddies are formed on the concave or side opposite a septal deviation as described in the Grutzenmacher [5] studies from the last decade, the *entire* nasopharynx and nasal cavities exhibit reduced airflow because all or most airflow is diverted through the mouth and oropharynx. The negative pressure generated by the lungs is still partially transmitted to the nasopharynx by an imperfect soft-palatal seal during states of partial or complete mouth-breathing. So, the degree of mouth-breathing in an individual exists predictably in a spectrum (Fig. 2.1), from a complete mouth-breather with co-existing physical nasal obstruction from deviation and valve collapse to an occasional and partial mouth-breather whose jaw only opens during the deepest stages of sleep when body muscle tone, including that of the jaw closing muscles (temporalis and masseter) are limp [6, 7]. As expected by reasoning, the degree, frequency, and severity of this mouth-breathing will determine what physical manifestations and degree of symptoms a patient will experience.

The negative pressure that subsequently exists in the nasal airway acts upon the nasal soft-tissue of the sidewalls, causing the sidewall and turbinate soft-tissue to expand toward the cavities' lumen during these states of low flow [8].

This concept of how air flow and pressure causes the luminal soft-tissue expansion (called fluid-structure interaction) in the engineering world, and shows the opposite cause and effect relationship that is conventionally accepted (i.e., that tissue enlargement causes airflow reduction) [9]. Figure 2.2 demonstrates on the left, how the negative pressure *extrinsically* draws the turbinate or other erectile tissue intra-luminally, while the right side demonstrates the conventional view that the turbinate (and other tissue) grows *intrinsically* from inflammation/allergy and is the source of obstruction.

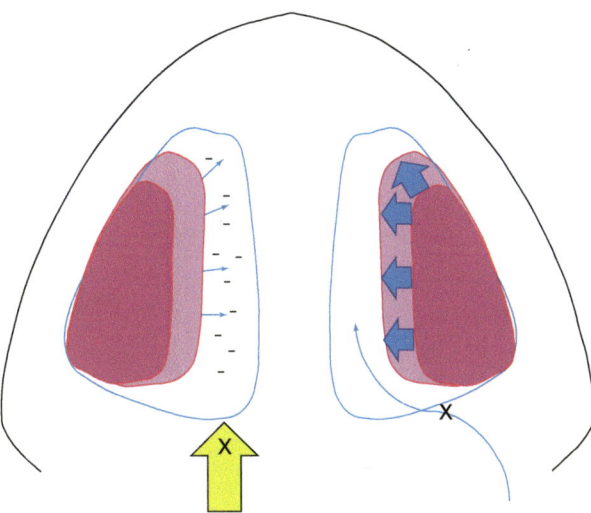

Fig. 2.2 Schematic of nasal inlet demonstrating on the left, how the negative pressure *extrinsically* draws the turbinate or other erectile tissue intra-luminally, while the right side demonstrates the conventional view that the turbinate (and other tissue) grows *intrinsically* from inflammation/ allergy, and is the source of obstruction. The yellow arrow with X indicates a lack of nasal airflow due to mouth-breathing, while in the opposite nostril, the turbinate is the source of obstruction

In reality, the inferior turbinates exist well inside the nasal inlet. And, despite what this consensus of experts concludes, the turbinate enlargement is not the *source* of the obstruction, but is likely primarily a compensatory response to nasal underuse and dead-space. In contrast, over-reduction, (or possibly any reduction) of the compensatory inferior turbinate enlargement has been shown to cause variations on what is known as "Empty nose syndrome," or intranasal turbulence and aerodynamic distortions [10, 11]. This concept is not dissimilar to the equivalent of a lake-type opening in the middle (not inlet) of a flowing river, that of course will not increase flow, instead creating more diffuse circular patterns of flow.

Several studies have examined this clinically, and in models, supporting the nasal underuse concept, albeit without a clear-cut randomized clinical trial, but with enough evidence to demonstrate its importance. Controlled studies showed a large placebo effect for turbinate reduction [12, 13]. Most studies on inferior turbinate surgery simply compare two different techniques, and typically find one is better than the other, although I personally remain cynical about the effectiveness of any reduction technique.

It is well accepted that negative pressure is generated in the nasopharynx during sleep, particularly in Obstructive Sleep Apnea (OSA) patients [14]. What remains unclear is what the significance of the pharyngeal negative pressure is, or more exactly, why it is more negative in OSA patients than in others. In order to test whether primary mouth-breathing, or nasal underuse could be responsible for this negative pressure exacerbation, we tested this using a non-anatomic model of a forked airway (Fig. 2.3).

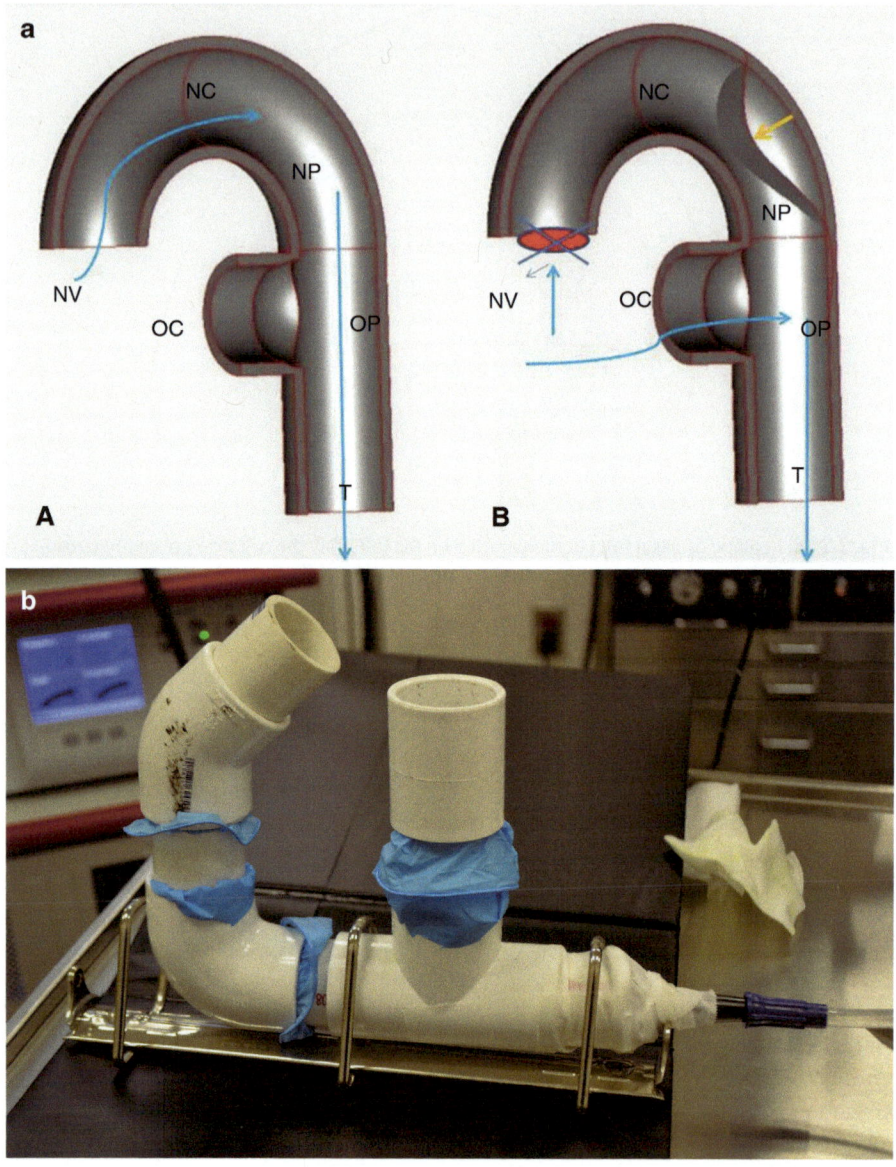

Fig. 2.3 A Non-anatomic model of a "forked" airway made of PVC (polyvinyl chloride) and lined with latex mucosa. (**a**) With the nasal passage opened, mucosa remains in place. (**b**) With the nasal passage occluded (red disk), negative pressure and dead-space occupies the nasal fork, drawing the mucosa intra-luminally at the approximate location of the adenoid (yellow arrow). Blue arrows are airflow. *NV* nasal valve, *NC* nasal cavity, *NP* nasopharynx, *OP* oropharynx, *OC* oral cavity, *T* Trachea and distal airway. B. Actual PVC forked non-anatomic model used for testing in Fig. 2.3. (©Reprinted with Permission from Sage Publishing [15])

In this "forked" tube model, the two forks representing the nasal and oral airways with a confluence in the pharynx was set to negative pressure simulating an inspiratory environment, as the airway would be subjected to during inspiration. The polyvinyl chloride (PVC) pipe, simulating the bony structure of the airway was lined with latex "mucosa" internally. During "nasal" fork breathing, the mucosa remained adjacent to the walls of the bony structure as expected, with easy airflow past the entire airway. However, during mouth-breathing, with limited nasal airway, the latex "mucosa" of the nasal cavity drew intra-luminally, substantially, in the region of the turbinates and adenoid, resembling the erectile tissue of these structures. But, as we have explained, the erectile tissue here does not emerge from its intrinsic growth, but is drawn outward by the intra-luminal build-up of negative pressure due to lack of nasal airflow [15].

I emphasize *forked* airway here in contrast to the conventional view of the airway and pharynx with regard to sleep disorders that typically uses a single tube, and with the known negative pressure involved, Bernoulli's law causes restriction and narrowing of the tube in its center by the distensible soft-tissue [16, 17]. Using this model that the internal soft-tissue is the cause and not result of obstruction, most researchers and clinicians thus justify the use of removal of tissue like the uvula, tonsils, adenoids, or shrinking the base of tongue, in order to limit the collapsible tissue "responsible" for the obstruction. Further, using this model, most consider that pharyngeal collapse during sleep is due to "crowding," although with reasoning, one must wonder why this "crowding" does not cause airway problems during the awake state. A three-pronged forked model, in a negative pressure can be expected to demonstrate a much different aerodynamic behavior, and its study reveals the flaws of the simple tube model that has been so often used.

In the forked airway model described above, we used a fiberoptic scope and recorded the mucosal motion using the video stroboscope. Even more than we expected, in the nasal underuse, mouth-breathing state, the mucosa stretched intra-luminally, resembling turbinate hypertrophy and septal tumescence in the "nasal cavity," and in the nasopharynx, at the curve where the nasopharynx and oropharynx meet, the tissue distended intra-luminally in a pattern that strongly resembled Waldeyer's ring of lymphoid tissue, particularly the adenoid in its posterior nasopharynx position. From this model, we hypothesized that the repeated mucosal intra-luminally directed stretching, as expected to be repeated over a night, or many nights of mouth-breathing in a human, would develop a submucosal inflammatory response as a result of extensive micro-traumas. It is this chronic inflammatory response that we believe most researchers refer to as rhinitis, turbinate hypertrophy, or adenotonsilitis that may be actually due to repeated baro-traumas than as an isolated primary inflammatory response as we imply with some variants of the "allergic rhinitis" variant. For a video of this latex and PVC model, see the video attachment for the scholarly article [15]. To further confirm (indirectly that baro-trauma had occurred in a submucosal fashion as opposed to primary inflammation, a study found that in uvular specimen from uvulopalatoplasty patients, elastin (the elastic structural support of this layer, was severely fragmented in a way not seen in similar inflammatory responses in gut mucosa [18].

Fig. 2.4 Elastin stain of uvular specimen demonstrating disorganization and disruption. (Reprinted with permission from Elsevier Publishing) Stupak and Park [20]

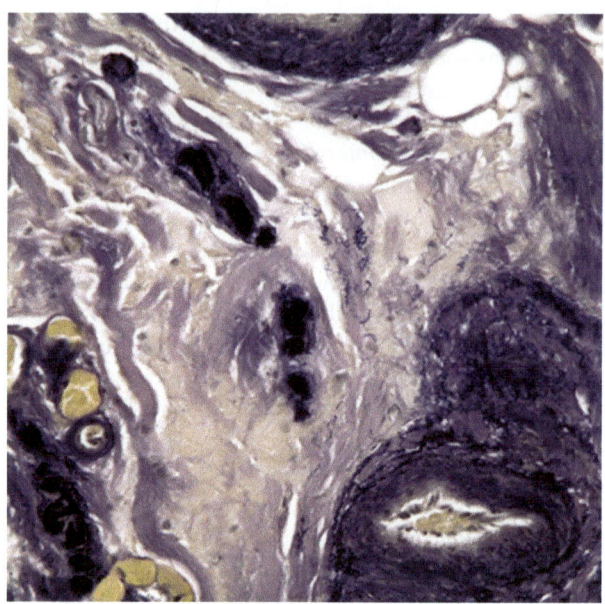

A pathologist, Maria Abadi, MD at our institution confirmed this anecdotally by staining several similar uvular specimen and finding a similar disruption of elastin protein (Fig. 2.4).

Just this basic absence of airflow in the nasal passages and nasopharynx during inspiration (negative pressure state) creates in both the model, and in physiologic sleep [14] a relative dead-space, or vacuum-like environment. Simple reasoning will predict that this state over the long term, from repeated negative pressure will induce a direct change to the mucosal lining of these chambers, as in the physical model. Further, one can predict that the degree of nasal underuse, or mouth-breathing, both frequency and severity, would correlate in a spectrum-like fashion with mucosal changes to these regions. Thus, the nasal branch of the forked airway, like the Starling resistor in the tube model, will have its soft walls drawn intra-luminally in proportion to the amount of negative pressure and dead-space [19].

This specific finding was corroborated clinically in a paper where a patient who had undergone three prior nasal surgeries for obstruction underwent isolated nasal inlet surgery, which assisted in the conversion of this patient from a primarily mouth-breather to a primarily nose-breather, even viewed in his published photographs (Fig. 2.5) [15]. Pre- and post-operative Computed Tomography (CT) analysis, using computational flow dynamics, and volumetric analysis was performed on this patient by a biomechanical engineer named David Wootton at Cooper Union University. Most interestingly, the patient showed a more than 40% improvement in volume, nasal resistance and airflow in the downstream *non-operated* sections of the nasal air passage. This downstream change, mostly occurring at the turbinate mucosa could only be explained by the improvement in upstream airflow at the nasal valve. An alternative hypothesis would of course include usage of decongestants by the patient at the time of the postoperative CT, but he denied this, and the degree of change was pronounced far beyond what would be expected by nasal sprays (Figs. 2.6 and 2.7). In the more obstructed nasal valve, a 24.6% change in the cross-sectional area of the valve resulted in a cavity cross-sectional area of 50.6% at the anterior portion of the maxillary sinus near the head of the inferior turbinate which progressively fell to a 40.7% increase by the posterior nasal cavity. The

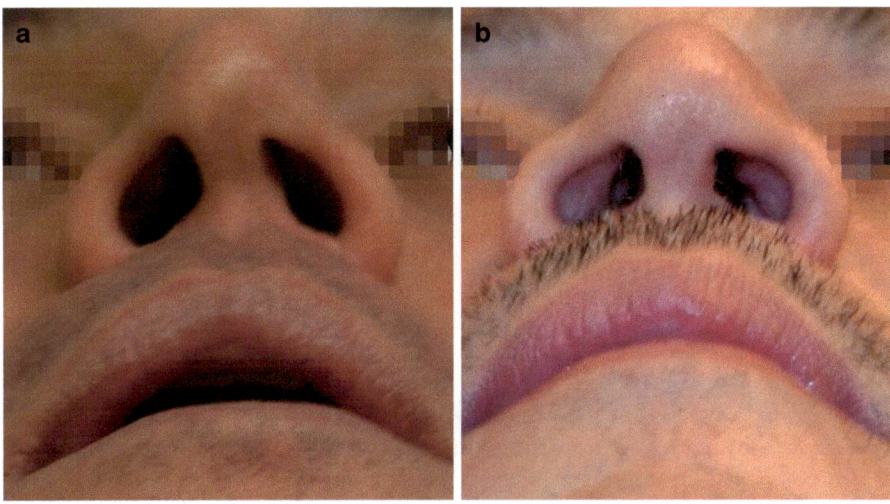

Fig. 2.5 Base view of the nose and nostrils. (**a**) Before reconstruction and (**b**) after reconstruction. (Reprinted with permission from Sage) Naughton et al. [15]

Fig. 2.6 Three–dimensional CT airway reconstruction of patient in Fig. 2.5, left before reconstruction and right after reconstruction

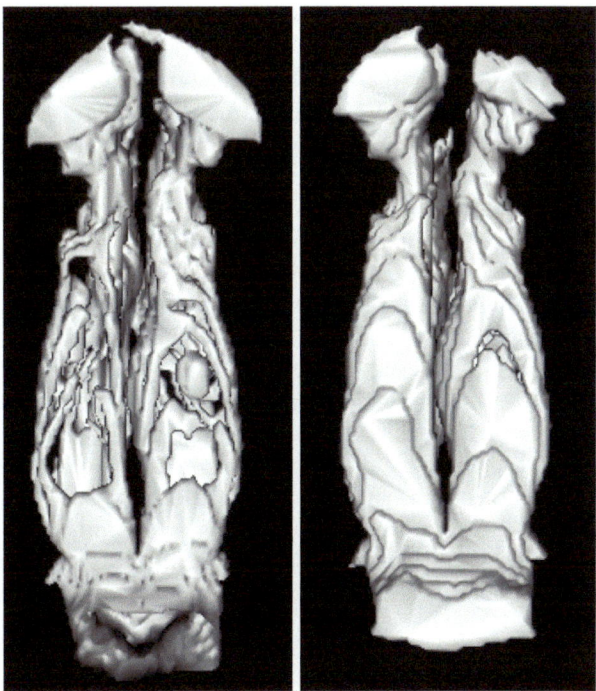

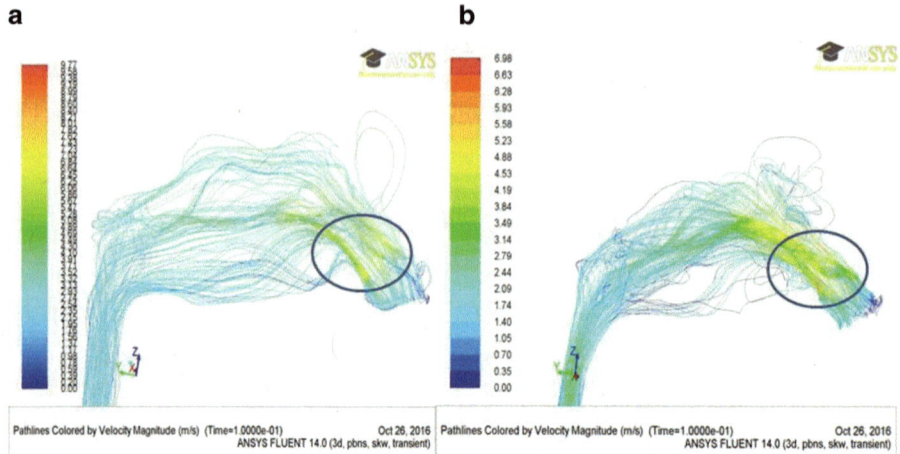

Fig. 2.7 Computational flow dynamics image of flow pathlines for patient in Fig. 2.5. (**a**) Before reconstruction and (**b**) after reconstruction

nasopharynx volume remained relatively constant with only minimal increase in surface area by 2.8%. This suggested that at least in this adult, the primary dead-space compensation occurred in the actual nasal cavity, mostly near the turbinates [15].

Putting this all together, it appears that tissue enlargement like turbinates, especially with "rhinitis" diagnoses may be less the cause of airway obstruction, requiring specific reduction existing than as a RESPONSE and physical compensation for the dead-space and reduced nasal airflow found in mouth-breathing and nasal underuse.

As you can see, possibly the greatest flaw in our understanding of nasal function and nasal surgery has been that thus far, we have as specialists failed to distinguish between true physical nasal obstruction and an *underuse* of an anatomically intact nasal airway. Both conditions, have nearly identical symptoms and complaints, but have vastly different causes and treatments. Further, while these two conditions can be easily confused for the other, more confusion arises in that many patients can have both conditions compounding each other, or at least co-existing, along the lines of the spectrum described above. Unfortunately, patients and individuals cannot distinguish between these disorders, so do not expect to see patients begin complaining of "nasal underuse" on their chief complaint—both conditions will still be described as blocked, congested, or stuffy by sufferers.

There is no specific diagnostic code for nasal underuse, but there is a mouth-breathing International Classification of Disease (ICD)-10 code R06. Simple "mouth-breathing," as a diagnosis or as a diagnosis code fails to fully encompass the clinical spectrum caused by underuse of the nose. Thus, to more accurately describe the cascade of symptoms and signs of this problem, we propose the term Nasal Underuse Syndrome (NUS). As described above, through an indirect analysis of medical and physiologic literature combined with some rational thought, we can glean the importance of this "disorder" and possibly estimate its prevalence, and even attempt to understand how this entity has been essentially missed and mislabeled for so long.

The first question most experienced readers will ask is "why is this important?" We have practiced long enough without making this distinction, so why should we start now? In my opinion, this distinction is the cornerstone of success versus failure in understanding the airway, and perhaps the greatest contributor to inefficient selection of procedures and waste of health-care expenditure.

Only physical obstructive entities like out of position cartilage can be mobilized in the airway to permit relief of nasal obstruction. In contrast, compensatory enlarged turbinates LOOK like they are the SOURCE of the obstruction, but are actually due to inadequate *use* of the nasal airway. This is why reducing the turbinates or doing a well-intentioned but limited septoplasty will not work sufficiently to resolve the problem. Again, the root cause of the "congestion" feeling in these patients is that they are partially or primarily using the mouth as their airway instead of their nasal passage, as summarized in the adjacent figure (Fig. 2.8) [20].

How over-reliance on the "NOSE" scale, the limited "allergic rhinitis" diagnosis, "standardization" of nasal and sinus treatments, misunderstanding of the nasal valve and routine acceptance of failure have contributed to our near-complete missing of NUS

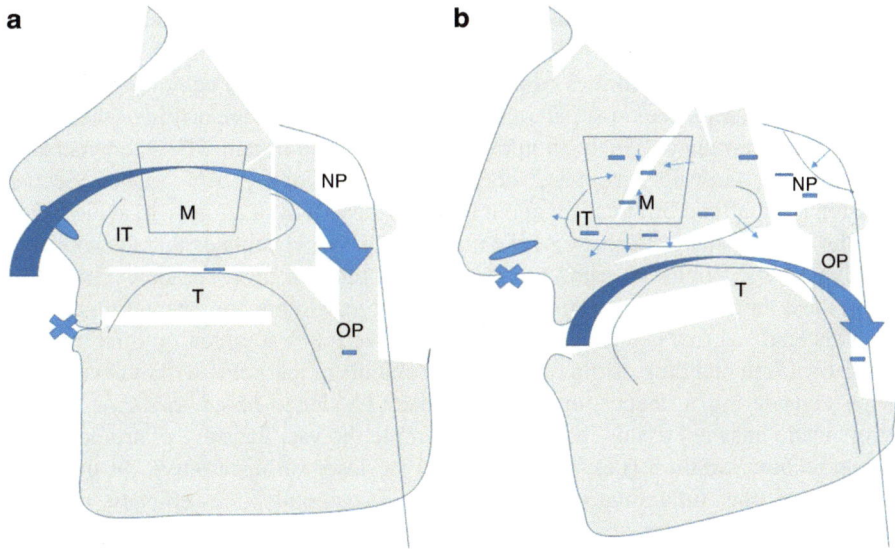

Fig. 2.8 Schematic of sagittal face during (**a**) pure nasal breathing and (**b**) pure mouth-breathing due to a musculoskeletal structure that predisposes to mouth-breathing. Large blue arrows indicate majority of airflow. Negative symbols indicate negative pressure, and X is the absence of flow. Small blue arrows indicate direction of intra-luminal mucosal stretching. *IT* inferior turbinate, *M* maxillary sinus, *T* tongue, *NP* nasopharynx, *OP* oropharynx. (Reprinted with permission from Elsevier) Stupak and Park [20]

Strategy without tactics is the slowest route to victory. Tactics without strategy is the noise before defeat.—Sun Tzu, Art of War

I have several well-respected rhinoplasty textbooks laid out in front of me in my office. I just spent the last while poring over them to understand how NUS (see previous section) could have been either missed or ignored for so long, when differentiating this problem from actual nasal obstruction. My conclusion, similar to that of Sun Tzu's when analyzing military operations (see above quote), is that we as providers and physicians focus chiefly on tactics (specific maneuvers) and almost never on strategy (grand goals). By this, I mean that we tend to think of differential diagnosis as lists, and treatments surgery as a series of steps that we can pick and choose, as though from a menu. The textbooks I reviewed are always "comprehensive," full of details, and list every type of problem that can exist in a nose, and give a laundry-list of solutions, leaving it to the practitioner to decide the tactic of choice. Unfortunately, this "tactical" focus leads us to think mostly about the small steps and about the multitude of variations in the procedure. It even prevents us from having a goal and strategy-oriented conversation with patients; instead, we focus upon offering a procedure and list possible risks and benefits. If you Google the term "attention to detail" and "plastic surgeon," you can also see that in the 1.6 million hits, the concept is heavily utilized to describe how we wish to be portrayed for our patients on our websites.

Instead, by focusing on questions about the bigger picture, like, what could be the root cause of this individual's problem and what will appropriately address the root cause? Thus, in the textbooks, there are chapters about turbinate enlargement and how these isolated entities can be treated (or ignored), but beyond a discussion of inflammation for the most part, a grand understanding of the origin of these entities is not entertained. "There should be little hesitation in removing the hyperplastic ends of the inferior turbinate," suggests *Essentials of Septorhinoplasty*, Second Edition [21], after a brief caveat about limiting the extent of surgery to avoid harming the "thermostat of the nose." Like many, he further speculates that the source of turbinate hypertrophy is from "a mucosal inflammation that spreads centrifugally from the ethmoid" and recommends ethmoid surgery to prevent or treat this.

This leads us to a deeper question. Why do we focus so much on inflammation as its own free-standing origin of so many problems in medicine without ever really even considering a deeper, underlying cause? Evidence based medicine usually gives us no answers to this. Instead, for example the vast majority of articles focus on technique variation (i.e., radiofrequency vs. laser turbinectomy), on the basic science of the inflammatory cascade, or occasionally the efficacy of anti-inflammatory sprays.

EBM and the current clinical research model are not structured to provide answers; instead, these appear to be just beneficial at establishing more details in the conventional models of entities like allergic rhinitis and turbinate enlargement.

Allergic rhinitis, a diagnosis deserving over 26,000 search hits on Pubmed at the time of this writing, is never subject to a re-analysis of its actual etiology. Instead, we accept that enlarged, pale, or "inflamed" turbinates are predominantly due to a primarily immune-mediated or allergic origin, despite this association pre-dating EBM. While there is clearly a seasonal hay-fever origin, we tend to lump nearly every other erythematous-looking nasal mucosal picture into the same category, possibly missing other origins of "inflammation," and usually we tend to lack the introspection to see daily that despite the EBM to the contrary that nasal steroid sprays and other measures are marginally helpful at best in reality. Even this usually does not trigger a search for alternative explanations, just more costly drug treatments or complex treatment devices, usually introduced by the pharmaceutical or device industries.

> The usual thing among men is that when they want something they will, without any reflection, leave that to hope, while they will employ the full force of reason in rejecting what they find unpalatable
> Thucydides, History of the Peloponnesian War, 5th Century BC

Thus, while we continue to hope that just a few technologic or pharmacologic tweaks will finally solve the nasal congestion problem in the absence of severe structural deformities, the unpleasant answer is that we may be barking up the wrong tree.

Over-Reliance on Subjective Outcome Measures: Why We Are Not Getting Reliable Feedback About Our Treatments

The chiefly used outcome measure considered to best measure degree of nasal obstruction is the NOSE (Nasal Obstruction Septoplasty Effectiveness aka Nasal Obstruction Symptom Evaluation) Instrument score [22].

While of course well-intentioned by its creators, the implementation and acceptance of this score as the primary "objective" measure for treatment of nasal obstruction has in reality done little but restrict our progress, by having such a weak measuring stick to evaluate our results with, and encouraging sensation to get in the way of objectivity.

Of course, the first and biggest flaw of this score is that, while "validated," it has very limited capacity to linearly correlate with degree of obstruction or nasal function. However, a study did show that while the scale cannot predict actual airflow, using a threshold cutoff, could permit it to distinguish between physical obstruction and NUS. This excellent study by Lipan et al. did identify a threshold of 30 on the 5–100 scale (five being no symptoms and 100 being most severe) that differentiates true obstruction from non-obstruction. This may correlate with the threshold between the symptomatic cascade of NUS versus actual nasal obstruction [23].

Either way, using a purely subjective measure to use as a surrogate for nasal function neglects an important point: *Patient experience will not correlate with actual flow*. For example, in a patient with severe obstruction, who has always had obstruction, has never experienced a better functioning nose. As this individual is perhaps stoic, they give themselves low scores for their obstruction, despite the obvious severe obstruction and forced mouth-breathing. In contrast, a patient with minimal obstruction and symptoms, but extensive concerns over their nasal issues gives themselves very elevated scores on their test, of course having never experienced a truly poorly functioning nose. Thus, when comparing the two patients, and then assuming many other patients will have varying degrees of similar problems, aggregates of this data will essentially be of minimal value.

Many experts will argue against the above paragraphs and will be quick to say that patient-based satisfaction outcomes are the most important, and after all, we are in this to make patients feel better. The flaw of this thinking is that while patient satisfaction IS important, it may not be the best way to measure functional improvements in airflow while we evaluate or compare techniques, or even evaluate pathophysiology. I will use an analogy to illustrate this point. Patients take pride in choosing their specialist, particularly for complex procedures like rhinoplasty, much like football fans have much pride in their teams. With a subpar, but not disastrous performance, the team's fans will still aggressively believe that their team has won or not committed a foul, regardless of the objective measures. The same holds true for many patients, who chose their surgeon for a reason, and without disaster, will primarily believe and support their surgeon, showing a benefit to surgery regardless of limited or subtle improvement. Only in disaster (obvious incompetence) do fans turn on the coaches and leaders and emotionally demand firing, and so on. Similarly, if patients could make their feelings known and attempt to reward or punish their doctor with varied NOSE scores. Thus, allowing subjectivity to determine the primary outcomes of our research is catamount to using emotion to evaluate a structural outcome. We will never learn how to do an operation or understand the root causes of the pathology using this outcome measure. Just as players and coaches will never learn to do their jobs better and have actual competition if we merely permit the loudest fans to determine the outcome of the game.

A recent review article in Journal of the American Medical Association (JAMA) Facial Plastic Surgery that highlights "Advances in diagnosis and treatment" of nasal airway obstruction [24], is a good example of how well-intentioned, but dated reliance on the conventional model of understanding of the airway and its associated faulty subjective nasal obstruction measures actually harms our understanding of how the nose interacts with the broader airway.

The "advances" article acknowledges the extent of nasal obstruction in the USA and divides the source of obstruction into physical obstruction, and allergic and vasomotor rhinitis, and acknowledges the confusion in the literature between diagnostic tests and actual "sensation of" breathing. They reviewed the literature for nasal obstruction for a 5 year period, but excluded all for consideration that involved, obstructive sleep apnea, sleep-disordered breathing, rhinitis, and any including patient's age below 14 in order to focus on surgically treated nasal obstruction. Again, while well-intentioned to keep their focus narrow, they miss the greater picture that the true importance of nasal obstruction and nasal underuse is that individuals are subsequently more *prone to mouth-breathing*. In the case of obstruction, the individuals are forced to mouth-breathe, while in the case of underuse (NUS), the congested feeling is a result of mouth-breathing. As we will discuss in a subsequent chapter, the best CURRENT diagnostic objective test for nocturnal mouth-breathing is the diagnostic sleep study. Essentially, as we will discuss at length in the next chapter, this is because mouth-breathing occurs due to a state of an unlocked upper and lower jaw set, releasing the tongue and possibly soft palate to collapse posteriorly, dynamically obstructing the lower airway during low tone states of sleep, and causing apneic events. Unfortunately, sleep studies also do not distinguish between obstruction and NUS, which is just one reason why the degree of nasal obstruction does not show correlation with OSA severity [25].

The article [24] then briefly reviews objective measures like acoustic rhinometry, rhinomanometry, and peak nasal inspiratory flow (PNIF). Due to the confounding factors that abound with these techniques, I agree with the authors that due to nostril distortion and effort-based measures, these are hardly worth discussing. PNIF, in addition to being severely effort base, has such a small measured difference between pathology and normal values that it is almost too subtle a system for any meaningful value. Computational flow dynamics using CT scan anatomy seems to actually predict airflow, but is so unwieldy, expensive, time consuming, and requiring substantial radiation to patients that it is hard to envision as a useful entity beyond esoteric research papers. I suppose as software and hardware continue to improve, one day this could be an efficient technology.

In contrast, in the best objective nasal airflow study that I have seen to date by Bailey et al. 2017 [26], the authors use a temperature probe to measure actual nasal airflow. The authors were surprised to find that while the probe reliably measured magnitude of inspiratory and expiratory airflow, the findings failed to correlate with NOSE or Visual analogue scale (VAS) scores, they refreshingly consider "that the NOSE and VAS scores, although universally used in the literature, are imperfect measures of subjective nasal patency."

The conclusions in the "advances" [24] paper largely echo the expert consensus, and "gold-standard" of our time, first stating that the value of the NOSE scale "cannot be overstated," and that the "NOSE scale is *outstanding* ... revealing the inconsistent findings of (objective) inter-measure correlation," and while necessary, that "structural measures are insufficient."

In reality, focus on patient sensation of airflow, and subjective scores as our primary measurement is possibly a way to explain why surgical techniques fail in many cases to make actual improvements. This focus on the subjective even provides a loophole to permit any surgical procedure, regardless of its lack of utility show "improvement," as we will discuss in Chap. 6.

Again, Bailey et al. [26], described above uncovered a useful system to measure nasal airflow in their conclusion, "Our observations suggest that two strategies could be used in future studies to clarify the role of nasal mucosal temperature in subjective nasal patency, namely [1] non-contact temperature sensors can be used to prevent mucosa irritation and [2] nasal mucosal temperature can be measured before and after an intervention, such as nasal surgery or exposure to cold air."

While the authors have hit upon a fantastic finding, focus upon the temperature of the mucosa itself maybe an imperfect target. In contrast to the accepted "belief" about nasal mucosal cooling, the key to measuring temperature as a surrogate for nasal airflow during nasal breathing may be measuring the *air* temperature at the nostril. Non-contact digital thermal imaging has a great potential to take this measurement. A simple thought experiment can be convincing:

For our experiment, let us assume in a perfectly functioning nose in a healthy individual that the air temperature in the lung approaches 37 °C and that air temperature in the room surrounding the nostril approaches room temperature of 27 °C. The room temperature air is essentially warmed by the entire pulmonary system during inspiration to rise to nearly body temperature when it reaches the base of our lungs. Then, this warmed air will be expired out through the nostrils still at approximately 37 °C. As this air dissipates into the environment, another inspiration will begin, with nostril air temperatures returning to 27° room temperature. Thus, for the sake of our model, we can assume that a perfectly efficient nasal airway will have a change in air temperature (ΔT) of approximately 10° between peak inspiration and expiration. The Bailey study (above) showed a ΔT that approximated this (27–34 °C) in deep breathing using an inserted probe. Any digital thermal imaging system will show a similar change in temperatures in an adequately functioning nose. On the other extreme, a nearly or completely closed nostril, that is either not used, or not able to be used will have a severely restricted ΔT because it does not exchange air between the lungs and the room. Closed nostrils on thermal imaging will show a very low ΔT as well as expected. Most patients have nostrils that can be expected to fall somewhere in between these two extremes, and a threshold can be identified where nasal airflow is adequate, or not. Thus, once this threshold is identified, a patient can be identified as having their nasal symptoms due to actual obstruction ΔT below the threshold, or NUS (ΔT above the threshold). The thermal imaging ΔT may be unlikely to directly correlate linearly with nasal airflow but will likely simply determine the cutoff between pathologic and non-pathologic airflow, as even this modality is effort and operator aiming dependent.

Our own preliminary data showed that measuring ΔT tracked nasal function, mostly with the "total ΔT," or sum of two nostrils, and with the worst performing nostril. In practicality one could very clearly see the temperature change with inspiration and expiration and this tracked with effort and obstruction. The device itself had good resolution, using the Seek ThermalPro™ ($450) in pinpoint mode, where a pointer in the device center gives a temperature read. The device is a very compact device that attaches to any mobile device.

Figures 2.9, 2.10, and 2.11 show the thermal imaging device, and normal functioning nostrils during inspiration and expiration, while Fig. 2.12 is a figure of one healthy nostril and a severely obstructed nostril in contrast).

The goal of the study was to establish a threshold using thermal imaging that separates functional from substantially obstructed noses using comparisons of thermal imaging and survey scores. Essentially, adult patients completed the NOSE survery. The Seek™ thermal imaging device was used to record the difference in

Fig. 2.9 Seek™ thermal imaging device and attachment for smartphone

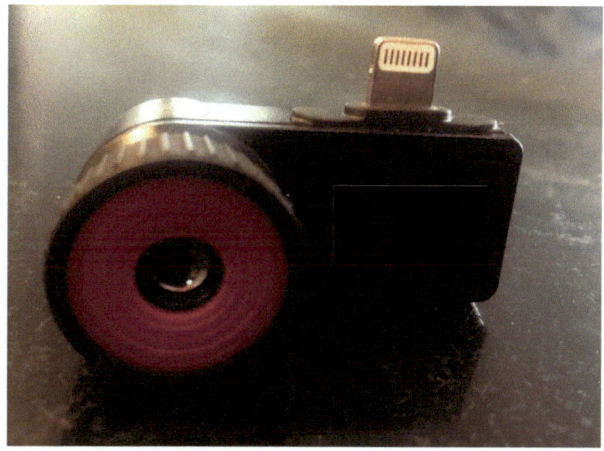

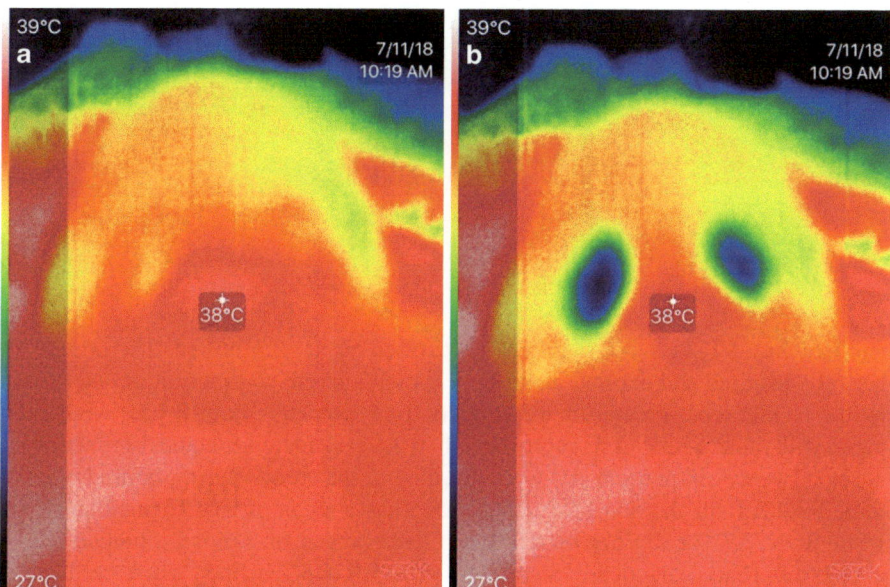

Fig. 2.10 (**a**) Image captured of base view of nose using thermal imaging device during expiration (showing lung-warmed air). (**b**) Same view, seconds later during inspiration (showing room temperature air)

Fig. 2.11 Thermal image demonstrating excellent contrast during inspiration from base view of nose, illustrating adequate nasal function

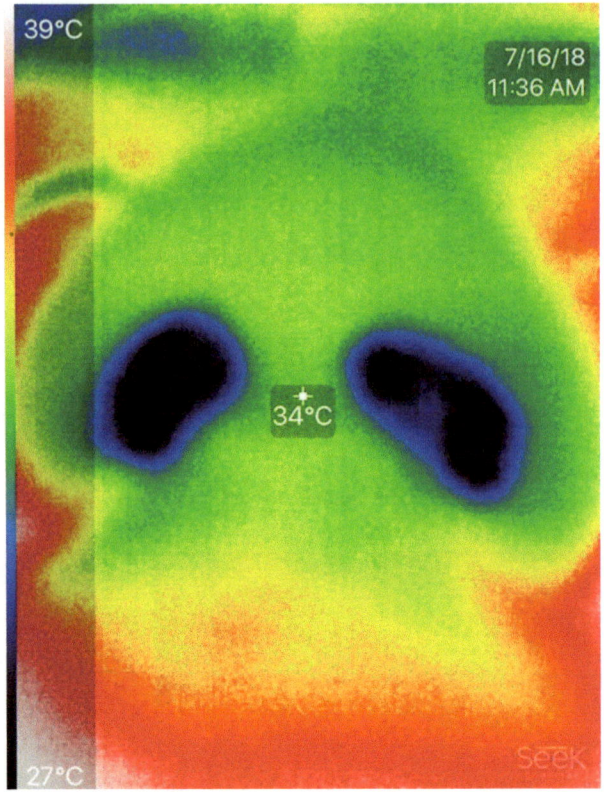

temperature (ΔT) between inspired and expired air at each nostril. The nostril ΔT between inspired and expired air of patients with severe obstruction as determined by the NOSE score greater than 30 (using the Lipan et al. cutoff) [23] were compared with those with NOSE scores less than 30 (considered adequately functioning noses). Twenty-six participants were enrolled in the study. During normal respiration, Total ΔT for the non-obstructed group has a mean of 9.0 °C (median 9 °C), while Total ΔT for the obstructed group had a mean of 7.69 °C (median 8 °C), a 17% difference statistically significant at $p = 0.045$. For the "worst performing nostril" tested, ΔT for the non-obstructed group had a mean/median of 4 °C, while the obstructed group had a mean of 3.23 °C (median 3 °C- 23.8% difference $p = 0.023$) (Figs. 2.13 and 2.14).

In addition, we constricted AND dilated the nostrils as part of the exam. Patients simply narrowed their nostrils with pinching, or the examiner performed the Cottle maneuver using disposable Q-tips. The nasal narrowing resulted in a severe and predictable reduction in ΔT, but the Cottle maneuver seemed to cause as much reduction in ΔT as an increase and its use did not cause a statistically significant increase. The Cottle maneuver or modified Cottle maneuver has been shown to be

Fig. 2.12 Image captured using thermal imaging device of a left-sided total obstruction, (right side of image) and right sided function (left side of screen) demonstrating the difference between pathology and normal function

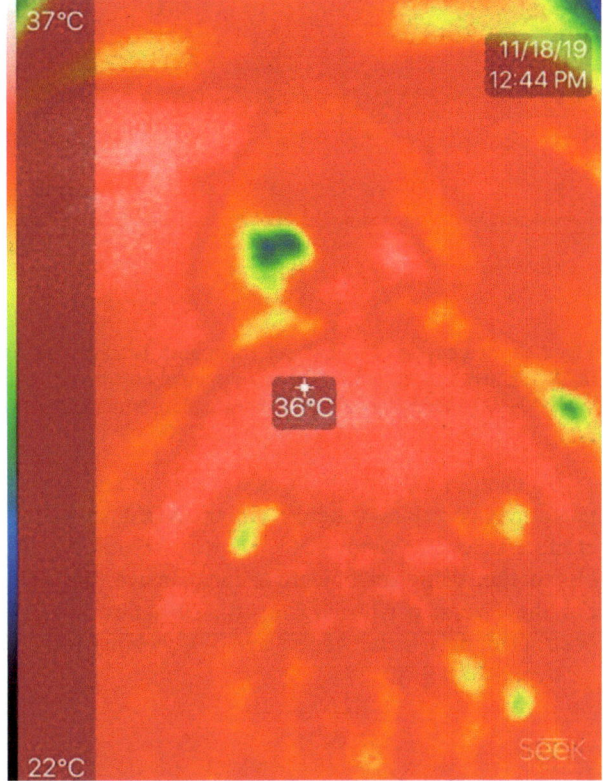

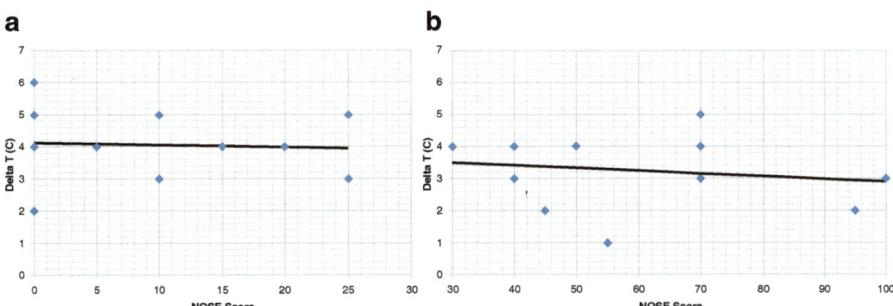

Fig. 2.13 Scatterplot of "worst performing nostril" ΔT plotted against NOSE scores (0–100). (**a**) NOSE score 0–25, indicating no substantial obstruction, with median ΔT of 4 °C. (**b**) NOSE score 30–100, indicating substantial obstruction, with median ΔT of 3 °C

fraught with inaccuracy and operator dependence [27], thus making this data generally inaccurate as a dilating tool. This was a major flaw in study design, and something we should have thought more about in advance, as this only created more confusion.

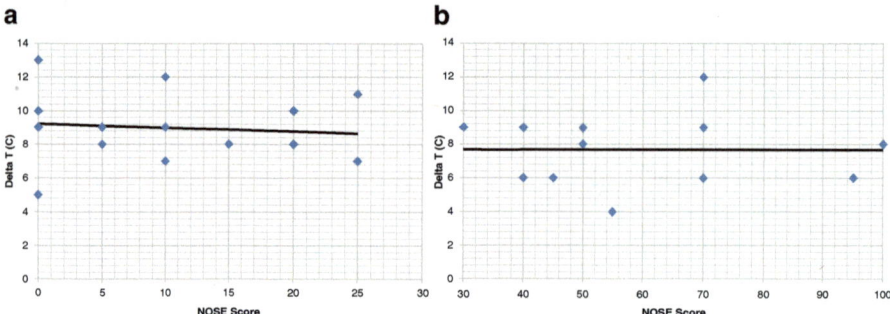

Fig. 2.14 Scatterplot of "total" ΔT (both nostrils added) plotted against NOSE scores (0–100). (a) NOSE score 0–25, indicating no substantial obstruction, with median ΔT of 9 °C. (b) NOSE score 30–100, indicating substantial obstruction, with median ΔT of 8 °C

By using a ΔT threshold as a cutoff of adequate and inadequate function that potentially correlates roughly with the NOSE score cutoff as described by the Lipan et al., article [23] (above 30), we may be able to discriminate NUS from classic obstruction using an objective, inexpensive, and non-nostril distorting measure. For the "worst performing nostril," this threshold between obstructed and non-obstructed, may lie between 3 and 4 °C, while for the sum of the two nostrils, it lies between 8 and 9 °C [28].

NUS Causing "Secondary Obstruction"

While we have taken great pains to explain and differentiate between NUS and true nasal obstruction, we must conclude by also noting the confusing place where the two overlap: *Secondary Obstruction*. In the view of the author, secondary obstruction is the case where the reactive changes of the intra-luminal soft-tissue has enlarged beyond the point of just serving as a sign of nasal underuse and has progressed sufficiently to cause actual obstruction. An example of this is what most call "polypoid change" of the turbinates, as opposed to a more limited turbinate "hypertrophy." As in the case of any intra-airway pathology, as we have discussed, the origin of this problem is mostly believed to be of primary inflammatory/allergic/infectious origin. However, a small amount of reasoning is required to realize that the polypoid change state is the severe response to the intra-nasal negative pressure caused by NUS and/or upstream obstruction at the nasal valve. In the case where the underuse and primary obstruction generates this more extreme negative pressure, the actual mucosa and its underlying lamina propria are irreversibly damaged, causing the tissue to have lost its elasticity, becoming floppy and space-occupying. This is not dissimilar to the waistband of athletic wear, that once stretched beyond a breaking point, loses its recoil and becomes permanently widened. This is supported by a histologic analysis showing disruption of the architecture of the lamina propria, specifically in patients diagnosed with chronic rhinosinusitis with polyposis [29].

Based on this line of thinking, although this is widely considered to be an inflammatory disorder, one could consider that the polyposis and related inflammation could be actually a form of *secondary* obstruction and is simply the manifestation of the inflammatory/fibrosis stage of wound healing from negative pressure related trauma and disruption of the nasal mucosal lining in NUS. While conventional treatments like turbinate reduction and polypectomy or FESS (Functional endoscopic sinus surgery) can be effective at reducing the severe *secondary* obstruction created by the stretched tissue, it is important to understand that these techniques due not address the root cause of the problem (NUS!) and will only be temporary solutions despite their invasiveness.

Conclusion

Physical nasal obstruction and NUS are completely different problems, both with very different treatments. True obstruction can only be treated by physical change, from surgery to nasal dilators, while NUS can only be treated by encouraging the jaw to remain closed.

The reasons for this failure are numerous, and include relying primarily on subjective outcome measures, and an anatomic misunderstanding of the nasal valve that incorporates the inferior turbinate into the nasal valve or primary resistor of the nose. In other words, by the flawed reasoning that assumes that the inferior turbinate is a primary source of obstruction, instead of enlarging *as a result* of NUS, we have convoluted the two disorders and further confused ourselves with an outcome system that does not easily correlate with any objective measure.

Most importantly, most consider nasal complaints to be linear in severity, from mild to severe, and the quest for an objective measure to match this linearity is in itself flawed. The best any individual can hope for with their nasal airway is not an excellent airway, but an *adequately* functioning nasal airway that is capable of functioning without oral supplemental flow. A more reasonable goal of NOSE scores, as identified by Lipan et al. is that a threshold is reached discriminating adequate from inadequate flow [23]. Similarly, in contrast to the goal of most nasal function diagnostic devices and questionnaires, thermal imaging (nostril ΔT) may be useful, not as a true linear quantitative measure of flow, but as a method to distinguish NUS from true obstruction by demonstrating simple ADEQUACY of nasal airflow, tested over several minutes of resting breathing. The subjective testing, the thermal imaging (pending further review), and physical exam demonstrating physical blockage by substantially misplaced nasal framework (see future chapters) can be considered together to help a clinician discriminate between the common NUS and the more rare obstruction requiring physical intervention. In reality, the only worthwhile objective is to convert mouth-breathing patients to primarily nasal breathing patients. In the cases where the nasal airway is adequate, patients can instead be counseled that although the nasal symptoms are real, they are actually due to underuse of the nasal airway, and strategies to discourage mouth-breathing and encourage nasal breathing.

Right now, the best existing surrogate for mouth-breathing is sleep apnea severity, the yet the conventional scale used to measure this, the apnea hypopnea index (AHI) is an imperfect measure, which has further confused the issue for several reasons. This is the subject of the next chapter.

References

1. Dowsett EB. Discussion on mouth breathing and nasal obstruction. Proc R Soc Med. 1932;25(8):1343–55.
2. Nunez DA, Bradley PJ. A randomised clinical trial of turbinectomy for compensatory turbinate hypertrophy in patients with anterior septal deviations. Clin Otolaryngol Allied Sci. 2000;25(6):495–8.
3. Illum P. Septoplasty and compensatory inferior turbinate hypertrophy: long-term results after randomized turbinoplasty. Eur Arch Otorhinolaryngol. 1997;254(Suppl 1):S89–92.
4. Sharhan SSA, Lee EJ, Hwang CS, Nam JS, Yoon JH, Kim CH, Cho HJ. Radiological comparison of inferior turbinate hypertrophy between allergic and non-allergic rhinitis: does allergy really augment turbinate hypertrophy? Eur Arch Otorhinolaryngol. 2018;275(4):923–9.
5. Grutzenmacher S, Robinson DM, Grafe K, Lang C, Mlynski G. First findings concerning airflow in noses with septal deviation and compensatory turbinate hypertrophy–a model study. ORL J Otorhinolaryngol Relat Spec. 2006;68(4):199–205.
6. Kato T, Masuda Y, Yoshida A, Morimoto T. Masseter EMG activity during sleep and sleep bruxism. Arch Ital Biol. 2011;149(4):478–91.
7. Ikawa Y, Mochizuki A, Katayama K, Kato T, Ikeda M, Abe Y, Nakamura S, Nakayama K, Wakabayashi N, Baba K, Inoue T. Effects of citalopram on jaw-closing muscle activity during sleep and wakefulness in mice. Neurosci Res. 2016;113:48–55.
8. Wang Y, Wang J, Liu Y, Yu S, Sun X, Li S, Shen S, Zhao W. Fluid-structure interaction modeling of upper airways before and after nasal surgery for obstructive sleep apnea. Int J Numer Method Biomed Eng. 2012;28(5):528–46.
9. Rhee JS, Weaver EM, Park SS, et al. Clinical consensus statement: diagnosis and management of nasal valve compromise. Otolaryngol Head Neck Surg. 2010;143(1):48–59.
10. Li C, Farag AA, Leach J, Deshpande B, Jacobowitz A, Kim K, Otto BA, Zhao K. Computational fluid dynamics and trigeminal sensory examinations of empty nose syndrome patients. Laryngoscope. 2017;127(6):E176–84.
11. Balakin BV, Farbu E, Kosinski P. Aerodynamic evaluation of the empty nose syndrome by means of computational fluid dynamics. Comput Methods Biomech Biomed Eng. 2017;20(14):1554–61.
12. de Moura BH, Migliavacca RO, Lima RK, et al. Partial inferior turbinectomy in rhinoseptoplasty has no effect in quality-of-life outcomes: a randomized clinical trial. Laryngoscope. 2018;128(1):57–63.
13. Harju T, Numminen J, Kivekäs I, Rautiainen M. A prospective, randomized, placebo-controlled study of inferior turbinate surgery. Laryngoscope. 2018;128(9):1997–2003.
14. Zang HR, Li LF, Zhou B, Li YC, Wang T, Han DM. Pharyngeal aerodynamic characteristics of obstructive sleep apnea/hypopnea syndrome patients. Chin Med J. 2012;125(17):3039–43.

15. Naughton JP, Lee AY, Ramos E, Wootton D, Stupak HD. Effect of nasal valve shape on downstream volume, airflow, and pressure drop: importance of the nasal valve revisited. Ann Otol Rhinol Laryngol. 2018;127(11):745–53.

16. Genta PR, Edwards BA, Sands SA, Owens RL, Butler JP, Loring SH, White DP, Wellman A. Tube law of the pharyngeal airway in sleeping patients with obstructive sleep apnea. Sleep. 2016;39(2):337–43.

17. Owens RL, Edwards BA, Sands SA, Butler JP, Eckert DJ, White DP, Malhotra A, Wellman A. The classical Starling resistor model often does not predict inspiratory airflow patterns in the human upper airway. J Appl Physiol. 2014;116(8):1105–12.

18. Sériès F, Chakir J, Boivin D. Influence of weight and sleep apnea status on immunologic and structural features of the uvula. Am J Respir Crit Care Med. 2004;170(10):1114–9.

19. McNicholas WT. The nose and OSA: variable nasal obstruction may be more important in pathophysiology than fixed obstruction. Eur Respir J. 2008;32(1):3–8.

20. Stupak HD, Park SY. Gravitational forces, negative pressure and facial structure in the genesis of airway dysfunction during sleep: a review of the paradigm. Sleep Med. 2018;51:125–32.

21. Behrbohm H, Tardy E. Essentials of septorhinoplasty, 2nd ed. Stuttgart; New York: Thieme; 2017.

22. Stewart MG, Witsell DL, Smith TL, et al. Development and validation of the Nasal obstructions symptom evaluation (NOSE) scale. Otolaryngol Head Neck Surg. 2004;130(20):157–63.

23. Lipen MJ, Most SM. Development of a severity classification system for subjective nasal obstruction. JAMA Facial Plast Surg. 2013;15(5):358–61.

24. Mohan S, Fuller JC, Ford SF, Lindsay RW. Diagnostic and therapeutic management of nasal airway obstruction: advances in diagnosis and treatment. JAMA Facial Plast Surg. 2018;20(5):409–18.

25. Leitzen KP, Brietzke SE, Lindsay RW. Correlation between nasal anatomy and objective obstructive sleep apnea severity. Otolaryngol Head Neck Surg. 2014;150(2):325–31.

26. Bailey RS, Casey KP, Pawar SS, Garcia GJ. Correlation of nasal mucosal temperature with subjective nasal patency in healthy individuals. JAMA Facial Plast Surg. 2017;19(1):46–52.

27. Bonaparte JP, Campbell R. A prospective cohort study assessing the clinical utility of the Cottle maneuver in nasal septal surgery. J Otolaryngol Head Neck Surg. 2018;47(1):45.

28. Jiang S, Davani A, Chen J, Stupak H. Thermal imaging as a potential measure of nasal airflow: a pilot study. Poster presentation at the 2019 american academy of facial plastic and reconstructive surgery spring meeting, Austin, Texas.

29. De Coster L, Eloy P, Ferdinande L, Taildeman J, Cuvelier CA, Watelet JB. Different types of tissue composition in inflammatory or reparative upper airway disorders. Rhinology. 2012;50(4):393–401.

Chapter 3
Nasal Function and Sleep Disorders

I find it more fitting to seek the truth of the matter rather than imaginary conceptions.
—Niccolo Machiavelli, *The Prince*

It appears to be convenient for both sleep surgeons and rhinoplasty surgeons that conventionally, that the nose, beyond a role in CPAP (continuous positive airway pressure) compliance appears to be uninvolved in the development of obstructive sleep apnea (OSA). This is because the typical rhinoplasty surgeon may not enjoy interpreting sleep studies, and the average sleep surgeon may not enjoy performing aesthetic rhinoplasty. The bad news for both, however, is that the nose and sleep *are* intimately related, both effecting the other, and are impossible to untangle, even if one wishes to not be disturbed by such trifles and inconveniences. But, as Machiavelli mentions in the quote above, we need to focus on reality, not what we hope reality to be.

In the previous chapter, we discussed how true nasal obstruction must be distinguished from the clinically similar appearing nasal underuse syndrome (NUS) in order to deliver efficient and appropriate care by best selecting candidates who will and will not benefit from surgery. By identifying that vague nasal symptoms can emerge from postural/tone/habitual mouth-breathing, and further, acknowledging that these symptoms/signs including "congestion" and turbinate hypertrophy stem from this, we can efficiently design treatment plans.

So, paradoxically, we can indirectly treat the nose in many cases by treating the nocturnally slack jaw. TW Huang and TH Young reported in their 2014 study that mouth opening itself may be implicated as the principle causative agent in OSA and sleep-disordered breathing (SDB) [1].

Much more has been written about how the nose and these sleep-breathing disorders are related, but most of this is targeted to how nasal treatments can affect sleep apnea. In contrast, while a few strong articles have described how mouth-breathing itself influences obstructive sleep apnea (OSA) only few articles have accurately described the mechanism of how mouth-breathing and sleep are related [2–4].

© Springer Nature Switzerland AG 2020
H. D. Stupak, *Rethinking Rhinoplasty and Facial Surgery*,
https://doi.org/10.1007/978-3-030-44674-1_3

Most clinicians tend to disregard mouth-breathing as a nuisance, and it is rarely considered except as a supplemental treatment during Continuous Positive Airway Pressure (CPAP) monitoring. In these cases, it is believed that there is an oral "leak" of the CPAP positive air pressure, thus a flimsy chin strap or mouth-closure device is recommended to improve the success of CPAP by preventing this "leak." In other words, mouth-breathing for sleep apnea is largely ignored.

Beyond this dismissal of mouth-breathing, the majority of articles and experts, *my own earlier articles included*, that relate nasal breathing with OSA tended to focus upon efficacy of surgery on the nasal airway for sleep, instead of focusing on the more important efficacy for prevention of mouth-breathing. Several errors of reasoning, as we will discuss further, are committed by promoting the belief that problems related to the nose are generally unrelated to OSA besides for the standard mantra that nasal surgery helps with CPAP compliance.

The origins of this line of thinking seemed to stem from a study by Friedman et al. [5], where, despite some symptomatic improvements, mean respiratory disturbance index (RDI) actually worsened from 31.6 to 39.5, despite an improvement in oxygen saturation nadir from 82.5% to 84.3%. The patients in this study did have a reduction in pressure requirements from CPAP. Koutsourelakis et al. followed this study with a randomized control trial and found similar outcomes [6].

Thus, as reported by Rosow and Stewart in 2010, "there is no evidence that patients with OSA will experience improvement in the defining objective measures of OSA— Apnea Hypopnea Index (AHI) or minimum oxygen saturation-after nasal surgery alone. This is consistent with the prevailing consensus that the obstruction in OSA is multifactorial, with multiple potential areas of pathologic anatomic obstruction" [7].

A meta-analysis of "nasal surgery" effects on OSA, by Ishii et al. [8], included ten studies and over 300 patients. This study unsurprisingly also showed only marginal improvement in sleep apnea parameters, concluding that aside from the standard "nasal surgery can improve CPAP" line, nasal surgery results in only slight or symptomatic improvement in sleep apnea severity and symptoms. While we usually assume that more studies and more patients will result in better information to guide our decisions, in this case, aggregating more data, while agreeing with contemporaneous literature, drifted our attention further from the reality of the true nasal-sleep interaction. Also, by lumping many variations of nasal surgery into one category, on many different types of patients, the researchers did not find much value in nasal treatment due to a missing of subtle nuances by mass aggregation of data:

First, the type of surgery performed in most of these studies is (the largely inadequate) sub-mucous resection of the septum and turbinate reduction. As we discussed in the previous chapter, the turbinates may not even be a cause of obstruction, but actually a compensatory feature of nasal underuse. Thus, removal of this tissue cannot be expected to relieve obstruction in general. Further, removal of a small portion of the posterior septum may be equally ineffective in improving the nasal airway. As we will explore in the chapter on the nasal valve, ignoring the anterior septum and nostrils while only focusing on the area of maximal deviation has only limited efficacy and cannot be expected to produce drastic improvements in the nasal airway. Third, nasal surgery will only be effective if the obstruction is *significant* in the first place, and then the obstruction must be substantially improved, including treatment of the L-strut and nostrils. In other words, of course septoplasty will have no benefit in improving sleep parameters if only mild septal deviation (not uncommon) was present in the first place. One could reason that only a surgery that more substantially improves the airway, that is a functional rhinoplasty that substantially enlarges the nasal inlet or nostril and that can be measured to improve the entire nasal airway from valve to pharynx could be expected to result in sleep parameter improvements. Very few of the studies evaluated utilized this type of surgery, thus the conclusions should have been that limited nasal surgery on a wide variety of patient types seems to be ineffective in treating OSA (but this does not mean that no nasal surgery treats some sleep patients when properly chosen).

Doctors most commonly get mixed up between absence of evidence and evidence of absence (with permission).—Nassim Nicholas Taleb

Perhaps the most confusing article of all on the topic was published during this period where the relation between the nose and sleep was most contested. In the article "Correlation between nasal anatomy and obstructive sleep apnea severity" [9], the general premise was to "determin[e] an association between nasal anatomic factors and OSAS as critical to determin[e] the appropriate management for patients with OSA." While no doubt well intentioned, the authors failed to note a reasoning error in their study. As in the quote above, finding a correlation between nasal anatomy and OSA could be supportive of a link between the two, *failure* to find a link does NOT mean that a link does not exist. This is a distinct error from, but not dissimilar to the conclusion that because a specific nasal "procedure" failed to improve OSA parameters, it must mean that *all* nasal surgery cannot be effective in treating OSA, or worse, that the nose is minimally involved in sleep breathing.

After this classic type II error of rejecting an association based on a lack of evidence, they do note the possibility of this error class, but only as a potential "limitation" in their statistical methodology, not as a reasoning error. Further, they decided to rely on a nasal anatomic worksheet that "had not been assessed in terms of validity or reliability … the fact that several components of the nasal anatomic worksheet correlated with the NOSE score strongly suggests appropriate validity" [9].

Lastly, they concluded by strongly stating that, "on the basis of the results of this study, the authors would not recommend turbinoplasty, septoplasty, or nasal valve correction as a primary treatment of OSA[S] even in patients with obvious turbinate hypertrophy, severe septal deviation, and/or nasal valve compromise." Further, they convincingly explain that "the study was designed to have 90% power to detect the association if one existed." I do completely agree with the authors about not being enthusiastic about turbinoplasty!

A casual reader of the literature at this time would thus have to assume the case to be closed … that there is little reason to further evaluate nasal breathing and its association with OSA. However, even further analysis shows why this statement is misleading.

The common trend in most of these studies is to use the "OSA is a multilevel problem" line to explain away any nasal/OSA interaction. Of course, as outlined in the previous chapter, none of these studies discriminated between patients with NUS, and primary true nasal obstruction (see prior chapter for explanation). Further, many of these studies included patients with high Body Mass Index (BMI) and many varied age parameters, in other words, patients of varied musculoskeletal tone. Decreased facial tone, as expected with age and increasing BMI can predispose to mouth-breathing, and thus sleep apnea [10]. Many of the nasal surgery and sleep parameters studies did not adequately stratify by BMI and age (surrogates for musculoskeletal tone).

The most important flaw of the "the nose can't be involved in sleep" literature trend, however, is the actual attempt to search for a link between nasal surgery and sleep parameters in the first place! In reality, nasal surgery or any nasal treatment *only* improves OSA parameters, when they convert a patient from a sleep-time mouth-breather to a sleep-time nasal breather. So, even a successful nasal airway surgery that improves nasal airflow will fail if the patient has persistent mouth-breathing due to jaw structure, habit, or tone. So, the underlying error in logic about the whole quest to link the nose to sleep apnea via pre- and post-surgery analysis was due to the assumption that nose breathing improves sleep by "opening" the airway. Instead, as we've discussed, even well-done and appropriate nasal surgery will *always* fail to adequately improve sleep apnea, even in patients with nasal obstruction if they remain as sleep-time mouth-breathers after surgery because of their musculoskeletal tone at the level of the jaw closing muscles. The more specific clinical questions we could be asking, then, are: Does substantially surgically open-ing the nasal airway in patients with good musculoskeletal tone (low age/BMI) improve OSA/SDB parameters or mouth-breathing? Or, can we combine nasal sur-gery in select patients with severe true primary nasal obstruction with mouth-closure techniques when their tone (age/BMI) is poor?

So, How Does Rhinoplasty/Nasal Valve Surgery Impact OSA?

In light of what I believed was an error to dismiss nasal surgery as a viable treatment of OSA, I initially focused on the reason for prior failure being inadequate surgery. On analysis of the existing data, as seen above, to me the logical conclusion was that the studies failed to incorporate treatment of the nasal valve, nostril, and specifically the deviated L-shaped strut of the septum. From my perspective, inadequacy of the procedures was the reason that "nose surgery" failed to treat sleep apnea. The radi-cal but anecdotal improvement in some patients' objective sleep parameters after isolated rhinoplasties convinced me enough to undertake a clinical study even though this improvement was inconsistent. In the study, conducted at the Albert Einstein College of Medicine, 26 consecutive clinic patients with nasal obstruction and OSA were treated with a variation on functional rhinoplasty (surgical details will be discussed in later chapters) [11].

The mean AHI pre-operatively of 24.7, dropped to a post-operative mean AHI of 16 (a 35% decrease, $p = 0.013$). Only nine of 26 patients were considered surgical successes, by the strict AHI definition, and six patients had worsening of their AHI despite reporting improvement in nasal obstruction. Oxygen saturation nadir improved from 84.5% to 87% ($p = 0.036$). NOSE scores showed a 63% improvement from pre- to post-operative improvement, reflecting specific improvement in nasal obstruction, but you already know what our thoughts are about over-reliance on this scale as the ultimate in measuring obstruction: Patients cannot compare their nasal airflow experience with that of others, as they have never experienced the other's nose, thus aggregated NOSE score data is inherently flawed. Nonetheless, the study explored the isolated performance of more aggressive nasal valve surgery on objective OSA parameters, while at least attempting to document the degree of nasal relief with these surveys [11]. A study from Turkey, also studying isolated functional rhinoplasty showed a similar improvement in AHI from 43.1 to 24.6 that resembled our results [12].

While intrigued and pleased that the functional rhinoplasty results were seemingly superior to that of conventional limited nasal surgery, I was also disappointed and puzzled as to why the results were not more successful and remained quite limited.

Subgroup analysis revealed some answers, but only with deeper understanding of this analysis much later, did we really understand WHY we had such limited success. When patients with Body Mass Index (BMI) greater than 30 were excluded, the overall AHI of the patients improved from 22.5 to 9.6 pre- to post-operatively, a 55.7% improvement, and surgical "success" improved to 50%. Increasing BMI and age were found to correlate most substantially with worsened OSA parameters, as previous studies have shown [13, 14].

With regard to sleep position during the tested night, supine position (as in other studies), was found to be apnea inducing [15]. In the patients whose overall AHI worsened during the course of the study (mostly with elevated BMI), more time was spent supine in the post-operative study, increasing from 59% of the night to 74% of the night, suggesting that perhaps the nasal surgery improved their breathing enough to spend more time in an apnea prone position. Along these same lines, supine AHI in the less than 30 BMI group improved most substantially, from 20 to 5.8 ($p = 0.0004$) [11].

So, the cause of the incomplete success from functional rhinoplasty in the treatment of OSA seemed to be related possibly to age, BMI, and possibly night-time sleep position. But, how could these factors be related to the airway? Was the pharynx just more floppy in these conditions, as the conventional answer would suggest, or was there more to it?

Fortunately, by considering these factors, we finally began to understand our critical mistake in understanding how the nose related to sleep. While correctly understanding that mouth-breathing was the prime culprit in OSA, we like many believed that mouth-breathing was purely *due to* nasal obstruction, more specifically, at the level of the nasal valve. Thus, by making the false assumption that mouth-breathing was DUE to nasal blockage, we nearly missed the true cause of the vast majority of OSA: reduced jaw closure tone. Jaw closure tone, as we later learned, seemed to be a product of age, BMI, and sleep position, the three factors we noted in our Plastic and Reconstructive Surgery (PRS) sleep paper [11] as hindering the success of functional rhinoplasty in the treatment of OSA. Could these three factors be responsible for exacerbating mouth-breathing even in the absence of nasal obstruction? How did these seemingly unrelated factors influence mouth-breathing? Why did tone matter, and is it just a minor factor compared to the generally agreed pharyngeal factors, or are these the most important variables?

To begin to look beyond just nasal surgery as a way to provide answers, we further analyzed these variables of sleep position, sleep stage (Rapid Eye Movement [REM]), BMI, age as surrogates of tone exerted on the airway, but we weren't sure how they fit together yet. We began by looking deeper at the sleep apnea parameters themselves, and as we had noted from the rhinoplasty study that when the amount of time spent in the most apnea inducing states, supine position [15], and REM stage [16] varied from pre- operative to post-operative studies, the *overall* AHI became much less useful. We also noted that some of the most obese patients with severely elevated BMI had nearly 0% of the night spent supine (as they were reportedly unable to) and had low percentages of the night spent in REM sleep. This correlates with the literature in general that elevated BMI patients had more varied responses to these states and may have been more responsive to gravitational forces as we shall see shortly [13, 14].

In response to a similar problem, Lee et al. [15] who had found that percent time spent in supine confounded sleep studies' overall AHI parameter. They developed a corrective measure to correct for the amount of time spent supine. We agreed with this and felt that overall AHI was too nonspecific to fully evaluate subtle alterations in nasal airflow without taking into account amount of time spent supine position or in REM sleep, particularly if improved nasal airflow "permitted" patients to spend more time supine. In other words, if a patient had much worse AHI during REM or supine sleep, and they varied from night to night or patient to patient the percentage of time spent in those states, it would skew the overall AHI substantially. For example, if a patient's supine AHI was 20, and lateral position AHI was five, the overall AHI would vary from approaching 20 if most of the night was spent supine, while approaching five if most of the night was spent in a lateral position. The same would hold true for REM sleep. Thus, we carried the work of Lee et al. further, and developed a scale that would take this variability out of the score, by assessing only sleep spent supine and in REM, which we called the "SUP-REMe" score [17].

By using only reasoning, using the AHI score during supine and REM sleep stages, the sleep score could be more comparable between patients, without the confounding variable of the amount of time spent in supine or REM sleep that could be highly variable. We also found a trend that the highest BMI patients had falsely low overall AHI as sometimes these most severely affected patients had no time spent supine and little in REM sleep. I believe that zero time spent supine and in REM sleep, despite a usually low overall AHI is an indicator of the most extreme disease, as these individuals do not have the airway anatomy capable of obtaining rest in these conditions. Thus, as Lee et al. identified [15], this could account for perceived worsening AHI after surgery, that we essentially improve these patients enough to post-operatively begin sleeping supine and entering REM stage, the apnea inducing states. There is no clinical evidence that SUP-REMe AHI is actually "better" than overall AHI, but it is essentially a more "fair" way to compare sleep studies by removing confounding variables.

So, what is the big picture message here? Despite that even extensive rhinoplasty can improve sleep parameters [11], sleep apnea severity correlates with NOSE scores [18] and nasal spirometry compared to oral spirometry in OSA patients is reduced [17, 19], the nose is only *PART* of mouth-breathing. The reason that the degree of actual nasal obstruction will not or only weakly correlate with OSA severity is that most mouth-breathing (surrogate for OSA) is not, or is only partly due to nasal obstruction, and is due more to jaw tone and posture (nasal underuse not obstruction). Thus, only nasal function studies or surveys that differentiated between NUS and true obstruction would correlate with OSA severity scores.

Can the relationship between nasal obstruction, tone (BMI × age) be reconciled then, if the measure of sleep apnea severity is controlled for sleep position (supine) and stage (REM)? Possibly, but not in a linear fashion as expected:

To explain, we will compare the diffuse scatterplot from the paper [9] that failed to find a correlation between nasal anatomy and OSA, and concluded that the two were unrelated. In contrast, we present a scatterplot (Fig. 3.1) [21] that contained a re-analysis from the rhinoplasty and OSA paper [11]. The analysis from the first scatterplot paper attempts to compare OSA severity (overall AHI), with a nasal anatomy score designed by the authors, and not surprisingly finds no correlation. As we discussed, this lack of correlation prompted the authors to conclude that nasal surgery cannot be useful in the treatment of OSA, a giant (flawed) leap in logic.

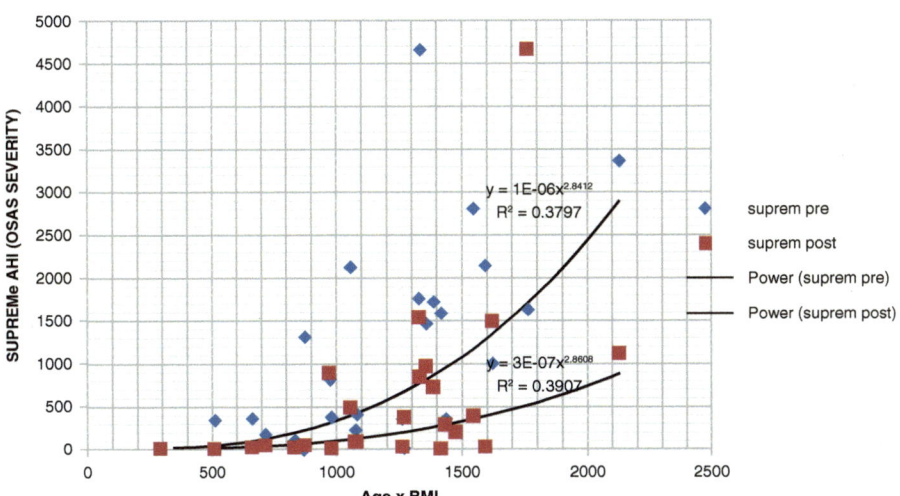

Fig. 3.1 Scatterplot of patients before (blue diamonds) and after (red squares) rhinoplasty for obstructive sleep apnea. The x-axis indicated facial tone (age × body mass index [BMI]), while the y-axis indicates sleep apnea severity (SUP-REMe Apnea-hypopnea index). The slope of the curve is what can be altered by surgery on an individual. (Reprinted with permission—Elsevier) Stupak and Park [20]

In contrast, using the data from a study of functional rhinoplasty on OSA [11], the Y-axis represented OSA severity using the SUP-REMe AHI score that removed the confounder of time spent in the apnea inducing states, and the X-axis represented mouth-closure "tone" using the product of BMI and age (BMI x age). Using this graph of OSA severity against tone, we plotted the pre- and post-operative functional rhinoplasty patients as a surrogate for nasal function, assuming that post-operative flow was closer to nasal adequacy.

Interestingly, one can see from this figure that the two patient populations sorted into two SEPARATE curves, the more vertically oriented curve consisting of patients with less adequate nasal function, while the more horizontally oriented curve representing the better functioning nasal airways. Both curves, you will note at higher "tone" become more vertical, similar to an exponential increase in slope, and suggesting that at poorer tone, OSA severity can become precipitously worse. More interestingly however is that while nasal obstruction does not have a linear correlation with OSA severity as suggested previously [9] nasal obstruction does have a relationship with OSA severity, as it determines WHICH curve of increasing tone one exists upon. This graph also suggests that an individual's nasal function or structure may determine an individual's OSA severity, by knowing the slope of the line that correlates with adequate or inadequate nasal breathing. Thus, instead of breaking OSA patients down by mild, moderate, or severe parameters, we may be better off determining an individual's slope, of the line determined by OSA severity plotted against "tone" (AgexBMI). Perhaps, there can be cutoffs dividing slope into mild, moderate, and severe obstruction that would allow us to understand that OSA severity will be different for the three nasal function groups at different "tones." Finally, we can see from the curves that OSA may actually be a lifelong progression of a condition, that is mild with all nasal function measures in good tone states, and progresses to worsened severity along different "life" curves with advancing age and BMI as determined by which anatomic curve one exists on. The slope or relationship of an individual's nasal function should determine the relationship of nasal function and OSA severity (Fig. 3.2). For example, with an inadequately

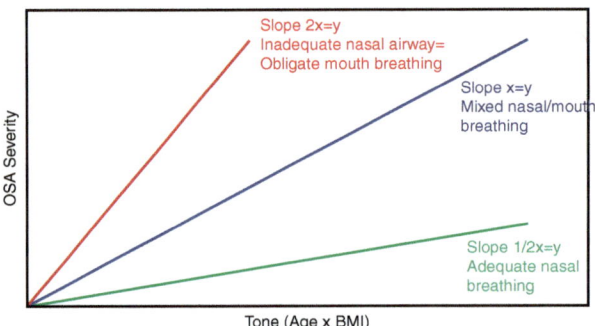

Fig. 3.2 Estimated curves of degree of mouth-breathing when plotting tone versus sleep apnea severity. Green indicates adequate nasal breathing most times, blue indicates mixed mouth and nose breathing, and red indicates obligate mouth-breathing. Only the slope varies between the individuals

functioning nose, an individual would exist on a steep vertical slope ($y = 2x$) and would develop more severe symptoms at a younger age or BMI. Conversely, a vertically flat slope would be the relationship for OSA severity to nasal function in those with adequately functioning noses, who would require substantial increases in age or BMI to develop the same symptoms. So, surgery to improve obstruction cannot cure OSA, but can only shift *which* curve we are on, as in from the steeper vertical curve to a flatter one, but surgery cannot change our tone! Likewise, this graph also explains why childhood OSA has a different cutoff for mild, moderate, and severe OSA than adult OSA in current literature.

But, what is the anatomic mechanism for these interactions? We will attempt to answer this in the next section by exploring HOW nasal obstruction and/or mouth-breathing causes sleep induced respiratory obstructions.

The mechanism of nasal airflow disturbances causing OSA, or AERODYNAMIC DIFFERENCES BETWEEN NASAL AND ORAL ROUTE OF BREATHING
Air on inspiration through the nose will impinge directly upon the pharyngeal wall.
—Proceedings of the Royal Society of Medicine, 1932

Surgeons interested in facial surgery are not usually too interested in the pharynx or sleep disorders. I think I could previously be included in this group as well. While the structures of the nose, maxilla, orbit, and mandible are appealing to me as structures to re-imagine and re-engineer, I was much less passionate about the soft tissues of the mouth and pharynx and even less so about the procedures to treat these areas.

Perhaps there is something that did not feel right about the concept of removing soft tissue that has collapsed into a lumen, or perhaps it was the restricted operating through a mouth-gag or endoscope that was less appealing. Regardless of the reason, we should conceive of the pharynx in OSA as less of the conventionally viewed "crowded" tube [21] that must be mechanically dilated through tissue removal or modification and more as a conduit that in the face of aerodynamic challenges sustains intermittent collapse.

In other words, it is not the "redundant" structures of the pharyngeal walls that are the source of collapse as we assume, but reduced upstream airflow during sleep-time inspiration that results in an insufficient column of air and skeletal structure to support the soft walls. This is not dissimilar to the concept we discussed related to the turbinates in the previous chapter. What is the significance of this alteration of viewpoint from intrinsic pharyngeal obstruction to the alternate viewpoint of external aerodynamic forces secondarily creating pharyngeal narrowing? The significance is substantial, and of course involves addressing the root source of the aerodynamic instability, which permits indirect management of the collapsing pharyngeal tissue that is less focused upon tissue removal or suspension. In Fig. 3.3, we can contrast the conventional view of intrinsically thickening walls with an external source of obstruction at the tube inlet that secondarily draws the soft walls inward during negative pressure buildup.

The reason patients do not suffer apneic episodes during the day, and have minimal pharyngeal airflow problems during waking is because the problem lies elsewhere. The pharynx only suffers from obstruction *secondarily* to airflow or lack of

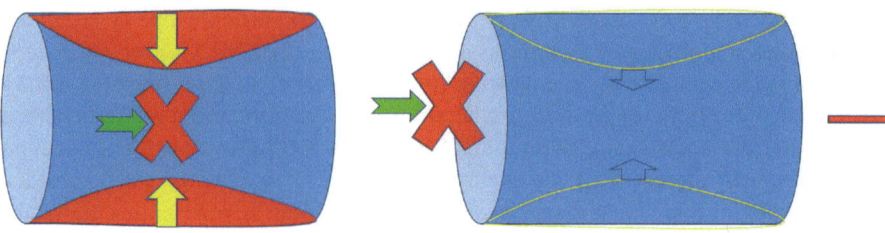

Fig. 3.3 A schematic contrast between the (left) conventional view of intrinsically thickening walls with (right) an external source of obstruction at the tube inlet that secondarily draws the soft walls inward during negative pressure buildup. Blue arrows indicate intra-luminal negative pressure drawing the walls inward due to obstruction (red X) at the nasal inlet. Yellow arrows indicate intrinsic wall thickening, which are the conventionally viewed sources of obstruction. Green arrows dictate direction of flow toward the red minus indicating negative pressure

airflow upstream at the lips and nostrils. Thus, the facial surgeon must study the pharynx in a realistic fashion to understand the true consequences of his/her work.

Start with a little home experiment: Close your lips and keep your jaws locked together. Now, while taking a deep breath through your nose, try to make a loud snoring sound. Not too impressive, right? Next, widely open your mouth, and similarly, attempt to make a loud snoring sound. That was much louder, right?

What was happening in this experiment? With a sealed oral cavity, the tongue and palate remain locked together, trapped in the oral cavity, with the tongue contacting the hard palate, and the soft palate in contact with the posterior tongue. With all of this mucosal contact, there is no airspace in the oral cavity, and via the sealed lips, no potential for outside airflow.

So, when chest cavity expansion creates a negative pressure environment in the pharynx to prepare for inspiration, a column of airflow from outside the nares is drawn into the nasal cavity, nasopharynx, and subsequently oropharynx to reverse the vacuum generated in this space to restore it to atmospheric pressure. So, not only are the palate and tongue trapped in the oral cavity, but a buttressing column of retro-lingual and retro-palatal atmospheric air "lift" these two structures in a direction directed toward the lips and away from the pharyngeal lumen, operating on a small scale the way CPAP is designed to. The absence of palatal and lingual motion toward the posterior pharyngeal walls is the lack of snoring, "laminar" airflow-sound you heard from part 1 of our experiment.

Now, with the open oral cavity, second portion of the experiment, the palate and tongue are unleased from mucosal contact and from a locked position between the jaws. When we generate our snoring sound (extreme negative pressure generated from chest wall expansion transmitted to the pharynx), the palate and tongue are free to be mobilized by aerodynamic forces. So, now to alleviate the negative pressure environment in the pharynx, a rush of airflow proceeds through the mouth, partially striking the anterior surfaces of the soft palate and tongue that drives these structures posteriorly toward the posterior pharyngeal wall, and partially closing off the nasopharynx. Thus, no column of retro-lingual and retro-palatal air flow can support these structures. Instead, the tongue and palate will vibrate violently against the posterior pharyngeal wall, creating partial airway obstruction, and the loud snoring sounds of our experiment. In addition, the oral airway is far less efficient in transmitting air than the nasal airway [22, 23].

What we have just illustrated is a simplification of the dramatic aerodynamic differences that are created between the oral route and nasal route of breathing, that has been demonstrated both in physiologic studies in the anesthesia literature evaluating the airway during sedation, and using fluid-structure interaction models [22, 24].

To explore this more in depth, please see Fig. 3.4a, b, models of the pharynx during mouth-open and mouth-closed states. When viewed in this sagittal cross-section, it is easy to see that the palate in particular, but also the tongue can be analogous to the cross-section of an airfoil (airplane wing or modern sail). These structures also experience differential air flow on their "top" (nasopharyngeal) and "bottom" (oral) surfaces (see orange line in Fig. 3.4 for airfoil surfaces), also similar to how the aerodynamic concept of "lift" applies to a wing. Like the concept of lift (determined by Bernoullian and Newtonian forces), the airfoil changes its orientation depending on the differential airflow between its surfaces (yellow arrow), influenced by a combination of muscle tone and airflow (green arrow). In many ways, these structures that exist at the intersection of the nasal, oral, and hypopharynx can be analyzed as airfoils subject to both intrinsic muscle activity as to aerodynamic forces that act upon them. An airfoil is defined by Wikipedia as the cross-sectional shape of a wing or sail subject. "An airfoil-shaped body moved through a fluid produces an aerodynamic force. The component of this force perpendicular to the direction of motion is called lift. The lift on an airfoil is primarily the result of its angle of attack and shape." Angle of attack in fluid dynamics is the angle of the air (or fluid) moving relative to the axis of the airfoil (Fig. 3.5).

For our purposes in understanding nasal versus oral aerodynamics in the pharynx, the cross-sectional view of the soft palate and tongue serve as "airfoils" subjected to variations in airflow. In essence, the muscle tone of the soft palate and

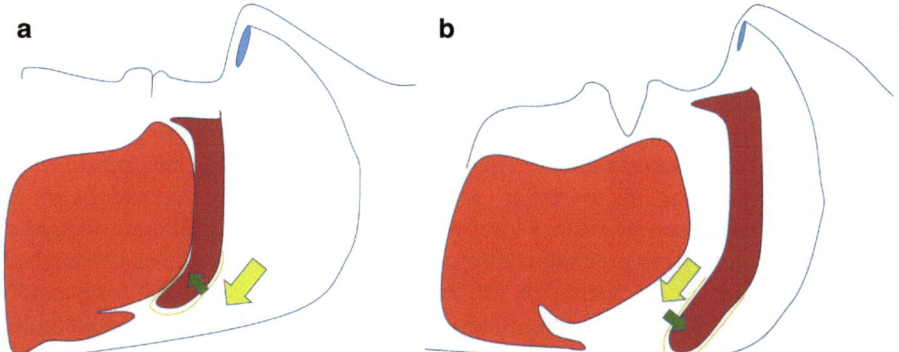

Fig. 3.4 Sagittal view of the face and airway cross-section. (**a**) Palate is lifted toward tongue (green arrow) on nasal breathing. (**b**) Palate is lifted toward nasopharynx (green arrow) on oral breathing. Yellow arrows indicate airflow direction. Orange indicates surface of airfoil

Fig. 3.5 Airfoil cross-
section demonstrating
"angle of attack," yellow
arrow relative to axis, and
direction of lift
(green arrow)

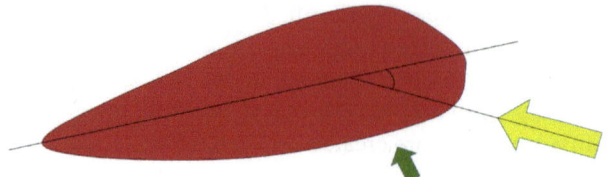

tongue determines airfoil cross-sectional shape, and the angle of attack is the angle
of the nasal or oral airflow orientation relative to where it contacts the cross-sectional
axis of the tongue or palate. The simplest explanation of lift generation utilizes
Newtonian physics, "The airflow changes direction as it passes the airfoil and follows a path that is curved downward. According to Newton's second law, this
change in flow direction requires a downward force applied to the air by the airfoil.
Then Newton's third law requires the air to exert an upward force on the airfoil; thus
a reaction force, lift, is generated opposite to the directional change. In the case of
an airplane wing, (or soft palate) the wing exerts a downward force on the air and
the air exerts an upward force on the wing. Most definitions of lift also incorporate
Bernoulli's principle and airflow speed, as do conventional understandings of
OSA. However, I believe that an in-depth explanation of how these forces apply
may only confuse our discussion as they apply more to very acute angles of attack
(like sailing upwind or close-hauled in modern sailing or with actual lift required for
airflight), where the airflow is nearly parallel to the airfoil. In our model, the more
perpendicular angles of attack of the air upon the soft palate and tongue functions
more like the sail of an archaic square-rigged sailing ship that could only sail down-
wind. The classic figure of the various "points of sail" used to teach sail position
relative to the wind can be helpful in better comprehending this concept. Regardless
of the theoretical explanations for lift, we will just focus on the lift itself to understand the clinical relevance.

Also according to Wikipedia, "It makes no difference whether the fluid is flowing
past a stationary body (our case) or the body is moving through a stationary volume
of fluid (an airplane wing or sail). Lift is the component of this force that is perpendicular to the oncoming flow direction. So, using the concept of the soft-palate and
tongue serving as airfoils, with muscle tone of these structures determining shape,
and nasal versus oral airflow determining the "angle of attack" of air upon the airfoil, we can begin to predict how different routes of respiration (nasal vs. oral) and
muscle tone (sleep vs. awake) can effect breathing efficiency and apneas.

The understanding that the tongue and palate can be thought of as airfoils whose
position is determined by various airflows is the basis for a model that can predict
how other factors, from gravitational forces, tone, to facial structure can exacerbate
sleep related airway disorders. We will analyze each one of these states separately
below, using our basic sagittal airfoil model and exposing it to different conditions.
This, in particular is how a rhinoplasty or facial surgeon can understand how these
complex factors can interact with the nasal airway in the real world.

Gravitational Forces

Let's begin with the most powerful and simplest force: Gravitational forces. Nearly 20 years ago, space shuttle STS-95 launched at the Kennedy Space Center in Florida. Aboard as a payload specialist, who also happened to be the first American in orbit, and the first US senator and the oldest individual to undergo spaceflight was John Glenn. While of course most known for his pioneering Mercury 7 spaceflight in the 1960s, and his political career, Glenn also participated directly in gaining knowledge about how gravity impacts OSA.

One fascinating article [25] shows how five astronauts, including the astronaut on STS-95, were subjected to sleep studies before and after flight, and in the near zero (micro-gravity) environment of space flight. Overall AHI was reduced by 55% in the microgravity (but normal air pressure) sleep studies, a statistically significant difference. On return to Earth, the AHI returned approximately to its pre-flight values.

This simple study demonstrated the powerful effect of gravitational forces upon the human airway. For those of us constrained from making orbital flights to cure our OSA, gravitational forces exert the most influence on our airway in the supine sleeping position, where the palate and tongue, although buoyed by retro-lingual and retro-palatal airflow, are drawn into a collapsed position against the posterior pharyngeal wall, increasing the likelihood of obstruction. The hinged mandible is also susceptible to the forces of gravity and is drawn posteriorly into an open position, thus also exacerbating the collapse by increasing mouth-breathing (Fig. 3.6—Gravitational forces on palate and tongue). Supine position has been well documented in the literature as an exacerbating factor in restricting the airway during sleep [26, 27].

Fig. 3.6 Sagittal view of the face and airway cross-section demonstrating gravitational forces in supine position

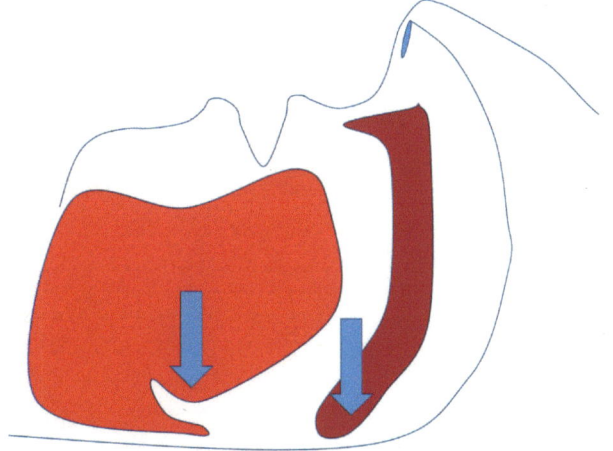

Tone/Airfoil Shape

What about when the airfoil-like structures (palate and tongue) are exposed to reduced musculoskeletal support (i.e. increased influence of gravity)? Adequate muscle tone in the palate and tongue (especially during wakefulness) applies essentially the opposite force from gravity, preventing pharyngeal collapse (Fig. 3.7). This, of course, is the key to why airway collapse generally occurs during sleep and sedation, and why stage of sleep (REM vs. nREM) matters. As you can see in the figure, loss of muscle tone will change the SHAPE of the palate and tongue (muscle-composed airfoils), creating a more "limp" structure, more prone to the influence of gravity and less able to resist maintaining a structured favorable posture. In addition, the jaw support or jaw closure structures become limp as well, exposing the palate and tongue airfoils to more oral surface airflow, which causes them to protrude posteriorly. Decreased tone of these structures can be due to diminished tone states of sleep, sedation from medications or alcohol, and in the long term from age or disease induced muscle atrophy. All of these factors can be additive, all present factors contributing to worsening airfoil shape and posture and worsening muscular jaw closure.

While we are discussing tone, we can briefly discuss the effect on our tongue and palate airfoil model of elevated Body Mass Index (BMI) or obesity. First, a team led by Raanen Arens at Montefiore shows us from Magnetic Resonance Imaging (MRI) studies of OSA, that is not just pharyngeal crowding, but misplaced structural position. This supports our airfoil model that shows that muscle position and airflow dynamics can affect the shape of the airway and relate to the severity and amount of collapse events [28].

But, there is also substantial MRI evidence that the tongue and possibly palate in OSA patients have a substantially higher fat content and lower muscle tone and stiffness than non-OSA patients [29–31].

Fig. 3.7 Sagittal view of the face and airway cross-section with yellow arrows demonstrating direction of muscle tone and lift

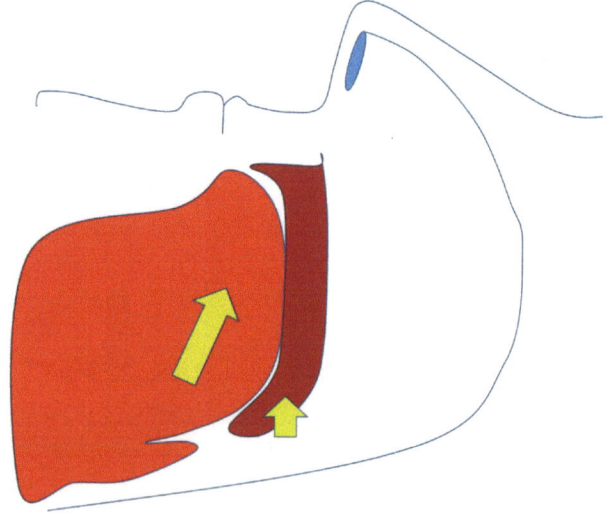

Ito et al. found also that it is not just tongue size being overly large, but being overly large compared to a small jaw "cage." In this situation, the tongue appears and functions as an overly large structure, but just appears relatively so compared to small upper and lower jaws [32].

These effects of the palate and particularly the tongue combine to alter the airfoil structure of the tongue in obesity states, making it overly large compared to the surrounding airspace, and pre-disposing to mouth-breathing and collapse. This would be analogous to insufficient wing lift design and under-powering in an aircraft, perhaps like the famous gigantic "Spruce Goose" designed by Howard Hughes that barely rose above the surface of the water in its Maiden and only test flight. Essentially, lift and tone fail to overwhelm gravitational forces.

Finally, elevated BMI states may involve overall poor muscle tone including weak jaw closing muscles. Like other reasons for limited tone of these muscles, this condition may predispose or exacerbate mouth-breathing, particularly during sleep states of diminished tone. In the next section, we will discuss the exact mechanism of actually how the open mouth can be the cause of obstruction, despite the conventional belief about the large caliber of the oral airway.

Airflow Angle of Attack/Zones of negative air pressure: How mouth-breathing specifically causes pharyngeal collapse

Whereas we have previously discussed how the angle of air striking an airfoil like the palate and tongue is called "the angle of attack," and that this angle can determine the relative position in space of the airfoil, we will now more deeply explore the specifics of this concept and how it relates to nasal versus mouth breathing. In one published study, we tested this concept using a rudimentary "windtunnel," testing these concepts with a palate-like airfoil exposed to various angles of attack [23].

If you look at the sagittal figure of the palate and tongue airfoils at a neutral resting position in the pharynx, these structures are essentially in an equilibrium state determined by muscle tone, gravitational forces and head position, as well as airflow currents and differential pressure in different regions of the pharynx.

Inspiration begins with negative pressure (relative to atmospheric pressure) generation in the chest via chest wall and diaphragm expansion. This vacuum or negative pressure is transmitted via the rigid trachea and larynx into the hypopharynx. In the ideal clinical scenario, the mouth is completely closed, with the tongue locked firmly between the upper and lower jaws, the dorsal tongue surface contacting the hard and soft palate. Because the mouth is closed, no air jet will pass via the oral cavity to neutralize the negative pressure, thus only negative pressure is transmitted from the pharynx to this region, further sealing the tight connection between the tongue and palate. Instead, a jet of air is drawn via the nostrils, through the nasal cavity and nasopharynx to the hypopharynx to neutralize the negative pressure. The jet of air strikes only the posterior palate and dorsal tongue, "lifting" the airfoils away from the posterior pharyngeal wall, and preventing airway collapse, even in low tone or unfavorable gravitational conditions (supine position). Because the air flows in a curved pattern from the inferiorly directed nostril, then chiefly over the inferior turbinate [33], it strikes the posterior palate and dorsal tongue at a near perpendicular favorable angle of attack to promote lift of these structures. The superior curvilinear surface of the inferior turbinate may even further assist in this lift process via a concept known as the Coanda effect. The Coanda effect is where a "moving stream of fluid in contact with a curved surface will tend to follow the curvature of the surface rather than continue traveling in a straight line" [34] (Fig. 3.8a). Thus, in this case maximizing the concentration of airflow at the optimal angle of attack on the palate, without diffusing this jet into other directions.

In contrast, in a primarily mouth-breathing model, the jet of an oral column of air will obliquely contact the ventral tongue of the open mouth at an acute angle and will contact the dorsal surface in a near parallel fashion. The jet will also perpendicularly contact the anterior surface of the palate. This angle of attack will cause the palate and tongue to "lift" posteriorly toward the posterior pharyngeal wall, thus partially occluding or obstructing the airway, and predisposing toward collapse (Fig. 3.8b).

While we conventionally tend to see a larger caliber nasal airway as superior to a narrower one, the relationship may not be as simple, and we may actually have the relationship incorrectly analyzed. Using these models of "angle of attack" upon airfoils, one can see that a *less* perpendicular angle of attack of the air jet from the nasal cavity, that strikes the palate in a more-or less parallel axis to the palate will exert less Newtonian force, and will achieve less "lift" of the palate and subsequently the tongue (as the palate itself will obstruct the jet from fully reaching the dorsal tongue) away from the posterior pharyngeal wall. This may be the case where a well-meaning surgeon partially removed an inferior turbinate as "obstructive."

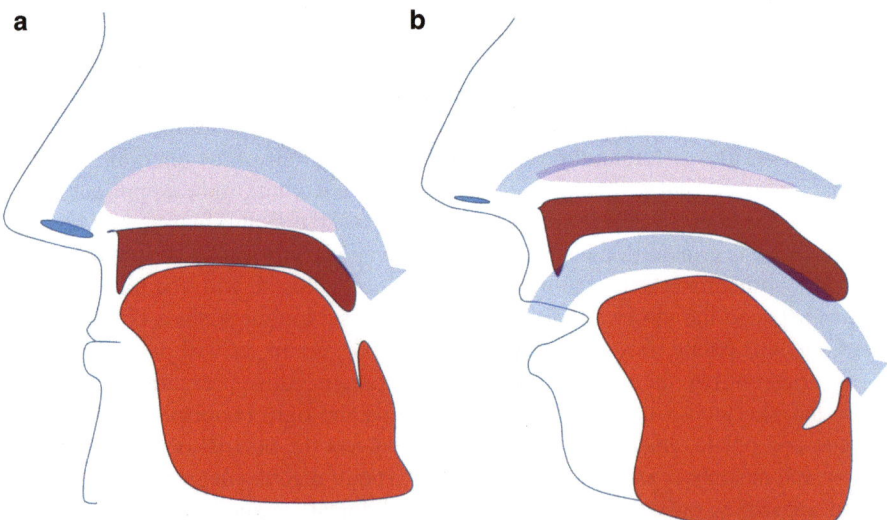

Fig. 3.8 Sagittal view of the face and airway cross-section demonstrating the Coanda effect (blue arrow) in the (**a**) nose breathing model and (**b**) mouth and nose breathing model

Without the presence of the turbinate's bulk, the inspiratory air jet directed from the nostril will not be directed over the turbinate, and then take a steep angle of attack into the nasopharynx, but instead, the inspiratory air jet may course along the floor of the nose, eventually striking the palate at an unfavorable "opening" angle of attack. This may be the phenomenon partially responsible for the condition known as "empty nose syndrome," where over-aggressive turbinate resection relative to the size of the nasal inlet creates a spectrum of negative nasal symptoms that do not match the enlarged nasal cavity. In addition, as previously discussed in the prior chapter, the absence of the turbinate (or a large septal perforation) creates vortices that may reduce the organized jet flow to reach the nasopharynx. This aerodynamic inefficiency explanation is a contrast to most conventional viewpoints that attribute the empty nose disease to loss of mucosal airflow sensation receptors.

Finally, with a mix of nasal and oral breathing routes open, one jet of atmospheric air will pass via the nostrils and eventually the nasopharynx contacting obliquely the posterior surface of the palate and dorsal surface of the tongue, finally passing the hypopharynx to neutralize the negative pressure. Simultaneously, an oral column of air will obliquely contact the ventral tongue at an acute angle as well as a parallel flow to the dorsal tongue, as well as the anterior surface of the palate. These two jets of air will in this example cause a neutralization of motion on the palate and tongue and will maintain the equilibrium of the neutral position in the airway. This of course may create a pharyngeal eco-system that matches neither pure nasal nor pure oral respiration, but has features of both, and may have a mixed clinical picture of healthy sleep-time respiration with occasional apneas.

While this chapter has carefully examined how nasal versus oral respiration interacts with physical forces like airflow jets, negative pressure, tongue size, and gravitational forces, it is easy to spot what we have thus far neglected: the influence of facial structure. This will be the topic of the next chapter.

References

1. Huang TW, Young TH. Novel porous oral patches for patients with mild obstructive sleep apnea and mouth breathing: a pilot study. Otolaryngol Head Neck Surg. 2015;152(2):369–73.
2. Lee SH, Choi JH, Shin C, Lee HM, Kwon SY, Lee SH. How does open-mouth breathing influence upper airway anatomy? Laryngoscope. 2007;117(6):1102–6.
3. Meurice JC, Marc I, Carrier G, Sériès F. Effects of mouth opening on upper airway collapsibility in normal sleeping subjects. Am J Respir Crit Care Med. 1996;153(1):255–9.
4. de Oliveira PW, Gregorio LL, Silva RS, Bittencourt LR, Tufik S, Gregório LC. Orofacial-cervical alterations in individuals with upper airway resistance syndrome. Braz J Otorhinolaryngol. 2016;82(4):377–84.
5. Friedman M, Tanyeri H, Lim JW, Landsberg R, Vaidyanathan K, Caldarelli D. Effect of improved nasal breathing on obstructive sleep apnea. Otolaryngol Head Neck Surg. 2000;122(1):71–4.
6. Koutsourelakis I, Georgoulopoulos G, Perraki E, Vagiakis E, Roussos C, Zakynthinos SG. Randomised trial of nasal surgery for fixed nasal obstruction in obstructive sleep apnoea. Eur Respir J. 2008;31(1):110–7.

7. Rosow DE, Stewart MG. Is nasal surgery an effective treatment for obstructive sleep apnea? Laryngoscope. 2010;120(8):1496–7.
8. Ishii L, Roxbury C, Godoy A, Ishman S, Ishii M. Does nasal surgery improve OSA in patients with nasal obstruction and OSA? A meta-analysis. Otolaryngol Head Neck Surg. 2015;153(3):326–33.
9. Leitzen KP, Brietzke SE, Lindsay RW. Correlation between nasal anatomy and objective obstructive sleep apnea severity. Otolaryngol Head Neck Surg. 2014;150(2):325–31.
10. Huang YS, Guilleminault C. Pediatric obstructive sleep apnea and the critical role of oral-facial growth: evidences. Front Neurol. 2013;3:184.
11. Shuaib SW, Undavia S, Lin J, Johnson CM Jr, Stupak HD. Can functional septorhinoplasty independently treat obstructive sleep apnea? Plast Reconstr Surg. 2015;135(6):1554–65.
12. Bican A, Kahraman A, Bora I, Kahveci R, Hakyemez B. What is the efficacy of nasal surgery in patients with obstructive sleep apnea syndrome? J Craniofac Surg. 2010;21(6):1801–6.
13. Ahlin S, Manco M, Panunzi S, Verrastro O, Giannetti G, Prete A, Guidone C, Berardino ADM, Viglietta L, Ferravante A, Mingrone G, Mormile F, Capristo E. A new sensitive and accurate model to predict moderate to severe obstructive sleep apnea in patients with obesity. Medicine (Baltimore). 2019;98(32):e16687.
14. Yeh PS, Lee YC, Lee WJ, Chen SB, Ho SJ, Peng WB, Tsao CC, Chiu HL. Clinical predictors of obstructive sleep apnea in Asian bariatric patients. Obes Surg. 2010;20(1):30–5. https://doi.org/10.1007/s11695-009-9854-2.
15. Lee CH, Shin HW, Han DH, Mo JH, Yoon IY, Chung S, Choi HG, Kim JW. The implication of sleep position in the evaluation of surgical outcomes in obstructive sleep apnea. Otolaryngol Head Neck Surg. 2009;140(4):531–5.
16. Kim SH, Yang CJ, Baek JT, Hyun SM, Kim CS, Lee SA, Chung YS. Does rapid eye movement sleep aggravate obstructive sleep apnea? Clin Exp Otorhinolaryngol. 2019;12(2):190–5.
17. Fastenberg JH, Fang CH, Patel VM, Lin J, Stupak HD. The use of handheld nasal spirometry to predict the presence of obstructive sleep apnea. Sleep Breath. 2018;22(1):79–84.
18. Ishii L, Godoy A, Ishman SL, Gourin CG, Ishii M. The nasal obstruction symptom evaluation survey as a screening tool for obstructive sleep apnea. Arch Otolaryngol Head Neck Surg. 2011;137(2):119–23.
19. Shepard JW Jr, Burger CD. Nasal and oral flow-volume loops in normal subjects and patients with obstructive sleep apnea. Am Rev Respir Dis. 1990;142(6 Pt 1):1288–93.
20. Stupak HD, Park SY. Gravitational forces, negative pressure and facial structure in the genesis of airway dysfunction during sleep: a review of the paradigm. Sleep Med. 2018;51:125–32.
21. Genta PR, Edwards BA, Sands SA, Owens RL, Butler JP, Loring SH, White DP, Wellman A. Tube law of the pharyngeal airway in sleeping patients with obstructive sleep apnea. Sleep. 2016;39(2):337–43.
22. Jian Y, Bao FP, Liang Y. Effectiveness of breathing through nasal and oral routes in unconscious apneic adult human subjects: a prospective randomized crossover trial. Anesthesiology. 2011;115(1):129–35.
23. Stupak HD. The human external nose and its evolutionary role in the prevention of obstructive sleep apnea. Otolaryngol Head Neck Surg. 2010;142(6):779–82.
24. Wang Y, Wang J, Liu Y, Yu S, Sun X, Li S, Shen S, Zhao W. Fluid-structure interaction modeling of upper airways before and after nasal surgery for obstructive sleep apnea. Int J Numer Method Biomed Eng. 2012;28(5):528–46.
25. Elliott AR, Shea SA, Dijk DJ, et al. Microgravity reduces sleep-disordered breathing in humans. Am J Respir Crit Care Med. 2001;164(3):478–85.
26. Kastoer C, Benoist LBL, Dieltjens M, Torensma B, de Vries LH, Vonk PE, Ravesloot MJL, de Vries N. Comparison of upper airway collapse patterns and its clinical significance: drug-induced sleep endoscopy in patients without obstructive sleep apnea, positional and non-positional obstructive sleep apnea. Sleep Breath. 2018;22(4):939–48.
27. Cartwright RD, Diaz F, Lloyd S. The effects of sleep posture and sleep stage on apnea frequency. Sleep. 1991;14(4):351–3.

28. Tong Y, Udupa JK, Sin S, Liu Z, Wileyto EP, Torigian DA, Arens R. MR image analytics to characterize the upper airway structure in obese children with obstructive sleep apnea syndrome. PLoS One. 2016;11(8):e0159327.

29. Brown EC, Cheng S, McKenzie DK, Butler JE, Gandevia SC, Bilston LE. Tongue stiffness is lower in patients with obstructive sleep apnea during wakefulness compared with matched control subjects. Sleep. 2015;38(4):537–44.

30. Turnbull CD, Wang SH, Manuel AR, Keenan BT, McIntyre AG, Schwab RJ, Stradling JR. Relationships between MRI fat distributions and sleep apnea and obesity hypoventilation syndrome in very obese patients. Sleep Breath. 2018;22(3):673–81.

31. Kim AM, Keenan BT, Jackson N, Chan EL, Staley B, Poptani H, Torigian DA, Pack I, Schwab RJ. Tongue fat and its relationship to obstructive sleep apnea. Sleep. 2014;37(10):1639–48.

32. Ito E, Tsuiki S, Maeda K, Okajima I, Inoue Y. Oropharyngeal crowding closely relates to aggravation of OSA. Chest. 2016;150(2):346–52.

33. Naughton JP, Lee AY, Ramos E, Wootton D, Stupak HD. Effect of nasal valve shape on downstream volume, airflow, and pressure drop: importance of the nasal valve revisited. Ann Otol Rhinol Laryngol. 2018;127(11):745–53.

34. www.formula1-dictionary.net.

Chapter 4
The Human Facial Skeleton: Influence on the Airway and Aesthetics? An Analysis of Cause/Effect Paradigms

Hominids typically haven't so much adapted to change, as they have accommodated to it.
—Ian Tattersall, Curator Emeritus of the Division of Anthropology, American Museum of Natural History (with permission)

My mentor and fellowship director, Calvin M. Johnson, Jr., MD, referred to the nasal septum as the "pedestal" of the tip tripod. The tripod/pedestal concept revolutionized rhinoplasty at the time, creating a paradigm for understanding that the external nose was not just a loose unintelligible collection of named cartilages, but that it had a dynamic structure, not unlike any other architectural structure. In honoring this advance of understanding, I think it can even be expanded upon.

A "pedestal" implies an inferior structure to the more important structure above—the tip or alar cartilages. Instead, I think one might conceive of the underlying structures that support the nose as the foundation (bony skeletal structure) and framework (cartilaginous septum) to portray their proper significance. A failure to recognize this and understand the critical importance of these support layers has resulted in confusion about surgical procedures. This foundation and framework, as in a building structure, are literally the substrate of the nose, but also are the figurative foundation of a revised concept of really understanding the engineering of rhinoplasty. Of course, the facial structure as foundation is not at all only existing to serve the nose, but I merely wish to impress upon the reader the importance of the facial and jaw structure to both nasal structure and function. An understanding of facial structure and dynamics could not be more critical to a rhinoplasty and facial surgeon. The key to this understanding begins with understanding how the *Homo sapiens* face differs from that of our ancestors.

© Springer Nature Switzerland AG 2020
H. D. Stupak, *Rethinking Rhinoplasty and Facial Surgery*,
https://doi.org/10.1007/978-3-030-44674-1_4

Evolution of the Human Face: Why This Matters Clinically

During my medical school and residency years, (and I think this has not changed much), there is little exposure or consideration of the subject of human evolution. Our training on this subject is largely confined to undergraduate biology courses, with more or less exposure depending on an individual's choice of majors or interest. In many ways, in retrospect, I consider this to be a flaw in our medical educational system. While I have no doubt that classes in subjects like biochemistry, histopathology, and physical exam are critical, they typically fail to provide a context for *why* we face certain medical problems by not understanding how problems which we call diseases may have arisen over the course of time in our human and pre-human (hominid) ancestors. In some ways, the perspective that ignores temporal development, instead only focusing upon the physical details of the disease, its associated symptoms, differential diagnosis and treatment, is another variation of the "compartmentalization" or conventionality blindness that we discussed in Chap. 1.

While I had the fortune of taking a few extra biology classes that emphasized evolutionary biology, I am not sure I had an opportunity to have a front-row seat view of the facial anatomy of a living human relative until nearly the end of my residency. In the midst of preparing for my move to New Orleans for fellowship, I received a call from my closest friend Karsten Munck late one night, and I expected that it was about the next day's case coverage. "We are going to be operating at the zoo tomorrow," he stated matter-of-factly to me in his typical sarcastic tone. "We are off the hook for the OR."

"Right," I replied with an equal amount of sarcasm. "I will pack the picnic lunch and let all the attendings know."

"Dr. Cheung said they already approved it, and we'll get lunch at the zoo," he said surprisingly maintaining a serious tone. I told him that I didn't have time for his nonsense, but he finally explained that our otology attending Dr. Steven Cheung, had actually been asked to assist with a sinus procedure for a silver-backed male gorilla named Kubi who was undergoing a partial lung resection for abscess by a UCSF (University of California at San Francisco) thoracic surgeon. The belief was that Kubi's sinuses were the cause of his lung infection, and we would be bringing endoscopic sinus surgery instruments to the zoo, and assisting with this procedure. The news article for this story and photos can be found at SFgate: (Fig. 4.1— CHRISTINA KOCI HERNANDEZ / San Francisco Chronicle / Polaris). https://www.sfgate.com/bayarea/article/SAN-FRANCISCO-Gorilla-s-life-in-human-hands-2781961.php

The gorilla was masterfully intubated by the physician and veterinary anesthesia teams with a massive endotracheal tube. I was amazed by the shear robustness of the gorilla's features. And while the endoscopic sinus anatomy did not look much different that our own besides a longer, more stretched appearing nasal cavity, we did note some important differences. First, our instruments were too weak to cut even through the usually flimsy bone like the uncinate process of the maxillary sinus,

Fig. 4.1 Veterinarians and UCSF physicians intubating Kubi. I am in the background wearing a facemask and looking on very curiously. (CHRISTINA KOCI HERNANDEZ / San Francisco Chronicle / Polaris—SF Gate, 2004)

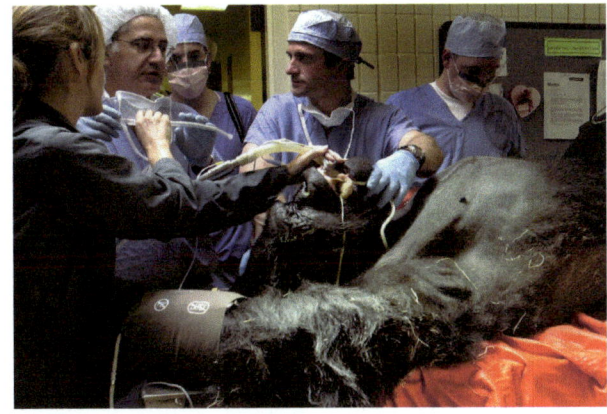

practically causing the instruments to crumble. We noted how powerfully thick this bone was compared to its *Homo sapiens* analog. Second, the gorilla, like most non-human simians, had almost no external nose structure beyond a flimsy, easily collapsible nasal valve, and had almost zero nasal tip or dorsal projection. I am not sure if our sinus surgery helped Kubi too much, despite our good intentions. The little we accomplished failed to reveal any obvious pathology. Sadly, Kubi died a few weeks after the procedure of a pulmonary complication. Even more sad and shockingly, a few years later so did my young and hilarious friend Karsten, also of a surgical complication, leaving behind a huge void.

However, this early view of the anatomy of our relatives may have stimulated me to consider more deeply how the dynamic evolutionary *Homo sapiens* facial structure impacts airway disorders and even aesthetics. Only shortly before the Kubi incident, a professor of otolaryngology and facial plastic surgery at the University of California at San Diego named Terence Davidson published an unusual paper in the journal *Sleep* in which he described the evolutionary loss of the ape-like "snout" over the course of hominid evolution from our earliest human simian ancestor as ultimately responsible for the disorder obstructive sleep apnea. He proposed, that as the evolutionary selective pressure for language increased, the previously protruding snout became more set-back into its current flat-faced position to permit the soft palate and tongue to more easily modulate sound into spoken language be being closer to the posterior pharyngeal wall [1]. And, as we discussed in the previous chapter, this increased approximation of these two muscular and collapsible organs to the posterior pharyngeal wall led to an increased predisposition to obstructive sleep apnea, as our model of collapse would predict especially when compared to our more ape-like ancestors (Figure 4.2).

Davidson's concept that natural selection for the acquisition of language via maxillary and mandibular retrusion resulted in the undesirable "side-effect" of OSA predisposition fascinated me tremendously. I was inspired personally to explore this concept further, and eventually published an article that proposed that the prominent human external nose developed similarly, as a counter-measure to the worsening

Fig. 4.2 Cross-sectional comparison of sagittal view of (**a**) human skull/airway and (**b**) chimpanzee skull and airway. (Reprinted with permission of Sage—Stupak [2])

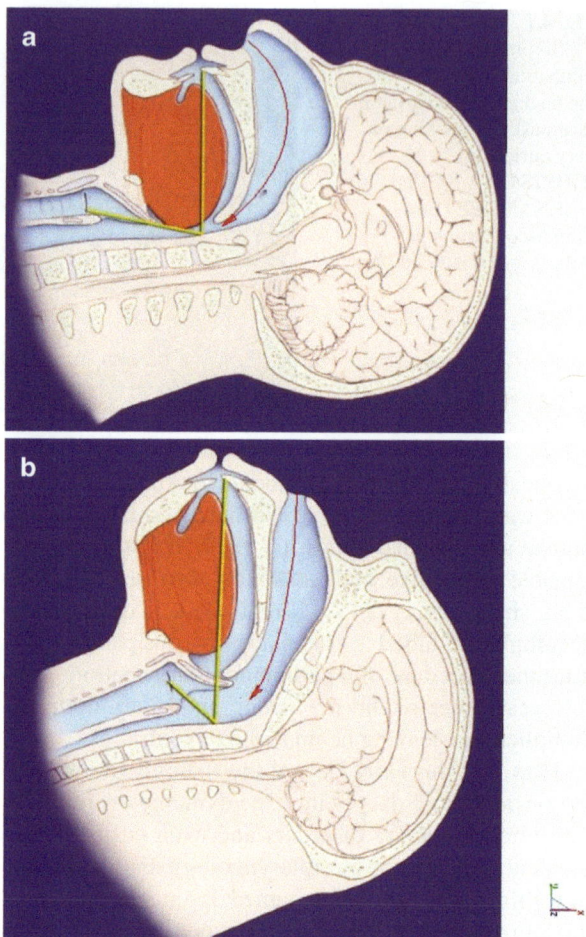

OSA of Davidson's model, that improved the angle of attack of air striking the palate [2]. In reality, both Davidson's proposal and my own from that era, while stimulating and satisfying, approach the truth, but not in a completely accurate way, because of their reliance on now-dated beliefs that evolution of traits requires only natural selection for selection. Later in the chapter, we will discuss how he work of Richard Prum helped change this perspective.

In reality, the observation that the facial snout has receded in the history of human evolution is not debatable, and is well-established by the anthropology literature, the fossil-record, and even gross observation. In the same study, using lateral photographs of hominid skulls, we used a protractor to measure the angle of the dorsum of the nasal bones relative to the plane of the maxilla. In the earliest hominids, the protruding nasal bones were almost non-existent and were nearly parallel to the plane of the protruding maxilla. As our ancestors approached modern facial structure, the nasal bones protruded more relative to the receded maxilla, and

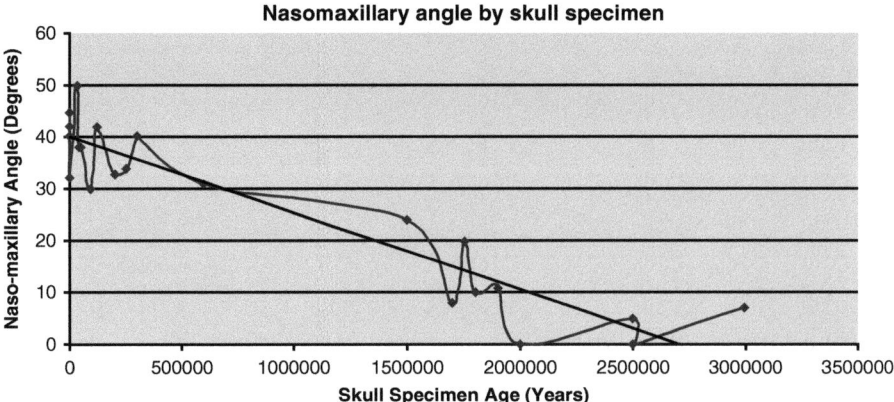

Fig. 4.3 Angle of the nasal bones relative to the plane of the maxilla from photographs of hominid skulls. The x-axis represents skull specimen age, with most modern skulls closest to zero. The y-axis represents naso-maxillary angle measured. (Reprinted with permission of Sage publishing—Stupak [2])

approached nearly 40 to 50 degrees from the maxilla, indicating a protuberant nose (Figure 4.3). While I proposed that the external nose "grew" for a purpose, I was gently and appropriately corrected in a letter to the editor that the nose simply grew externally essentially as the maxilla shrunk [3]. *How* this recognized anatomic observation of the shrinking maxilla and protruding nose inter-plays with sleep apnea, aesthetics, and the acquisition of language *is* much more controversial, which leads us to a discussion of its clinical relevance, and the controversy of cause and effect.

The Facial Skeleton, Aesthetics, and the Airway: Is the Conventional Cause and Effect Correct?

> Man is descended from a hairy, tailed quadruped, probably arboreal in its habits.
> ——Charles Darwin

The conventional view of how facial structure impacts the airway during sleep is illustrated in Fig. 4.4a. In summary, this traditional view considers that a vague inciting "inflammatory/allergic" event (like adenoid growth or turbinate hypertrophy) causes narrowing of the pharyngeal airway. This narrowing of the airway during development in turn causes the facial skeleton to develop incompletely, creating the subtle "adenoid facies" phenotype. As noted in the slide, septal deviation, turbinate hypertrophy, and nasal obstruction are an unrelated phenomenon, only randomly occurring in the same patient.

The adenoid face, defined by Elluru [4] as "a long, thin face with malar hypoplasia, high-arched palate, narrow maxillary arch, and angle class II malocclusion,"

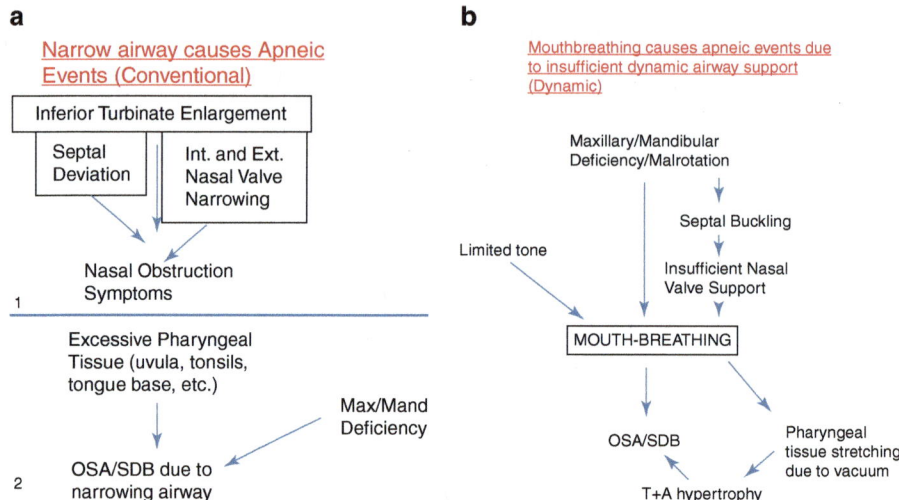

Fig. 4.4 Causal diagram for the interaction of the facial skeleton, airway, and pharyngeal tissue. (**a**) The "conventional" viewpoint causal diagram that shows a number of anatomic factors that can combine to cause nasal obstruction. The structures located within the pharynx are only related to this as the "multi-level" causes of narrow airway and sleep apnea. (**b**) In contrast, the causal diagram that asserts that facial structure causes mouth-breathing which results in pharyngeal tissue growth and sleep disorders is presented

creates additional narrowing of the airway because of skeletal deficiency. According to the conventional view, these patients thus have a compounded narrow airway, that is treated conventionally first by adeno-tonsillectomy, to "create space." Then, if indicated, as adults with a persistent sleep disorder, to have additional airway "widening" by either soft tissue removal (turbinectomy and uvulopalatopharyngoplasty) or bony expansion (maxilla-mandibular advancement). Concurrent nasal obstruction, in the unfortunate patients who also have this problem can have further airway enlargement with a septoplasty, turbinate reduction, or the placement of airway-dilating grafts. It is also commonly accepted that an early and effective adenoidectomy would prevent the development of the cascade, as this inflammatory structure is the root cause [4]. Many, if not most practitioners operate within this framework of understanding, and see little risk in following the accepted pathway, despite the works of skeptics [5–7].

While a neatly packaged algorithm that encourages inter-specialty collaboration and surgery, there are several distinct flaws and clear fallacies in this reasoning, despite their long-held acceptance.

In a recent article published in Sleep Medicine (2018), we attempted to rationally discuss these fallacies using a dissection of the literature, and to provide an alternative, logic-based order of events (Fig. 4.4b) [8].

Refuting these long-held beliefs by the majority is not an easy task. As EJ Dierks put in 2005 Archives Otolaryngology (OTO)/Head and Neck Surgery (HNS) opinion, a prospective clinical trial investigating this concept's cause and effect in twins would be both impractical and unethical [5]. Instead, we are forced to work on the problem indirectly, through observation, modeling, and reasoning. The lifetime body of work from the recently late Stanford sleep researcher Christian Guilleminault along with many colleagues has made great strides in questioning these fallacies through a combination of clinical studies and indirect analysis. In his work, he essentially has found that a subclinical bony structural problem is the primary inciting event in this cascade, with eventual mouth-breathing and sleep apnea as downstream events.

We will address these nearly institutional fallacies in the remainder of this chapter, as we discuss the alternate pathway of how the facial structure, the airway, and sleep interact.

Fallacy 1: The Adenoid Develops Due to a Vague Inflammatory Process

During the twentieth century, a good deal of work was committed to demonstrating the commonly accepted belief that the adenoid was the true villain in the process of development of fore-shortened faces. Perhaps some of the motivation behind this was for specialists to provide some concrete explanation to themselves and their patients for the clearly occurring facial phenomenon that satisfied the desire to be proactive by encouraging the removal of a very visual, palpable, and removable organ. The term of "adenoid facies" was coined by CV Tomes in 1872 and adopted in the 1930's by prominent orthodontists [9]. Evidence was provided for this concept in the early 1980s that seemed to "settle" the cause and effect issue. Rhesus monkeys, in studies conducted by Harvold, Tomer, and Vargervik demonstrated facial deformities with nostril plugs [10–12]. These studies were quoted throughout the subsequent literature to justify the use of adenoidectomy and implied that the cause and effect question of the adenoid and the adenoid face was settled. Undoubtedly, these concepts when relayed to parents of children being considered for adeno-tonsillar surgery were an impetus to proceed. What parent could risk being the cause of their child's facial deformity, or even vague unattractiveness?

But, did the use of nostril plugs in monkeys really replicate the development of the adenoid facies in these disorders? Of course not. First, the adenoid is quite different in location than the nasal valve or nostril. It is substantially further downstream and is almost never completely occluding of the nasopharynx. In addition to the plugs having almost nothing in common with adenoids, the studies and related clinical studies of the time almost completely failed to effectively measure cause and effect. Second, the few facial "structural" changes that *were* documented in the study after plugging were not actual structural changes! The monkeys simply changed their jaw posture to a resting open-mouth posture, thus elongating their facial length. Clinically, the concept that adenoidectomy would relieve nasal obstruction and restore proper growth was primarily championed by Sten Linder-Aronson, Professor and Chairman of the Orthodontic Department of the Karolinska

Institute in Sweden. Through several publications between his thesis in 1970 followed through 2018, Linder-Aronson proposed that adenoidectomy improved maxillary incisor plane, restored horizontal growth, and better mandibular growth [13].

In one letter, he criticized one author for questioning the adenoid/face association by announcing that "reviews of the kind published by O'Ryan and her colleagues fail to contribute to a deeper understanding of an *apparently* controversial topic. Unfortunately they only serve to create further confusion" [14].

In a 2006 study, another similar study suggests that "it would appear that there is a cause and effect relationship between nasal airway obstruction and dentofacial development, and that early treatment of children with OSA in order to normalize the mode of breathing is indicated," further suggesting after the results of a 17 patient study that "early treatment of OSA was successful and dentofacial morphology was normalized after adeno-tonsillectomy" [15]. While the authors do acknowledge to some degree that the interaction is complex, the proponents of this treatment do not see that cause and effect cannot be established by these limited observation studies and does recognize that the association of the adenoid and the facial deformity does not actually support the causality proposed. The obvious flaw in these limited studies is that although facial structure measurements may have "normalized," there is absolutely zero reason to attribute this to the adenoid removal. In other words, we all know that between the mean age of five in the 17 patients, there is no doubt that all of the patients experienced facial growth. This, as we will see later in the chapter is the real reason that very few adults have adenoid tissue, and that with or without adenoid surgery, faces will grow from childhood size to eventual adult size, regardless of sophisticated measurement techniques. As we will see when we discuss the mechanism of how mouth-breathing, the adenoid, and facial size relate, the adenoid is more of an "innocent bystander" (with the exception of the secondarily completely occluding structure) that more likely actually appears DUE to mouth-breathing and facial structural abnormalities, and not vice-versa. For example, while an overwhelming international consensus of papers with extensive data [16–31] describes an association of adenoid size and cephalometry, there is absolutely zero evidence of a cause-effect relationship of adenoid→facial abnormality!

This is analogous to other spurious examples of causality as when the association of growing shoe size in children and concurrent increase in academic knowledge is documented, which are of course unrelated but trend upward in a parallel fashion.

I find that I am struck by the sheer forcefulness of the insistence that the adenoid serves as the inciting agent in causing facial growth anomalies. After extensive literature review, it becomes evident that some specialties support this concept more than others. One paper states that "the craniofacial structure before, and its change after adeno-tonsillectomy, in patients with large adenoids and tonsils (classically, regarded as mouth breathing patients) are not only caused by a mechanistic alteration in the muscular balance and head and tongue position due to the change in the mode of breathing but also caused by a more complex sequence of epigenetic events. Because of abnormal nocturnal secretion of GH and its mediators in children with obstructed breathing, mandibular ramus growth is less than that in healthy subjects" [32].

Table 4.1 The fallacies of the conventional facial structure→sleep disorder paradigm:

1. Unknown/vague inflammation cascade induces adenoid growth.
2. The adenoid is the inciting cause of nasal obstruction during development.
3. Nasal obstruction from the adenoid causes facial deformity "adenoid facies."
4. The sleep-breathing disorders are caused simply by restricted airway caliber (either soft tissue obstruction or narrowed bony structure).

Perhaps it is related to fallacy number four (Table 4.1 above), the belief that the function of the airway is strictly related to its caliber, instead the deeper understanding of a more dynamic concept related to route of breathing. Thus, viewing the larger adenoid on dental plain films in children must have prompted individuals to conclude that the airway is "obstructed" by the adenoid, and ascribed cause to this visible structure (although this obstruction should have been present at both day and night, not just during sleep to hold up to validity, not to mention the huge variability in adenoid size in practice that almost never correlates directly with the degree of symptoms.)

In contrast, as early as 1932, in a paper from the Proceedings of Royal Society written by a British otolaryngologist and oral surgeon (Warwick James and Somerville Hastings), it has been clear that the insignificant adenoid plays almost no role in the process:

"Contrary to the generally accepted view, we are of opinion that nasal obstruction is rarely caused by adenoids. Too often in the past cases of children with lips apart have been diagnosed as 'adenoids' and hurried off to operation; it is not surprising that some adenoids have been found, as adenoid tissue is present in the nasopharynx of most children. It is true that in a few cases the lymphoid tissue of the nasopharynx is so much increased in amount that it blocks the airway. Most of the children, however, who are diagnosed as cases of 'adenoids' and benefited by operation have a mass of lymphoid tissue in the nasopharynx of such a size that it could not possibly cause any obstruction. We have been impressed by the fact that in very few of the cases we have seen with open mouth is the airway in any part of the nose or nasopharynx less than that through the open glottis. It is very difficult to see, therefore, how real obstruction could be caused by the adenoids. Moreover, in very many cases the open-mouth habit continues, in spite of the removal of adenoids, unless the child is instructed and trained otherwise" [7].

Only after carefully reading the conclusions of papers on the adenoid topic, and moving beyond the abundance of "data" that stir the controversy, it is not difficult to see that "the data" tend to support more intervention. One author, in a review of the topic notes in his final statement: "Finally, it is noteworthy that in many cases, the growth acceleration [from adenotonsillectomy] is not sufficient to solve the already formed malocclusion and skeletal discrepancy, and therefore, orthodontic treatment is also indicated" [32].

Of course, this phenomenon is universal in medicine, and not isolated in this segment of the literature. I believe the literature as a whole is also subconsciously devoted to the processing of data to increase or justifying the use of favored surgical procedures using easily manipulated outcome measures like satisfaction surveys or ratings scales and promoting dated (and never questioned) cause/effect models. A recent example of this is a recent paper that creates a statistical model using clinical assumptions of surgical success rates, recommending the addition of turbinate reduction as a standard cost-effective measure to adeno-tonsillectomy procedures for sleep disordered breathing in children, citing added benefit to society [33]. Thus, the study essentially uses a computer model to "double-down" on the limited tactics described in the two previous chapters. The fallacy is based on the mistaken assumption that two unreliable procedures performed together will make a better operation.

Of course, there are many exceptions to this, as there is fortunately the occasional study that questions the utility of accepted procedures and long-standing paradigms, but these are more the exception than the rule. However, I cynically believe that the cause and effect "controversy" focused upon the adenoid has been at best a distraction from the actual causes of limited facial growth.

The late Christian Guilleminault, a psychiatrist by training, and eminent sleep researcher, did not have the burden of the usually unmentioned conflict of interest of conducting research that supports one's financial reimbursement from favorite procedures, as he is neither surgeon nor orthodontist. Over a lifetime of research, he proposes a simpler and more reasonable cause and effect relationship, that subtle deficiencies or imperfections in facial musculoskeletal structure and growth are the cause of mouth-breathing and OSA. The adenoid and tonsil, in this case, simply are "fellow-travelers," making *very inconsistent* appearances from this perspective and are likely not of as great importance as previously suggested. Logical analysis of the tremendous variability of the size and presence or absence of these structures in both healthy and severe cases argues strongly for their lack of importance, despite the varied prominence of the tonsil on pharyngeal exam [34, 35]. If crowding by excess prominence of the structures was the cause of the sleep disturbance, the severity MUST correlate with the size of the structures. Thus, by demonstrating that size and severity do not correlate, the data essentially shows that crowding by these structures is not the cause of the disease. And, obstructive objects should be obstructive all of the time, not just during sleep.

And as James and Hastings noted in 1932: The term "adenoid facies" has been used to describe a particular facial appearance in children and adults in which most of the characteristics [already defined above] are pronounced. Such a facial appearance may be present without adenoids, and without any history of their ever having been removed" [7].

Even the accepted wisdom about the origins of the tonsil and adenoid (Fallacy # 2—origins of the vague inflammatory process), and their role in OSA treatment can be taken into serious questioning, even beyond their supposed effect on facial structure. The current established paradigm consists of a vague inflammatory or infectious process triggering the growth of adenotonsillar tissue [36]. While this concept is deeply ingrained in our concept of modern medicine, a more thoughtful analysis may prompt one to question how and why. There are several obvious inconsistencies in this concept. First, in a pharynx filled with micro-organisms, why do only some organisms cause lymphoid hypertrophy in only certain individuals? Is there a specific biofilm, [37, 38] bacteria, [36] immune response, or immature immune system at fault that we just have not fully discovered yet? Why do some allergic individuals have extensive tonsils, while others have none?

In general, there is no consistent or logical established explanation that convincingly explains how the tissues of Waldeyer's ring develop, and certainly there is no reason to think in reality (despite the prolonged "controversy") that this tissue plays any role in maxilla-mandibular development. Despite the historical longevity and broad acceptance of the infectious/inflammatory concept of origins of the tissue, linked in a vague way to an unfavorable pharyngeal environment, one can at least see the utility in digging deeper into root causes that may pre-dispose to these infection or inflammation responses [39].

Further, although at least in children adeno-tonsillectomy is viewed as the "standard of care" first step in treating mouth-breathing, facial deformity, nasal obstruction and even behavioral problems related to pediatric OSA, the overall success and results of this procedure have recently been substantially called into question. With an at best roughly 40–60% chance of achieving success by most published studies in the short run, especially with obesity the overall results of this procedure are not satisfactory enough to prevent further investigation into its utility [40]. In addition, a very recent and very large study suggests that the procedure conversely is associated with long-term negative health effects. In this study, in Denmark, over one million children with and without adenoid/tonsil surgery were followed for up to 20 years after surgery. The study found that the surgery group had a two to threefold increase in respiratory problems later in life. The study, conducted by non-surgeons, attributed the increased respiratory problems as a result of undergoing surgery. However, similar to the bias of the surgical literature, which implies that improvements after surgery are due to the removal of the tonsil and adenoid, they imply that the respiratory and infectious problems these patients face in the long run are due to the removal of these tissues as well. The reasoning error that both the pro- and anti-surgery groups fail to recognize is of course that the mouth-breathing in these patients is independent of surgery. In other words, in the patients who "improve" after adeno-tonsillectomy, in the long run, it is actually because they experienced increase and growth in their facial structure, and they were able to at least partially transition to primarily nasal breathing. Those that failed to transition to primarily nasal breathing after tonsillectomy are considered "failures," but the surgery was simply an unrelated red-herring, and these patients were doomed to continue to mouth-breathe anyway, due to more severe facial structural problems or tone problems like obesity or other syndromes. On the other side of the coin, while in the Byars study it appears that the long-term respiratory problems are due to a lack of tonsils and adenoids from surgery, in reality, this cohort of mouth-breathers who were selected by physicians and parents for surgery due to a snoring and sleep apnea profile, would of course have had an increased risk of a lifetime of respiratory problems with or without surgery [41]. For example, in the traditional entity of "post-obstructive pulmonary edema" that suggests that by removing the tonsils, this relief of the obstruction can cause rapid pulmonary edema upon extubation. Of course, the root problem (mouth-breathing related pharyngeal obstruction) has not actually been relieved, instead only the visual manifestation of persistent mouth-breathing removed (the tonsils) is now reduced. Thus, the concept could be renamed "still-obstructed pulmonary edema," in the setting of these patients having limited tolerance for sedative anesthetics due to severe OSA. With the addition of sedation and thus further diminishment of tone, the aerodynamic collapse is exacerbated, and high intra-thoracic negative pressures can result without the use of an adequate chin-thrust. There is some real risk in adeno-tonsillectomy, with a recent study reporting up to 12% complication rates in a California inpatient study [42].

Of course, there are also risks (not easily quantified by the literature) for the failure of modern medicine to have completely misunderstood the concept of mouth-breathing, mistakenly believing that these structures are the source of mouth-breathing, and not a side-effect of it. These risks include misinformation, inefficient care, and unnecessary surgery, and of course most importantly that effective jaw closure strategies are never discussed.

Second, adeno-tonsillectomy "success" rates are comparable to the success of simple observation. In the literature, incomplete resolution of OSA after adeno-tonsillectomy occurs in a large portion of patients as mentioned above. Thus, approximately half of patients fail to improve in the long run. Similarly, a Cochrane database study showed normalization of polysomnograms in 49% of patients within 7 months without adeno-tonsillectomy [43]. When considering the data as a whole, "suggests that nearly half of children do not fully respond to tonsillectomy with regards to OSA; and that another half of children have transient OSA that would have responded to just watchful waiting. One cannot help but wonder if the complete responders to surgery are a similar cohort that would have responded to time, while the surgical failures are the same as those that do not respond to time either. At the very least, this opens the door to further consideration of the treatment paradigm and careful patient selection." [8]

Now that we have discussed the four conventional facial structure and airway fallacies, and considered the conventional pathway at length, we will now pivot to describe the alternative approach of facial and airway development. Many of the foundational clinical observations for this pathway were described first in the modern literature by Christian Guilleminault and colleagues. This alternate chain of events consists of: Facial musculoskeletal abnormality (subclinical) →Nasal disuse and underuse→Mouth-breathing and eventual adenotonsillar development→further musculoskeletal compensatory changes to structure (posture) (See Fig. 4.4b) [44, 45].

As you can see, this reverses the order of events from the primary inflammatory generated adenoid as the initiating culprit, instead proposing that simple variation in facial musculoskeletal structure serves as the inciting cause. This structural problem predisposes to nasal under-use and mouth-breathing, which in turn promotes the development of pharyngeal negative pressure (See Chap. 2) and eventual secondary development of the reactive tissues of Waldeyer's ring and further compensatory facial musculoskeletal changes. This is not necessarily new information, but a "rediscovery" of information from the distant past, presented now in the age of evidence-based medicine. From works dating back to the nineteenth and earlier twentieth century, subtle (subclinical/nonsyndromic) facial structural variations have been understood to be the potential source of mouth-breathing [46, 47].

More recent authors led by Guilleminault demonstrated that 93.3% of children with OSA had co-existing facial/structural features (including high-arched palate, septal deformity and petite maxilla/mandible) and of course they considered whether the facial problems were indeed the root cause. Later, these authors identified that the key finding in patients with sleep disordered breathing was mouth-breathing, in association with facial anomalies [45, 48]. These clinical studies, when considered together suggest that skeletal variations themselves and subsequently the oral route of breathing may be the primary inciting factors in stimulating adenotonsillar growth via mucosal dryness and irritation. In addition, a night of baro-trauma, induced on rats by researchers in Spain demonstrated a directly resulting and severe inflammatory response, with modulators found sometimes over tenfold relative to that of normal rats [49].

While mostly in the right direction, these studies also implied that children with size-limited craniofacial features combined with adenotonsillar hypertrophy had worse OSA because of a constricted airway due to combined bony and tissue problems. In our discussion of airway and mouth-breathing aerodynamics in Chap. 3, we have shown why simple "airway constriction" is not completely accurate.

Summarized in more detail from an article in Sleep Medicine: (1) Maxillary/ mandibular structural variation/size limitation predisposes to nasal obstruction and mouth-breathing; (2) negative nasopharyngeal pressure/mucosal creates wall stress in Waldeyer's ring; (3) repeated micro-seromas due to intra-luminal mucosal causes stretching with loss of elasticity; (4) eventual submucosal inflammation with lymphoid hypertrophy results; (5) adaptation to chronic mouth-breathing result as an altered equilibrium of mouth opening closing muscle groups [8].

A Shrinking "Snout"...or How Diminishing Facial Structure Specifically Causes Mouth-Breathing

Civilized man of today possesses a smaller face with less defined features than the more primitive type. It would seem probable that diminished use of the muscles of mastication is mainly responsible for this. —Proceedings of the Royal Society of Medicine (1932)

Before we discuss the "what" and "how" of this newer perspective, we will begin with the "why." There is no doubt that over the course of the historical development of *Homo sapiens*, that our structural facial bones, primarily the maxilla and mandible (collectively referred to as the snout of most primates) have been steadily receding as mentioned in the beginning of the chapter. The ape-like snout of the *Australopithecus africanus* was more protrusive than the more recent than the flatter-faced *Homo erectus*, which was in turn more protruding than the snouts of more recent Homo species like *Homo sapiens neanderthalis*. This fact is not disputed by primatologists, paleontologists, or even clinicians [1–3]. What IS greatly debated is why. To many, particularly in the dental community, this process is due to the reduced loading on our jaws as the requirement for near constant chewing and biting has diminished as our innovations have reduced the need for these actions. Most refer to the acquisition of these innovations, as "processing of food." Processing in its earliest from was the advent of fire and cooking to facilitate the digestion process. Removal of tougher elements of food via culinary tools that did not require teeth furthered this process. Of course, modern processing of grains and meats has taken the load off of our jaws in a recently accelerated fashion since the industrial revolution. The proponents of this concept believe that this dietary alteration, away from hard nuts, tough meats, and sinewy vegetables has removed the strain and load from our maxilla and mandible, thus causing them to partially atrophy. While this of course makes some sense, one would wonder if a child was fed exclusively on a pre-modern diet if he/she would develop an ape-like snout. This seems unlikely to me, although with a completely un-processed diet, there may have been less selective pressure to maintain a protruding and larger upper and lower jaw, so it is likely part of the picture [50].

Along similar lines of thinking, the "gracilization" hypothesis has emerged as a likely mechanism for the diminution of facial bones over the course of human and hominid history. In this concept, scientists have observed that the entire skeleton of hominid ancestors has diminished over time, including the maxilla and mandible. They contend that the bones have become in modern humans more slender and delicate than past species due to behavioral changes, with a highly active foraging/hunting life slowly transitioning to a more sedentary, agricultural and technology driven lifestyle in modern *Homo sapiens*, requiring less robust skeletal support. These processes may be accelerating in recent centuries, with rapid changes in technology driven innovation in agriculture and transportation. As I sit at my desk in the early morning, typing this manuscript, sipping liquid coffee, I cannot help but wonder about the contrast of how distant ancestors would be using similar early hours to physically struggle to find sources of food and clean water, sometimes failing in the process [51].

A further explanation of this concept is provided by the ornithologist Richard Prum from Yale University. We are accustomed, when considering natural selection and the evolution concept to identify a "selective advantage" to a physical adaptation. In this case, we assume that the gracilization of our skeletons has the advantage of reducing biologic energy needs in an environment that does not require thick bones. Prum, argues that this is actually not usually the case. He explains that the null hypothesis (no proof of difference required), for understanding the evolution of traits should not be the environmental adaptation model (i.e., selection of traits conferring specific advantages) we are so accustomed to considering Instead, he argues that traits are arbitrarily selected based upon Darwinian "sexual selection" via a model known as the Lande-Kirkpatrick mechanism [52]. In other words, he proposes that without obvious evidence of an alternative hypothesis, the progressively shrinking human maxilla and mandible are simply occurring due to mating preferences. In a 2002 psychology paper entitled "Testosterone increases perceived dominance but not attractiveness in human males" by Swaddle and Rierson, this concept is further supported. In this study, female test subjects were shown photographs of male faces with variable levels of testosterone-mediated facial size. Instead of selecting the most dominant male faces, or most dominant masculine forms, with the most prominent facial features, females preferred faces influenced by moderate levels of testosterone. Further agreeing with Prum, they honestly admit, "Even if some researchers insist on evolutionary interpretations, we cannot find evidence for directional selection to reduce or increase testosterone through female preferences" thus fulfilling Prum's null hypothesis concept [53]. The wildly successful Disney film, "Beauty and the Beast," its story based on folk tale shows how this concept is embedded in our collective conscience. In the story, well-known to most, Belle, the lead female protagonist receives a marriage proposal from Gaston, the ultra-masculine, large featured alpha male, who is clearly the dominant male in the village. Despite his unmistakable dominance, she finds him unattractive, and instead prefers a "beast," who when finally tamed under her guidance, is transformed into a delicately featured, but handsome young prince. This fable may illustrate how female sexual selection may have been slowly shaping the diminishing average *Homo sapiens* face from its thick ape-like origins, to its more slender current form. Thus, in ape societies where mating decisions are determined by dominance and inter-male competition exclusively, like that of gorillas, aggression and hyper-male features may be most advantageous. However, with a near complete role of female selection permitted, as obviously is the case in *Homo sapiens*, the larger mandible and its associated features of aggression become less important, and thus offspring of these less hyper-males inherit progressively smaller jaws. This may also explain the progressive reduction in inter-species violence and improved socialization witnessed over the same time period. Perhaps it also explains why our sinus surgery instruments were inadequate for Kubi the gorilla's maxillary structures (see earlier in the chapter).

Regardless of the reason, the shrinking snout causes OSA-like symptoms not just because of a narrower caliber airway, but because it causes mouth-breathing during sleep due to structural reasons. A high-arched, narrow palate is associated with OSA [54, 55]. But, a more recent study showed specifically an association between the gonial angle (the angle of mandibular ramus to body) and tongue collapse in OSA [56].

The gonial angle (a surrogate for the sagittal angle of the mandibular body to skull-base), which is well-known to be influenced by testosterone/hormone levels, may be the key anatomic factor in determining a predisposition to mouth-breathing in humans, and could be the starting point of the alternative hypothesis for adenoid/facial interaction [57].

Thus, an evolutionarily pre-determined obtuse or wider gonial angle, compared to the nearly right angle of the most simian jaws may be the initiating factor in the path toward mouth-breathing and OSA. Looking at figure (Fig. 4.5), a sagittal view of the intersection of the mandibular body and ramus (gonial angle), you can see a 90 degree (ideal) gonial angle on the left, and an obtuse (less favorable) gonial angle of the mandible on the right. Let's use this model for a thought experiment: In an upright position, imagine that in a situation of zero muscle tone, the hinged condylar joint will allow the ramus of the mandible to "hang" like a plumb line in the vector of earth's gravitational pull, assuming the mandibular body is not weighted

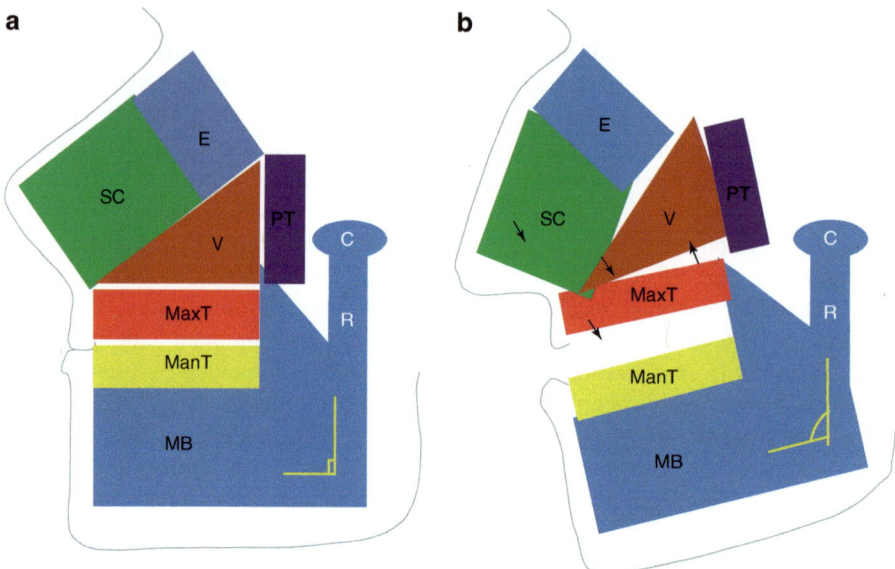

Fig. 4.5 Sagittal schematic view of the components of the facial skeleton. (**a**) In a favorable tone/structure position including acute gonial angle and encouraging nasal breathing. (**b**). In a less-favorable rotation of structures, beginning with obtuse gonial angle, each structure affecting the next that predisposes to subtle deformity and mouth-breathing. E = ethmoid, SC = septal cartilage, V = vomer, PT = pterygoid plate, MaxT = maxillary teeth, ManT = mandibular teeth, MB = mandibular body, R = ramus. Yellow angle signifies gonial angle, and black arrows signify direction of malposition of components

excessively to alter this. In the left model, with the 90 degree or less gonial angle, the occlusal surfaces of the teeth will remain in the closed position, or a position that favors the nasal route of breathing. In contrast, in the right-sided picture, with an obtuse gonial angle, perhaps 120 degrees, when the ramus hangs like a plumb line, the obtuse angle predisposes the mouth to remain open, and thus the open mouth inadvertently becomes the primary route of respiration. The obtuse gonial angle, unfavorable to mouth closure when vertically oriented, also creates greater strain on the equilibrium of the jaw opening and closure muscles when supine. In other words, the achievement of jaw closure of the more acute gonial angles tends to require greater force, and further promoting mouth-breathing in the obtuse gonial angle individuals (Figs. 4.6 and 4.7 – open sourced from Springer Nature) [58].·

In essence an increased gonial angle increases the sagittal distance from the skull base to mandibular body thus increasing required "work" for the jaw closure muscles like the masseter. The masseter muscle, inserted at the zygomatic arch and the body of the mandible will thus require more force for jaw closure when the gonial angle is more obtuse, (body is further from the arch). According to the physics formula for Work [Work (W) = Force (F) × Distance (D)], the masseter muscle would be required to do more Work, moving the body of the mandible a longer distance (D) to close the jaw, assuming the occlusal plane and weight of the mandible were consistent in the

MALES

Small muscle CSA   Intermediate muscle CSA   Large muscle CSA

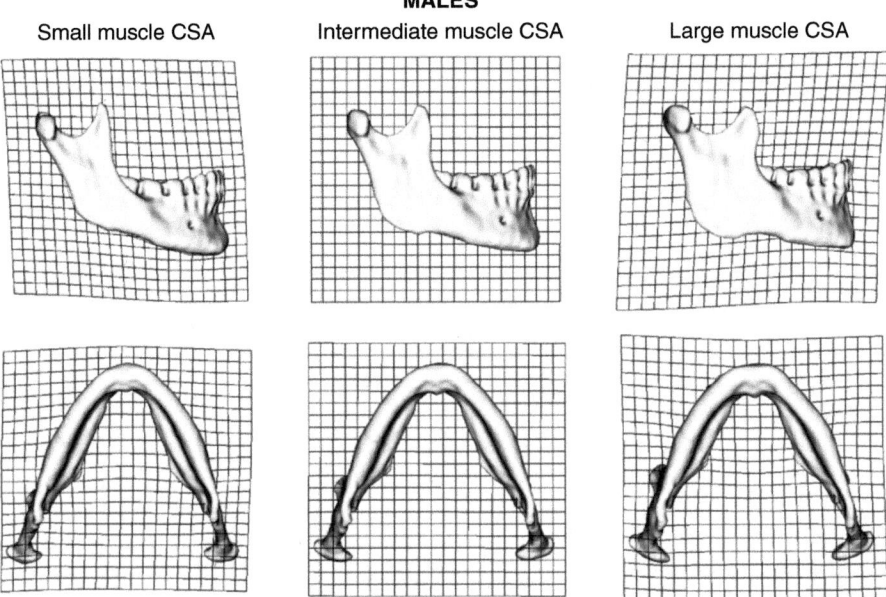

Fig. 4.6 Mandibular gonial angle dependent on muscle mass—males. (Reprinted with permission Springer—Tunis et al. [58])

FEMALES

Small muscle CSA   Intermediate muscle CSA   Large muscle CSA

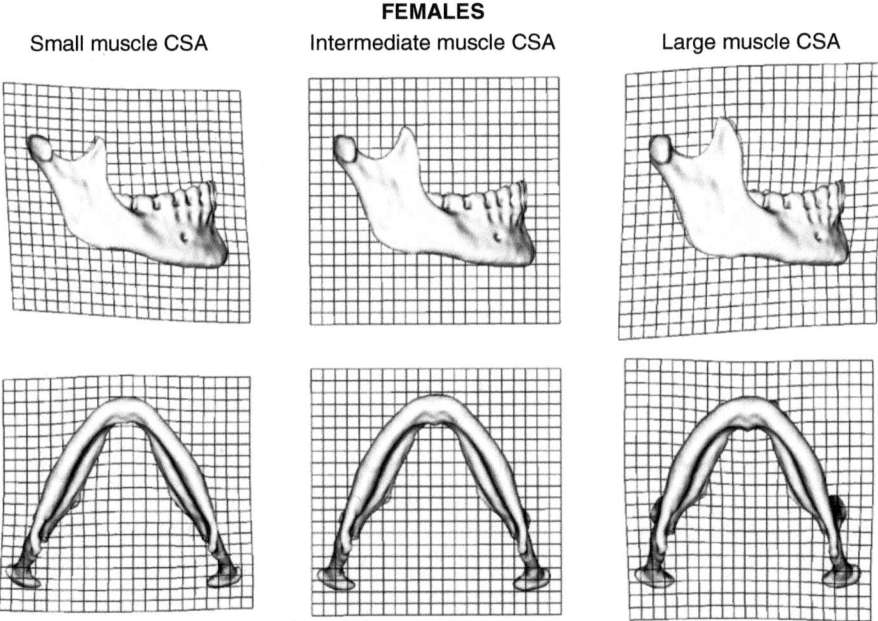

Fig. 4.7 Mandibular gonial angle dependent on muscle mass—females. (Reprinted with permission Springer—Tunis et al. [58])

acute and obtuse models. This increased requirement of work essentially during sleep may make the obtuse gonial angle patient more likely to maintain an open-mouthed posture. Actually, any maxillary or mandibular structure that creates increased Work (W) of jaw closure in the musculoskeletal equilibrium, from various malocclusions to other structural abnormalities will have similar results.

So, this initial premise of even a subtle predisposition to mouth-breathing via musculoskeletal posture, where extreme forms would be considered syndromic, is the inciting event in this alternate chain of events [8, 59]. In response to the tilting of the mandibular body relative to the ramus, the maxillary occlusal surface rotates from the Frankfort plane in a corresponding fashion to become parallel to the mandibular body, causing retro-clination of the maxillary anterior teeth (incisors). Like a stack of blocks tilting due to movement at the bottom-most, this rotation of the maxillary dental occlusal plane causes a high-arched palate, with telescoping of the roof of the mouth into the nasal cavity, which in turn promotes rotation of the vomer and ethmoid in a parallel trajectory. Similar to tectonic plates in geology, the shifting of these nasal septal components cause overlap and bending, which becomes a complex septal deviation. Further, the intrusion of the bony palate and maxillary crest deeper into the nasal cavity causes further warping of the growing septal cartilage, which growth inferiorly from an ethmoid origin [60] and external extrusion of the dorsal and caudal septum into the lip and creating a dorsal fullness, the classic nasal deformity associated with a retro-gnathic jaw [61]. The understanding of this condition, where nasal and septal components are rotated out of their ideal position to various degrees will form the foundation for our treatment strategies that we will outline in subsequent chapters at length. As we will discuss, this condition creates inadequate space for the septum, which buckles during development, and in turn does not provide enough support for the nostrils to maintain patency. Thus, the patients with varying degrees of this mandibular position will have their tendency to mouth-breathing compounded by the additional presence of actual nasal obstruction due to septal crumpling and valve narrowing.

The mouth-open posture is even further compounded over the course of development by further factors. The maxillary arch narrowing noted above creates a high vaulted palate, which not only intrudes on the nasal cavity from below, but creates inadequate space for the normal-sized tongue to reside. This also has been shown to be associated with OSA [55]. In cases of high BMI, the tongue is even larger than normal, and the masticatory tone less favorable [62]. So, a large tongue in the setting of a narrow "cage" of the maxillary and mandibular dental arch creates a setting of not an "over-crowded" airway, but one with a tendency to "pop-open" like an overstuffed hard suitcase [63, 64]. Finally, once an individual is set on the path to mouth-breathing, they will, as described in the "conventional pathway" experience further compensatory changes to facilitate chronic mouth-breathing, possibly with alterations in lip tone and further dental changes. This explains why even with anatomic correction, a tendency to continue mouth-breathing persists in many until corrective muscular retraining therapy.

Finally, as we discussed in the previous chapter, a tendency toward mouth-breathing sets up an environment of negative pressure and dryness in the

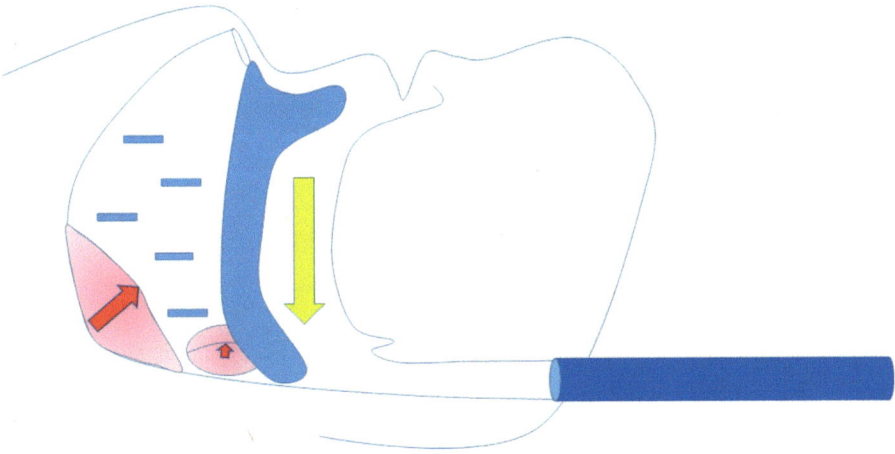

Fig. 4.8 Sagittal view of the airway demonstrating how negative pressure in the nasopharynx can generate tonsillar growth

pharynx. This negative pressure, found in model studies to localize in the area of Waldeyer's ring[65], may from repeated trauma or dehydration create a reactive inflammatory set-up [50] for the concurrent development of adeno-tonsillar tissue. This lymphoid appearing tissue may actually be an inflammatory or immune response to the unfavorable pharyngeal environment created by chronic mouth-breathing (Fig. 4.8). As expected, with the pubertal growth of the facial skeleton in the majority of individuals, this tissue tends to subside or disappear with the proportional reduction in mouth-breathing tendency. In patients who do not experience enough musculoskeletal growth to convert to nasal route of breathing, mouth-breathing and OSA will persist, as will adeno-tonsillar tissue concurrently, although the lymph tissue is NOT the cause of the condition, but a fellow-traveler. Thus, at long last, we understand that the adenoid is not the primary cause of the facial deformity, but more likely, the face is the cause of the adenoid enlargement.

So, why should a rhinoplasty or facial surgeon care about things like pediatric facial development and adenoid hypertrophy? You just want to skip all of this buildup, and learn the maneuvers involved in rhinoplasty with the pretty pictures of spreader grafts "expertly" laid into position? Let us follow the advice of Machiavelli, in understanding the environment in which we intend to operate, that we may achieve better results as surgeons and teachers: One "must also learn the nature of the terrain, and know how mountains slope, how valleys open, how plains lie, and understand the nature of rivers and swamps; and he(/she) should devote much attention to such activities." Napoleon Bonaparte, comfortable in the superior tactical ability of his army, fatally failed to recognize the terrain and weather challenges in his Russian invasion, resulting in his eventual defeat. Let us lead our patients with a better knowledge of the human terrain. We summarize all of the forces acting upon the face, nose, and airway that we have covered in Fig. 4.9. As we move into part

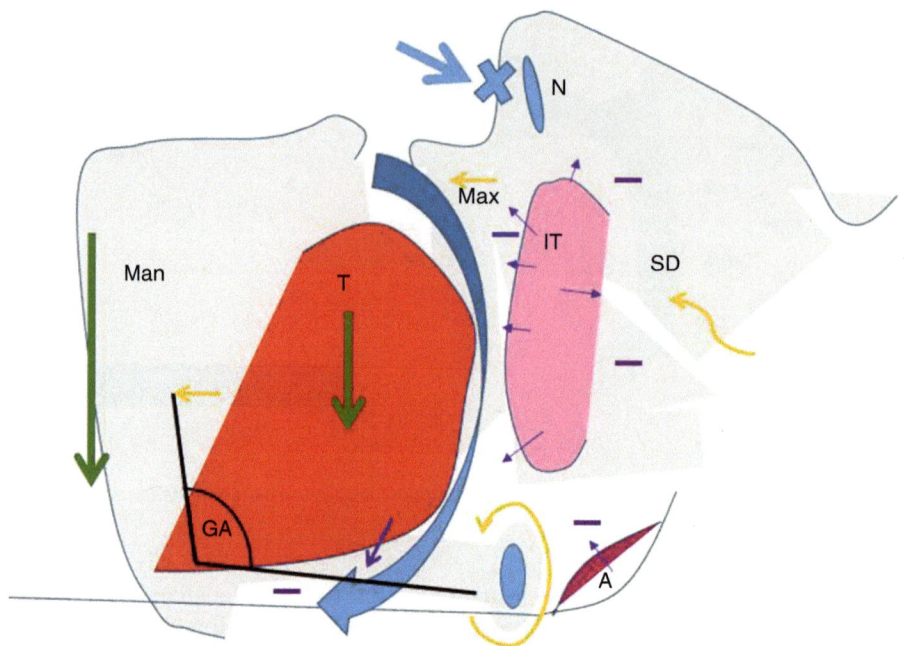

Fig. 4.9 Graphical representation of the forces of facial structure (yellow arrows), gravity (green arrows) and negative pressure (purple minus signs and arrows)on the airway. Man = mandible, GA = gonial angle, A = adenoid, Max = maxilla, SD = septal deviation, and IT = inferior turbinate. The blue arrow indicates airflow through the mouth, and blue X indicates nasal airway failure. The purple arrows indicate mucosal stretching toward the lumen. (Reprinted with permission from Elsevier—Stupak and Park [8])

two, treatment strategies, we understand why we have spent so much time building a solid understanding of the dynamics of our working environment.

References

1. Davidson TM. The Great Leap Forward: the anatomic basis for the acquisition of speech and obstructive sleep apnea. Sleep Med. 2003;4(3):185–94.
2. Stupak HD. The human external nose and its evolutionary role in the prevention of obstructive sleep apnea. Otolaryngol Head Neck Surg. 2010;142(6):779–82.
3. Mladina R, Skitarelić NB, Skitarelić NP. Letter to: the human external nose and its evolutionary role in the prevention of obstructive sleep apnea. Otolaryngol Head Neck Surg. 2010;143:712.. author reply 712–3
4. Elluru RG. Adenoid facies and nasal airway obstruction: cause and effect? Arch Otolaryngol Head Neck Surg. 2005;131(10):919–20.
5. Dierks E. No convincing premise for efficacy of prophylactic Adenotonsillar ablation. Arch Otolaryngol Head Neck Surg. 2005;131(10):918.

6. Huang YS, Guilleminault C. Pediatric obstructive sleep apnea and the critical role of oral-facial growth: evidences. Front Neurol. 2013;3:184.
7. Dowsett EB. Discussion on mouth breathing and nasal obstruction. Proceedings of the Royal Society of Medicine. Section of Odontology, April, 1932. p. 1343–55.
8. Stupak HD, Park SY. Gravitational forces, negative pressure and facial structure in the genesis of airway dysfunction during sleep: a review of the paradigm. Sleep Med. 2018;51:125–32.
9. Williams and Mahoney – "The effect of enlarged adenoids on a developing malocclusion". 2010, Revista latinomericana de otrodoncia y odontopediatria.
10. Vargervik K, Miller AJ, Chierici G, Harvold E, Tomer BS. Morphologic response to changes in neuromuscular patterns experimentally induced by altered modes of respiration. Am J Orthod. 1984;85(2):115–24.
11. Tomer BS, Harvold EP. Primate experiments on mandibular growth direction. Am J Orthod. 1982;82(2):114–9.
12. Harvold EP, Tomer BS, Vargervik K, Chierici G. Primate experiments on oral respiration. Am J Orthod. 1981;79(4):359–72.
13. Linder-Aronson S. The impact of adenotonsillectomy on the dentofacial development of obstructed children. Eur J Orthod. 2018;40(4):451.
14. Linder-Aronson S. The relation between nasorespiratory function and dentofacial morphology. Am J Orthod. 1983;83(5):443–4.
15. Zettergren-Wijk L, Forsberg CM, Linder-Aronson S. Changes in dentofacial morphology after adeno-/tonsillectomy in young children with obstructive sleep apnoea–a 5-year follow-up study. Eur J Orthod. 2006;28(4):319–26.
16. Koca CF, Erdem T, Bayındır T. The effect of adenoid hypertrophy on maxillofacial development: an objective photographic analysis. J Otolaryngol Head Neck Surg. 2016;45(1):48.
17. Farid MM, Metwalli N. Computed tomographic evaluation of mouth breathers among paediatric patients. Dentomaxillofac Radiol. 2010;39(1):1e10.
18. Basheer B, Hegde S, Bhat SS, et al. Influence of mouth breathing on the dentofacial growth of children: a cephalometric study. J Int Oral Health. 2014;6(6):50e5.
19. Masaaki S, Taiji F, Akira S, et al. Relationship between oral flow patterns, nasal obstruction, and respiratory events during sleep. J Clin Sleep Med. 2015;11(8):855e60.
20. Ali AA, Richmond S, Popa H, et al. The influence of snoring, mouth breathing and apnoea on facial morphology in late childhood: a three-dimensional study. BMJ Open. 2015;5(9):e009027.
21. Stellzig-Eisenhauer A, Meyer-Marcotty P. Interaction between otorhinolaryngology and orthodontics: correlation between the nasopharyngeal airway and the craniofacial complex. GMS Curr Top Otorhinolaryngol Head Neck Surg. 2010;9:04.
22. Fernando M, Feres N, Muniz TS, et al. Craniofacial skeletal pattern: is it really correlated with the degree of adenoid obstruction? Dental Press J Orthod. 2015;20(4):68e75.
23. Oh K, Kim M, Youn J, et al. Three-dimensional evaluation of the relationship between nasopharyngeal airway shape and adenoid size in children. Korean J Orthod. 2013;43(4):160e7.
24. Juliano ML, Machado MA, Bizari L, et al. Polysomnographic findings are associated with cephalometric measurements in mouth-breathing children. J Clin Sleep Med. 2009;5(6):554e61.
25. Grewal N, Alkesh V, Godhane L. Lateral cephalometry: a simple and economical clinical guide for assessment of nasopharyngeal free airway space in mouth breathers. Contemp Clin Dent. 2010;1(2):66e9.
26. Adedeji TO, Amusa BY, Aremu AA. Correlation between adenoidal nasopharyngeal ratio and symptoms of enlarged adenoids in children with adenoidal hypertrophy. Afr J Paediatr Surg. 2016;13(1):14e9.
27. Ritzel RA, Berwig LC, Toniolo da Silva MA, et al. Correlation between nasopharyngoscopy and cephalometry in the diagnosis of hyperplasia of the pharyngeal tonsils. Int Arch Otorhinolaryngol. 2012;16(2):209e16.
28. Grippaudo C, Paolantonio EP, Antonini G, et al. Association between oral habits, mouth breathing and malocclusion. Acta Otorhinolaryngol Ital. 2016;36(5):386e94.

29. Ucar FI, Ekizer A, Uysal T. Comparison of craniofacial morphology, head posture and hyoid bone position with different breathing patterns. Saudi Dent J. 2012;24(3e4):135e41.
30. de Sousa Michels D, da Mota Silveira Rodrigues A, Nakanishi M, et al. Nasal involvement in obstructive sleep apnea syndrome. Int J Otolaryngol. 2014;2014:717419.
31. Gupta N, Gupta SD, Varshney S, et al. Orthodontic treatment after adenoidectomy patients: effect on jaw relations in sagittal plane. Indian J Otolaryngol Head Neck Surg. 2009;61(2):153e6.
32. Peltomäki T. The effect of mode of breathing on craniofacial growth–revisited. Eur J Orthod. 2007;29(5):426–9.
33. Baik G, Brietzke SE. Cost benefit and utility decision analysis of turbinoplasty with adenotonsillectomy for pediatric sleep-disordered breathing. Otolaryngol Head Neck Surg. 2019;161(2):343–7.
34. Tang A, Benke JR, Cohen AP, Ishman SL. Influence of tonsillar size on OSA improvement in children undergoing adenotonsillectomy. Otolaryngol Head Neck Surg. 2015;153(2):281–5.
35. Nolan J, Brietzke SE. Systematic review of pediatric tonsil size and polysomnogram-measured obstructive sleep apnea severity. Otolaryngol Head Neck Surg. 2011;144(6):844–50.
36. Zautner AE, Krause M, Stropahl G, et al. Intracellular persisting Staphylococcus aureus is the major pathogen in recurrent tonsillitis. PLoS One. 2010;5(3):e9452.
37. Szalmás A, Papp Z, Csomor P, Kónya J, Sziklai I, Szekanecz Z, Karosi T. Microbiological profile of adenoid hypertrophy correlates to clinical diagnosis in children. Biomed Res Int. 2013;2013:629607.
38. Szalmas A, Papp Z, Csomor P, et al. Bacteriology of symptomatic adenoids in children. N Am J Med Sci. 2013;5(2):113e8.
39. Ruben RJ. The adenoid: its history and a cautionary tale. Laryngoscope. 2017;127(Suppl. 2):S13e28.. Review
40. Scheffler P, Wolter NE, Narang I, Amin R, Holler T, Ishman SL, Propst EJ. Surgery for obstructive sleep apnea in obese children: literature review and meta-analysis. Otolaryngol Head Neck Surg. 2019;160(6):985–92.
41. Byars SG, Stearns SC, Boomsma JJ. Association of long-term risk of respiratory, allergic, and infectious diseases with removal of adenoids and tonsils in childhood. JAMA Otolaryngol Head Neck Surg. 2018;144(7):594–603.
42. Lawlor CM, Riley CA, Carter JM, Rodriguez KH. Association between age and weight as risk factors for complication after tonsillectomy in healthy children. JAMA Otolaryngol Head Neck Surg. 2018;144(5):399–405.
43. Venekamp RP, Hearne BJ, Chandrasekharan D, Blackshaw H, Lim J, Schilder AG. Tonsillectomy or adenotonsillectomy versus non-surgical management for obstructive sleep-disordered breathing in children. Cochrane Database Syst Rev. 2015;10:CD011165.
44. Guilleminault C, Akhtar F. Pediatric sleep-disordered breathing: new evidence on its development. Sleep Med Rev. 2015;24:46–56.
45. Lee SY, Guilleminault C, Chiu HY, Sullivan SS. Mouth breathing, "nasal disuse," and pediatric sleep-disordered breathing. Sleep Breath. 2015;19(4):1257–64.
46. Catlin G. Shut your mouth and save your life. London, England: Paternoster House; 1891. p. 25e35.
47. Price W. Nutrition and physical degeneration: a comparison of primitive and modern diets and their effects. J Am Med Assoc. 1940;114(26):2589.
48. Zicari AM, Marzia D, Occasi F. Cephalometric pattern and nasal patency in children with primary snoring: the evidence of a direct correlation. PLoS One. 2014;9(10):e111675.
49. Almendros I, Carreras A, Ramírez J, Montserrat JM, Navajas D, Farré R. Upper airway collapse and reopening induce inflammation in a sleep apnoea model. Eur Respir J. 2008;32(2):399–404.
50. Vinyard CJ, Taylor AB, Teaford MF, Glander KE, Ravosa MJ, Rossie JB, Ryan TM, Williams SH. Are we looking for loads in all the right places? New research directions for studying the masticatory apparatus of New World monkeys. Anat Rec (Hoboken). 2011;294(12):2140–57.
51. Chirchir H, Kivell TL, Ruff CB, Hublin JJ, Carlson KJ, Zipfel B, Richmond BG. Recent origin of low trabecular bone density in modern humans. Proc Natl Acad Sci U S A. 2015;112(2):366–71.

52. Prum RO. The Lande–Kirkpatrick mechanism is the null model of evolution by intersexual selection: implications for meaning, honesty, and design in intersexual signals. Evolution. 2010;64(11):3085–100.
53. Swaddle JP, Reierson GW. Testosterone increases perceived dominance but not attractiveness in human males. The Royal Society Proceedings, May 2002 Wrangham, R. The goodness paradox. Pantheon 2019.
54. Johal A, Conaghan C. Maxillary morphology in obstructive sleep apnea: a cephalometric and model study. Angle Orthod. 2004;74(5):648–56.
55. Kim JH, Guilleminault C. The nasomaxillary complex, the mandible, and sleep-disordered breathing. Sleep Breath. 2011;15(2):185–93.
56. Anderson S, Alsufyani N, Isaac A, Gazzaz M, El-Hakim H. Correlation between gonial angle and dynamic tongue collapse in children with snoring/sleep disordered breathing – an exploratory pilot study. J Otolaryngol Head Neck Surg. 2018;47(1):41. https://doi.org/10.1186/s40463-018-0285-8.. Malhotra, J Indian Soc Pedod Dent, 2012
57. Lefevre CE, Lewis GJ, Perrett DI, Penke L. Telling facial metrics: facial width is associated with testosterone levels in men. Evol Hum Behav. 2013;34(4):273–9.
58. Tunis TS, Pokhojaev A, Sarig R, O'Higgins P, May H. Human mandibular shape is associated with masticatory muscle force. Sci Rep. 2018;8:Article number: 6042.
59. Crupi P, Portelli M, Matarese G, Nucera R, Militi A, Mazza M, Cordasco G. Correlations between cephalic posture and facial type in patients suffering from breathing obstructive syndrome. Eur J Paediatr Dent. 2007;8(2):77–82.
60. Hartman CH. Nasal septal deviation and craniofacial asymmetries. MS (Master of Science) thesis, University of Iowa, 2015. http://ir.uiowa.edu/etd/1620.
61. Stupak HD, Weinstock M. Bony/Cartilaginous Mismatch: a radiologic investigation into the etiology of tension nose deformity. Plast Reconstr Surg. 2018;141:312–21.
62. Kezirian EJ. Does my tongue look fat? Sleep. 2014;37(10):1583–4.
63. Ito E, Tsuiki S, Maeda K, Okajima I, Inoue Y. Oropharyngeal crowding closely relates to aggravation of OSA. Chest. 2016;150(2):346–52.
64. Kim AM, Keenan BT, Jackson N, Chan EL, Staley B, Poptani H, Torigian DA, Pack AI, Schwab RJ. Tongue fat and its relationship to obstructive sleep apnea. Sleep. 2014;37(10):1639–48.
65. Naughton JP, Lee AY, Ramos E, Wootton D, Stupak HD. Effect of nasal valve shape on downstream volume, airflow, and pressure drop: importance of the nasal valve revisited. Ann Otol Rhinol Laryngol. 2018;127(11):745–53.

Part II
Rhinoplasty Strategy and Tactics

Chapter 5

A Structural Model to Systematically Understand Nasal Framework: The Rhinoplasty Compass™

"Human subtlety will never devise an invention more beautiful, more simple or more direct than does nature because in her inventions nothing is lacking, and nothing is superfluous."—Leonardo da Vinci.

Most rhinoplasty textbooks tend to break down the chapters devoted to rhinoplasty maneuvers by subsection of the nose, for example, including a section on the "middle third" of the nose, and will discuss how to perform various tactics like "spreader grafts" and how these prevent the "inverted-V" deformity. In general, this step-wise and list-type thinking confuses cause and effect and gives the surgeon a false sense of confidence that if they reliably and predictably follow a step as shown in the text, then the result will be as the text predicts as well. Only a little real-world experience will show that reliably following text or course descriptions have little bearing on the end result of a better breathing and looking patient. However, like birds that repeatedly smash into windows not being familiar with the concept of glass, clinicians and even teachers tend to repeat this flawed analysis of cause and effect that has limited bearing on reality.

In a popular contemporary textbook chapter, I am struck by a diagram that shows six progressive stages of cephalic trim, labeled A through F, where F is a near complete removal or destruction of the lateral crura of the alar cartilages, narrowed down to 2–3 mm, and divided in half in its center. In each successive diagram, a progressively thicker arrow is pointing in the superior or cephalic direction, directly implying that the more aggressive destruction of the lateral crura will result in rotation or even shortening of the nose. In reality, each successive figure only is destroying the lateral support for the alar rim as the lateral crura is progressively compromised, and while rotation or shortening can be a side-effect of this destruction in some cases, the reader is misled into believing that this is the most efficient way to shorten a nose.[1]

---

[1] As we will discuss later, the release of the lateral crura of the alar cartilages from its attachment to the framework at the septum and upper lateral fusion via the inter-cartilaginous incision itself *can* release the inferior directed tip cartilages in a cephalic direction, but this does not require any trim, thus observers of the rotation mistakenly ascribed the removal of alar cartilages to being the source of rotation.

© Springer Nature Switzerland AG 2020
H. D. Stupak, *Rethinking Rhinoplasty and Facial Surgery*,
https://doi.org/10.1007/978-3-030-44674-1_5

Just as completing a paint-by-number does not make you an artist, executing textbook steps in a rhinoplasty procedure does not make you a reliable sculptor/ engineer of function or aesthetics.

The arbitrary anatomic division of the nose into parts, each part with a recommended respective repairing maneuver, is also partly responsible for why current rhinoplasty frequently results in failure: compartmentalization. Of course, on first glance it sounds reasonable to break the nose into parts, then to discuss the problems with each part as though they were isolated subdivisions. In reality, however, the nose is much more or a unified, cohesive structure, and the novice that believes that they can follow a step-wise "cookbook recipe" treating each part of the nose separately will be in for an unpleasant surprise. I encountered this situation as a resident myself, of course lacking enough wisdom to realize this until later.

In this unfortunate situation, while I was completing my residency with a Veterans Affairs (VA) rotation, I had the opportunity to attend a regional rhinoplasty course. The course, featuring a cadaver lab, excelled at providing this segmental approach to rhinoplasty, empowering the attendee to diagnose each separate deformity of the nose and come up with a corresponding series of steps (featuring various named sutures and grafts.) Brimming with new-found confidence, and having tested my new skills in the lab, we identified a patient in the VA clinic who was requesting a functional rhinoplasty. A very young attending was staffing the clinic, and kindly agreed to staff the case, knowing that I was planning on a facial plastic surgery fellowship and had some knowledge. The surgery itself proceeded just like the steps we learned in the course, with a harvest of septal grafts, avoidance of the L-strut, then open rhinoplasty approach to facilitate grafts and sutures. Placing the spreader grafts, batten grafts, tip grafts, and domal sutures and performing the limited cephalic trim was just as it had been during the cadaver lab. As we closed, I could not help but notice that the patient's nose looked rather thickened and clunky, but disregarded this observation, placing tape, and re-assuring myself that in a year (as we had learned in the course), the nose would return to normal, and all of the grafts would be a huge positive for the patient. That night, I gave myself a pat on the back for having really performed a rhinoplasty, and so successfully!

While the patient experienced no "complications," a short time after surgery, I changed rotations to another hospital and never saw the patient again. One of my co-residents did let me know that even a few months later, her nose was wide and thick, and she breathed hardly better than before, and she was quite unhappy with her result. I again re-assured myself that I had completed all of the appropriate steps and that things would get better over time (which they probably did not).

It was not until fellowship with the legendary Calvin M. Johnson, Jr in New Orleans, that I was taught to have a more global understanding of nasal aesthetics and function. The compartmentalized view that I had initially grasped, while seemingly benevolent, was quite destructive, replacing empathy and structural sense with step-wise tactics and poor strategy. I believe this is partially responsible for many poor results in rhinoplasty today: a false reliance on maneuvers that sound great, but in truth are illogical and mostly lack rigorous cause-and effect analysis. We will analyze many of these procedures in later chapters (Fig. 5.1).

Fig. 5.1 Dynamic triangular prism model (DTPM). Pink indicates the foundation/substrate, golden yellow represents the framework, and blue shows the canopy layer, here consisting of the paired medial and lateral crura of the alar cartilage

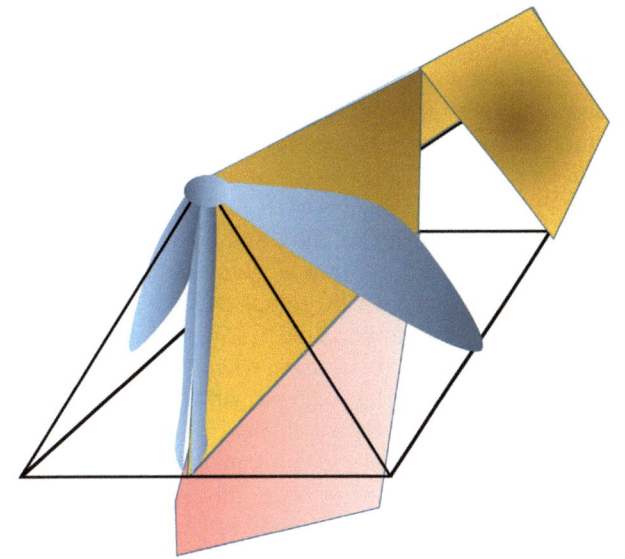

In order to consider the nose more as a single unit, and that overall aesthetic and functional results are inseparable from the framework, we will attempt to discuss the nose as a unified framework structure, with the tip cartilages playing only a supportive and secondary role. From my perspective, this is an evolution of the tripod/pedestal concept from Jack Anderson and Calvin Johnson, that while an amazing advance for its time, is overly "tip"-centric and misleading about a lack of septal importance, as we discussed in the beginning of Chap 4. In contrast, here we will divide the nasal anatomy into *the Foundation/Substrate* (facial bones, septal bones with their nourishing mucosa – similar to the underlying earth or soil that supports an architectural or botanical structure with its roots), the *Framework* (the septum and attached nasal bones), and finally, the *Canopy* (the superficial tip cartilages and skin). (Fig. 5.1 – pink is foundation/substrate, yellow is framework, and blue is the canopy layer, while the black spring represents the *scroll* that is simply the support strut attaching crura to framework.) If you notice similarities with a tent, or triangular prism, you are correct. From my perspective, the most efficient way to consider both the functional and aesthetic anatomy of the nose is as this three-layered, tent-shaped triangular prism. Most importantly, we have modified this layered structure of thinking from the tripod/pedestal model in order to change the emphasis. By considering the tripod to be the ultimate structure of importance, resting on a simple (implied much less important) pedestal, excessive attention is paid to the superficial tip structures that in reality should be more ignored, tolerated as-is, or in some cases subtly modified to match the underlying structure. While not usually discussed at rhinoplasty courses or in typical texts, the dated-looking over-operated looking rhinoplasty with a narrowed or over-structured tip is pervasive in the United States, particularly in affluent areas. While this may have been considered attractive at some point, a strong preference for more natural and appropriate appearances is a more recent trend, although there are still those relatively rare individuals who desire an operated-looking "pointy" tip. In many ways, the over-focus on the tip may be due to its easy accessibility and approach via the massively popular open rhinoplasty approach, and the over-emphasis in these educational models. Instead, the *framework* of septal super-structure is largely minimized as an accessory to the tripod, while the opposite is actually the case. Even well-regarded articles in the literature cannot help but focus upon tip-under-rotation and dorsal humps as *unrelated entities* (compart-mentalization) and as the utmost in aesthetics [1], largely ignoring that in reality that in the bigger picture septal oversize, with caudal and dorsal extrusion, is responsible for both perceived problems as we will discuss later in the chapter. This is equivalent to discussing what type of paint, nails, planks, and roof are used in the repair of a collapsed barn, while ignoring the fact that the chief goal has to be restoration of the barn's frame!

By re-analyzing how to think about our procedure, rhinoplasty, we can under-stand how to communicate about this more efficiently to our patients, and more-so how to use strategy to plan more efficient modification. So, while facial surgeons like to be known in their marketing materials for their "attention to detail," I suggest you de-focus your lens on the components, and zoom-out to the perspective of the sculptor and artist, getting the big picture perspective, perhaps emphasizing creative imagination over the rote step regurgitation that we are usually encouraged to emu-late. Calvin Johnson gave me my first perspective in this concept.

Are the septums of human noses really just "deviated"? Deviation implies a sin-gle shift, like a simple divergence off of a straight line. Anyone who has even dab-bled in septoplasty knows this is never the case. In reality, the pathologic septum is a twisted, gnarled mess that seems to defy rules and is always a challenge even with experience. The only really easy septoplasties are the ones that probably did not need to be performed. But, what can be the cause of this problem? Most, ascribe the problem to remote traumas and frequently create a biased cause and effect narrative around the trauma and its aftermath. In reality, most people experience nasal trauma during their lives but have limited deviation, and usually the severity of the described trauma fails to correlate with the degree of deformity. Can we find an alternative answer by studying nature? Let's begin by discussing the root of the majority of nasal problems: The Framework.

We discussed at length in the previous chapter that there may be evolutionary pressure toward a shrinking maxilla and mandible and spoke mostly how this prob-lem contributes to mouth-breathing and subtle facial aesthetic deficiencies. But, the receded maxilla has consequences for the nasal structure that causes many to seek rhinoplasty, septoplasty, or related procedures as well: The smaller maxilla has resulted in a relatively larger, and more prominent nose, due to external extrusion of the size-conserved nasal septum.

In the most extreme clinical example of this species-wide development, this phe-nomenon is known as the "tension nose deformity." This was first described by Calvin Johnson in a landmark *Plastic and Reconstructive Surgery* journal article as a condition where the tip of the nose is protruding, and the lip is shortened and rounded. Johnson and Godin used the term "tension nose deformity" to "connote a high nasal dorsum, with stretching of the skin and soft tissue of the nose over a highly arched and narrow nasal vault" with "anterior and sometimes inferior displacement of the nasal tip cartilages." [2] In the paper, the authors attribute the deformity to an *overgrown* septal cartilage that grows into the upper lip.

I still remember the moment during my fellowship when Dr. Johnson described this to me during surgery as one of the highlights of my entire education. I found the concept to be both intriguing, but also puzzling ... and still do. While the clinical observation and the described treatment rank to me among the most important but unheralded achievements in the history of rhinoplasty surgery, the description of the disorder is largely incomplete. First, the consideration of the concept as a "deformity," while conventional in the medical literature is misleading, particularly for conventional surgeons who prefer fixed concepts like a "classic" deformity. Even an expert reviewer in a paper on the topic that I wrote felt compelled to criticize that a photograph did not have a "classic deformity," in other words he/she felt that the photograph that I was presenting was not severe enough to be characterized as the deformity to be worthy of presenting. Once I explained in response that while considered as a "classic deformity," in reality, *tension nose* is actually part of a clinical spectrum of problems. Further, by considering the problem to be a "deformity" it not only implies it is a fixed severe problem, but also a relatively rare problem. In other words, by linking the clinical variations of the caudal septum and lip to a "deformity," the actual problem becomes condemned to the obscurity of syndromes. For the purposes of this chapter, we will inclusively use the term "tension nose," to include any excessive external septum (dorsally or caudally) that stretches adjacent soft tissue regardless of the severity, including simple septal deviation. This disorder is anything but obscure, but in reality it is the nasal manifestation of the *most severe* version of the maxillary recession that has progressed over the course of *Homo sapiens* history. While Lee et al. describe the "excessive septum" in their description of the over-projected nose [3], the true nature of the true causes of non-traumatic septal deviation, primary dorsal humps, and *tension nose* deformity remains elusive. Septal deviation and deflection has been thought to arise from nasal septal deformity that is either intrinsic to the septum itself or related to direct trauma to the septum. Johnson and Godin note that tension nose deformity is caused by excessive *growth* of the septal cartilage in a sagittal manner, whereas Behrbohm and Tardy refer to the cause as septal "hyperplasia" without citing histologic evidence [2, 4].

With actual measurement, however, multiple studies have shown that septal cartilage size is generally similar (well conserved in size) among humans, with cadaveric and radiologic surface areas varying from 650 to 845 mm [5–7]. Ironically, most of these studies were conducted for the purposes of maximizing the grafts which could be harvested from the noses of people of different ethnicities.

Further supporting this concept, rather than variation is septal size, septal deviation is shown to be associated with deficiencies or deformities of the maxilla, suggesting that abnormalities of the septum are attributable to extrinsic forces acting on the septum as opposed to intrinsic septal problems as conventionally accepted [5, 8, 9].

A doctoral thesis from the University of Iowa showed that the septal cartilage itself appears to originate from the ethmoid perpendicular plate, growing infero-anteriorly toward the maxillary crest and nasal spine [5, 10], forming the structural "keel" for the lower external nose. Finally, it has been proposed by Mladina and Krajina that the prominence of this lower external nose found in humans relative to simian and hominid ancestors is attributable to an extrusion of septal cartilage externally from the progressively shortening maxilla over the course of human evolution, as we discussed earlier [5, 11].

So, how does this extruding septal framework create septal deviation and nasal prominence (tension nose)? The answer again can be found by observing the natural world. Once, when visiting Mount Hood in Oregon, I found I was struck by the similarity of mountain shapes with the apex of the bony septal deviation found at the intersection point of the vomer, maxillary crest, ethmoid, and quadrangular cartilage. As seen in Fig. 5.2, if any number of these components are out of position, even by rotation, they will all compete to exist in the sagittal midline [12, 13]. Because only one structure can occupy the midline position, the structures will overlap, buckle, deviate, and bend, sometimes to an apical point in severe cases, creating great frustration and challenge for many a septal surgeon (present company included) very similar to mountain formation. In mountain formation, convergence of tectonic plates will cause one to over-ride the other, and a peak can be formed with multiple points of overlap, like the nasal septum. As we will discuss later, the peak of the deviated septum, commonly seen as the most pathologic portion that needs removal, is just the "tip of the iceberg" compared to the root cause mismatch of the septal aperture to cartilage size, just as the peaked mountain-top is just the manifestation of the root cause of misplaced and over-riding tectonic plates (Fig. 5.3a, b).

One could further infer, then, that a pathologically small maxilla could induce *over*-extrusion of cartilage, or induce space-limited cartilage and bone bending and twisting. As expected, some studies have shown an association of septal deviation and reduced midface height [14, 15].

Thus, our alternative hypothesis to the "overgrown septum" concept is that the septal quadrangular cartilage size itself is relatively conserved consistently between individuals, but a reduction in the size of the sagittal bony enclosure space (ethmoid plate and vomer/maxillary crest) for the septum results in "septal crowding" during its infero-anterior growth. As the cartilaginous septum has insufficient space to occupy, it will crumple or buckle (septal deviation), (Fig. 5.4a–c) or over-extrude externally in a dorsal or caudal direction (causing a tension nose deformity). It is the degree of nasal floor and maxillary bony space deficiency during septal growth or the extent of the mismatch between cartilaginous and sagittal bony septal aperture that may determine the degree of the resultant deformities, creating a clinical spectrum of variation.

Our hypothesis was supported by a study published in *Plastic and Reconstructive Surgery* where we studied sagittal computed tomography (CT) scans of the bony septum. Pathologic and non-pathologic CTs were sorted into two groups. Those exhibiting dorsal and caudal excess (tension nose) were considered pathologic and compared with those with "normal" sized noses. As expected, the perimeter and

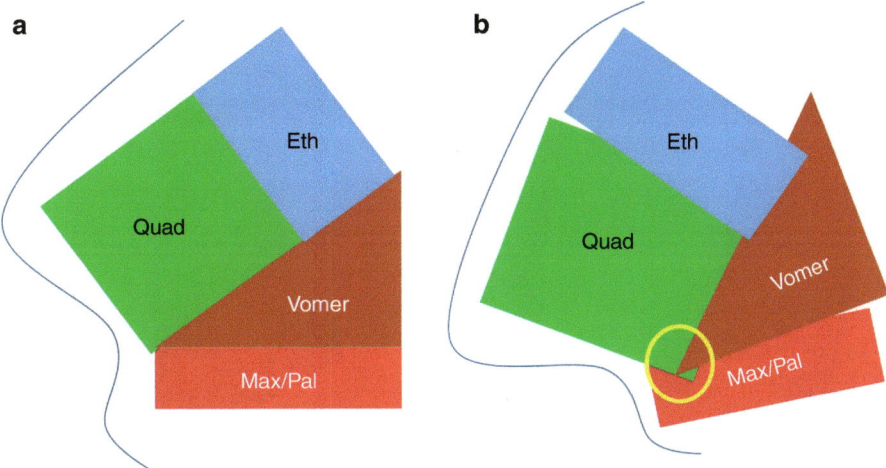

Fig. 5.2 Sagittal view of the nasal septal components schematic. (**a**) Normal septal component position without overlap. (**b**) Rotated premaxilla or high-arched palate causes rotation and overriding of septal components, peaking in the yellow circle creating buckling and deviation

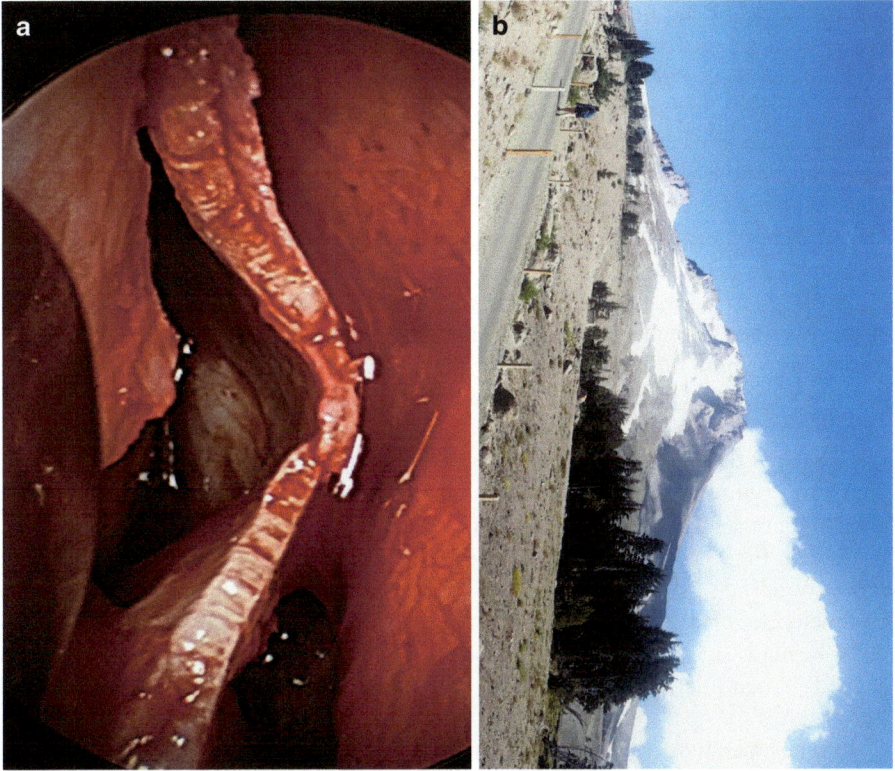

Fig. 5.3 (**a**) Endoscopic view of the peak over-riding region of septal elements after release of the quadrangular cartilages. (**b**) Similar pattern of over-riding tectonic plates created the mountain ranges of the American West

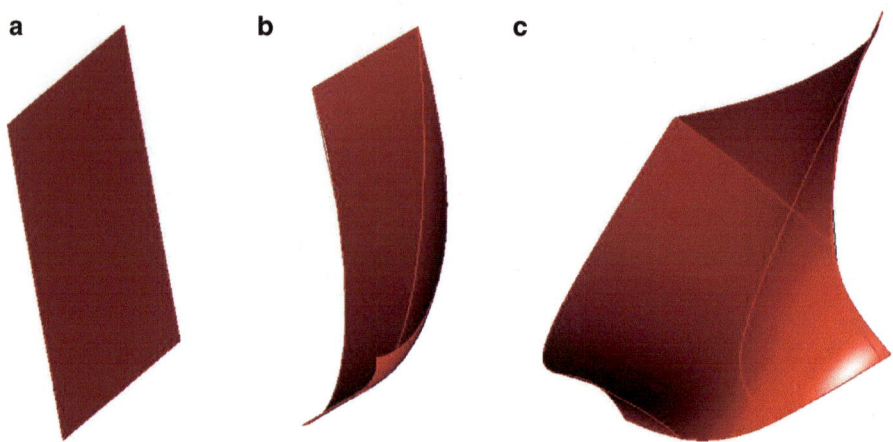

Fig. 5.4 (**a**) Computer assisted design representation (CAD) of non-buckled nasal septum. (**b**) CAD view of extrinsically caused septal buckling in the caudal region (supero-inferior buckling). (**c**) CAD view of extrinsically caused septal severe buckling (both antero-posterior and supero-inferior buckling)

surface areas of the quadrangular cartilage itself between the two groups were nearly *the same*, without statistical difference between the two groups. However, the tension nose group had a statistically significant reduction in bony septal aperture perimeter compared with controls ($p < 0.01$) and a more pronounced extruded external portion of the septum compared with their internal septal size. They also had a substantially higher rate of septal deviation than controls. This supports the idea that a mismatch between a small bony septal aperture and a normal sized septal quadrangular cartilage may be responsible for caudal, upper lip, dorsal hump, and septal deviation [5] (Fig. 5.5).

In the same study, we measured four pathologic patient's intraoperative photographs demonstrating the caudal cartilaginous septal excess that extended caudally to the nasal spine *after* release of the caudal cartilaginous nasal septum from its maxillary crest and nasal spine attachments. By releasing the entire inferior septum from its attachments FULLY from the nasal spine, maxillary crest, and vomer, the full length of the septum is realized, and the septum no longer is forced to be crumpled into a tight space. The septum then usually extends into one nostril or the other depending on its existing bony superior attachments at the ethmoid and nasal bones. As seen in Fig. 5.6, the septum is straighter due to its elastic capacity to recoil, but now protruding through one nostril. NOTE: A full transfixion incision is required to complete the release. One can easily measure how much septal excess exists caudally beyond, the natural end-point of the columella. In many cases, this excess exceeds a centimeter, accounting for the severity of some near maximal septal deviations.

In the same study, the excess beyond the nasal aperture or sill, or caudal to the nasal spine, was measured and recorded and correlated with bony measurement.

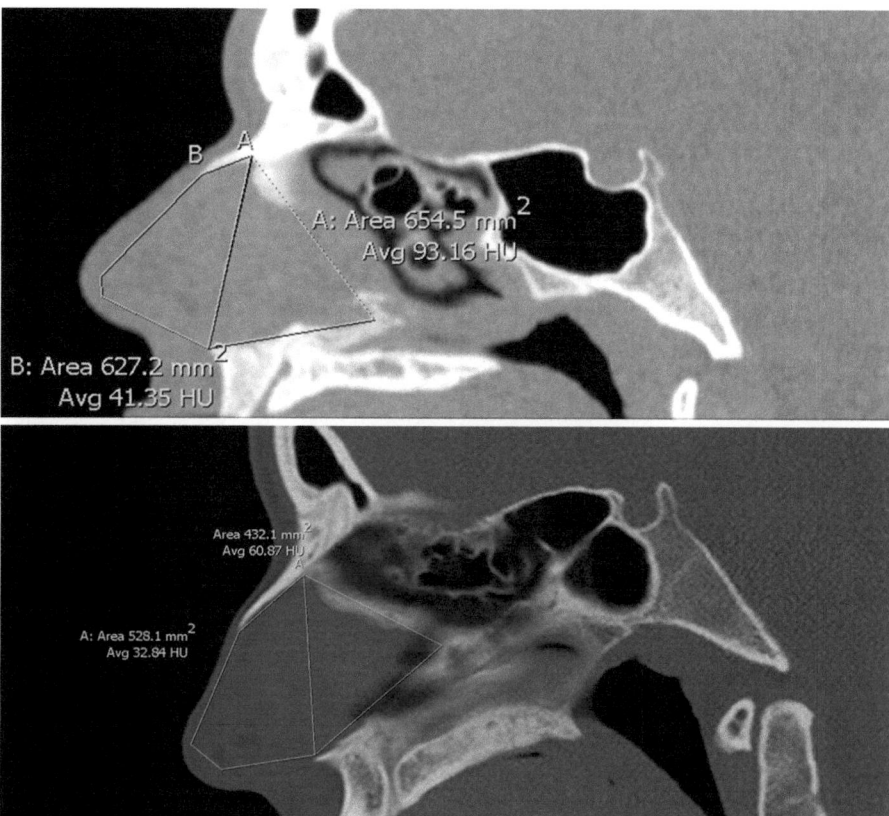

Fig. 5.5 Sagittal CT views of nasal septal measurement. The upper image is of a "normal" nose, without deviation and excess extrusion. The bony aperture measures 654 mm², while the external septum measures 627.2 mm². In contrast, with tension nose deformity and deviation, the septal aperture measures only 432.1 mm², while the external portion measures 528.1 mm². Notice the elevation of the hard palate in the bottom image relative to the top matching Fig. 5.2. (Reprinted with permission Wolters-Kluwer – Stupak, HD. Weinstock M. Bony/Cartilaginous Mismatch: A radiologic investigation into the etiology of tension nose deformity. Plastic and Reconstructive Surgery. 2018)

The measurements of caudal excess from the nasal spine (mean, 6.25 mm) trended toward correlation with their radiologic counterparts (mean, 7 mm), suggesting physical and radiologic correlation (Fig. 5.6).

The mechanism of this important diminishment of the maxilla and subsequently of the septal aperture, further causing the smaller oral cage as discussed in Chap. 4, and but more relevantly to our discussion, causing the extrusion and twisting of the septum may be in part directly due to the orientation of the independent bone known as the premaxilla. This bone, also known as the inter-maxilla, incorporates the upper incisor teeth, nasal spine, maxillary crest, and anterior hard palate. Interestingly, this concept was in essence first proposed by the famous statesman and iconic author

Fig. 5.6 Intra-operative photograph measuring caudal septal excess in millimeters. (Reprinted with permission Wolters-Kluwer – Stupak, HD. Weinstock M. Bony/Cartilaginous Mismatch: A radiologic investigation into the etiology of tension nose deformity. Plastic and Reconstructive Surgery. 2018)

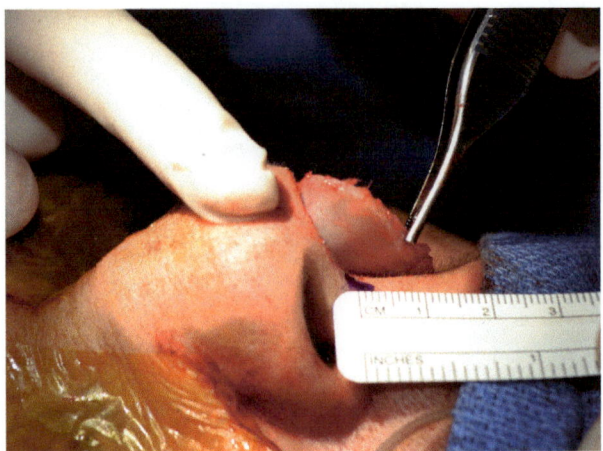

Johann Wolfgang von Goethe, who presciently suggested in the eighteenth century that the size and position of the premaxilla was what separated humans from apes [16].

So, in a follow-up to our bony aperture study, we investigated mis-orientation of the premaxilla as the actual specific mechanism of the diminished septal aperture that causes the *extrinsic* septal cartilage deviation and extrusion. This is in contrast to the common misconception that septal deviations and excess are intrinsic (i.e., hyperplasia or bent requiring scoring). In this study, we evaluated the CT scans of 68 patients, investigating the relationship of the axis of the premaxilla to the horizontal skullbase. We hypothesized that a more vertical premaxilla relative to the skullbase/horizontal would create a smaller bony septal aperture, and thus would have more septal deviation and bony extrusion (tension nose) findings (Figs. 5.7 and 5.8). When comparing the extremes of premaxillary rotation, specifically those greater than 87 degrees (Mean 91.7 degrees, SD 5.1) and less than 77 degrees (Mean 70.7 degrees, SD 3.6), differences were pronounced with regard to caudal septal excess and septal deviation in the axial plane and were statistically significant. Figures 5.9 and 5.10 show a radiologically normal and vertically malpositioned premaxilla relative to the skullbase [12].

Thus far, it may sound to the casual reader that this is a rare, simple problem, (i.e., tension nose deformity). In reality, this is not the case: The mismatch of the bony septal aperture (sagittal plane) to the quadrangular cartilage is very common, nearly pervasive! Remember in the last chapter how we discussed how there is a species-wide trend for a shrinking snout (maxilla and mandible), just to different degrees over many millenia? The reason for the existence of the prominent human external nose is the extrusion of the septal cartilage from within a progressively shortening maxilla. Beyond providing a rigid framework for the nostril opening, the external nose may have evolved for no other specific purpose except that the maxilla was evolving to be shorter, and in essence the prominent nose is just an attractive and sometimes unattractive side effect of this

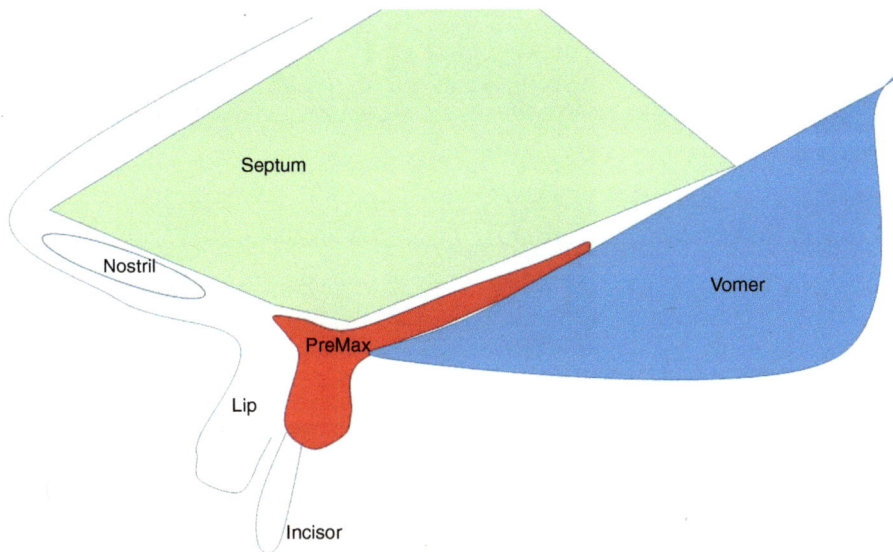

Fig. 5.7 Sagittal view of the three-pronged premaxilla (PreMax) and its surrounding structures in an ideal state. (Reprinted with permission Springer Nature – Hyman et al. [12])

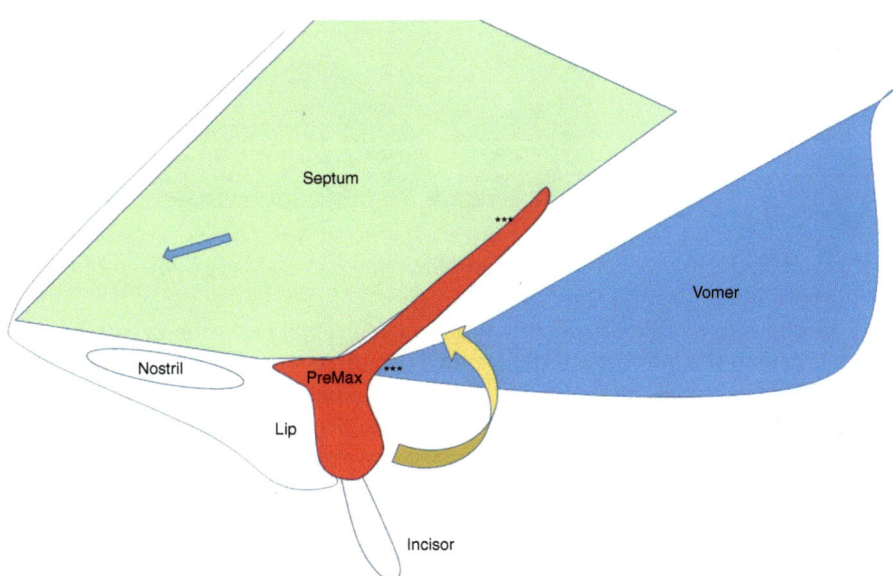

Fig. 5.8 Sagittal view of the three-pronged premaxilla (PreMax), and its surrounding structures in a rotated state, with retro-clining of the incisors, septal extrusion and tension nose, and arched palate. (Reprinted with permission Springer Nature – [12])

Fig. 5.9 Sagittal CT scan of the nasal septum with an adequate bony septal aperture and position of the premaxilla, permitting the neutral septal structure

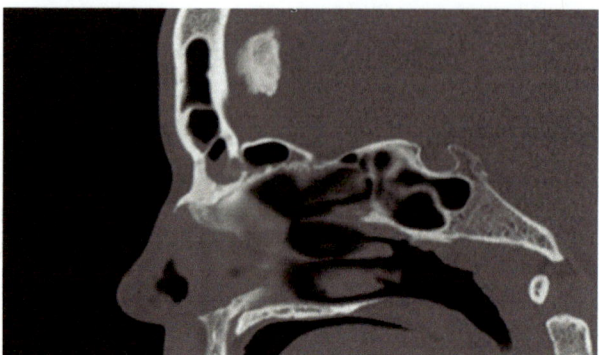

Fig. 5.10 Sagittal CT scan of the nasal septum with a limited bony septal aperture and unfavorable position of the premaxilla, causing elevated arched palate, and tension nose

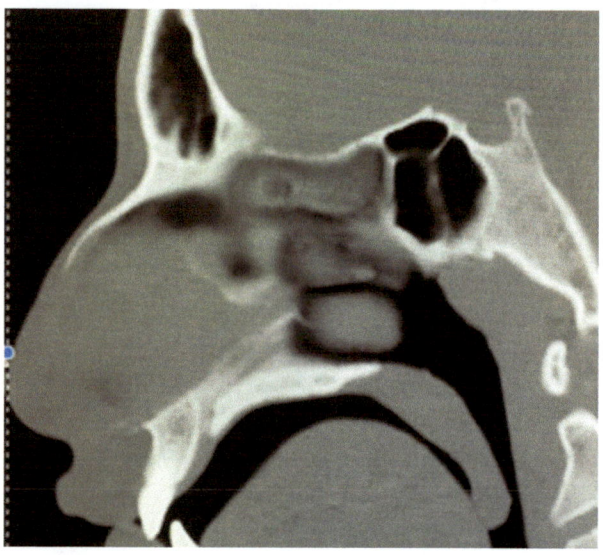

phenomenon (despite what myself and others have mistakenly conjectured about its purpose in the past) [17].

This condition of maxillary shrinking, causing septal extrusion in extreme versions accounts for most septal deformities (traumatic also occurs, but less commonly than you think), dorsal humps and fullness, non-postoperative "polly-beak," and even nasal valve collapse. Interestingly, almost all non-postoperative dorsal and caudal issues can be related to external septal extrusion, including severe nasal deviation, nasal asymmetry, "middle vault" narrowing, caudal deviation, and even nasal valve collapse. Even deformities we ascribe to the tip cartilages or tripod are actually primarily due to this problem, despite conventional wisdom and education. Finally, even seemingly unrelated aesthetic problems like facial asymmetry or chin retrusion can be perceived as more pronounced due to marked extrusion and severe axis deviation of the quadrangular cartilage. Because the septum is the indirect cause of many of these problems, treatment strategies can be adjusted where instead of direct treatments to the nasal tripod, middle vault, or mandible, indirect solutions addressing the septal size can be considered. In the next section, we will use a tent-shaped (triangular prism) model to explain how broad-reaching this problem really is, and how the under-sized bony septal aperture

How the *Framework* Layer Causes Functional and Aesthetic Problems?

In terms of temporary domiciles, the igloo is perhaps the most interesting structure. It really has no internal framework, but like the keystone of an arch, is elegantly dependent on all of its components essentially leaning against each other in a sort of controlled state of collapse. In contrast, the classic camping tent is completely reliant on its framework and the tension of its fabric or skin layer. The triangular prism-shaped tent, as we discussed before is an excellent way to visualize how the framework affects the fabric, skin, or fly layers, even though to an uninitiated external observer, the structural flaws will seem to reside in the superficial structures themselves, as they are the components that look narrowed, weak, or distorted. From my perspective, again it is this compartmentalization that has caused our paradigms of treatment in rhinoplasty to be flawed, as when we see narrowed nasal walls, we seek to add bulk to these structures with grafts, while in truth, the walls are narrowed by an oversized framework, much like a hiking tent with an overly tall framework from a parts mix-up, that would have overly narrowed walls. (Fig. 5.11) The solution to the problem would not necessarily involve treatment to the walls themselves, but to re-sizing and repositioning the framework, thus indirect solutions

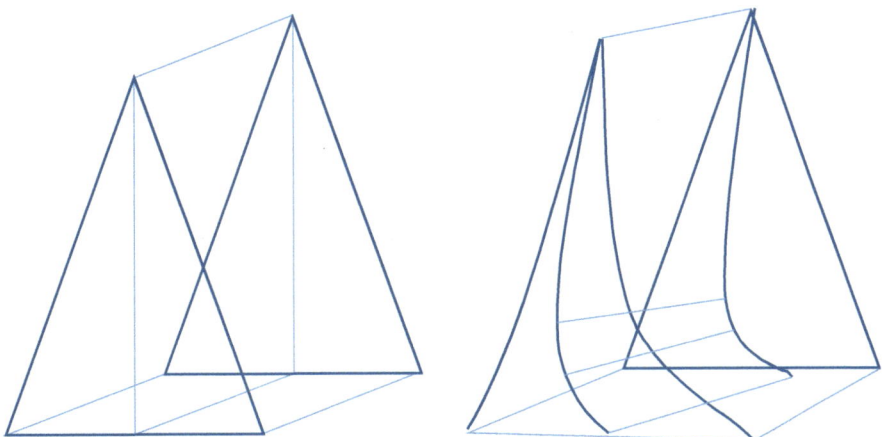

Fig. 5.11 Triangular prism with central support schematic. On the left is an adequately sized central support structure. On the right is an oversized central support structure that indirectly narrows the lateral walls. As in the nose, there is nothing intrinsically wrong with these walls

to the aesthetic and functional problem. We will discuss patterns of how the framework can impact the overall nasal structure using our dynamic triangular prism model (DTPM).

One other misconception must be cleared up before we can fully discuss this model: Our concept of the nasal valve.

Rethinking the Nasal Valve

First, among surgeons and patients there is a concept that somehow aesthetic and functional concepts are completely divorced from one another. I have heard of many situations where a pair of physicians combine to perform aesthetic and functional rhinoplasty as separate procedures. This sounds good from a division of labor perspective (especially to unsuspecting patients) and also from a reimbursement perspective. But from a structural perspective this is a terrible idea, as it simply demonstrates a lack of understanding that the two procedures are completely interwoven, and in most cases one in the same, despite the arbitrariness created by insurance companies and administrators as we will see shortly.

Second, our textbook concept of a separate internal and external nasal valve is misleading and incorrect, despite its broad concept buy-in and usage by authorities and so-called "experts." In the traditional view, the internal nasal valve is the narrowest point in the airway, bound by the inferior turbinate, the upper lateral cartilage, and the nasal septum. The external valve is essentially the space just inside the nostril opening. Most "authorities" consider the internal valve to be most important and gear most treatments to this space as it is "the narrowest space in the airway" that must be opened. In reality, the two-valve concept is so primitive and limited, that I think that the propagation of the concept is actually responsible for poorly designed and misguided treatments. The outcome measures for the internal valve include caliber measures, and the famous 15 degree upper lateral cartilage to the septal angle. Of course these measures are useless and have no bearing on actual airflow or symptoms. The angle can be confounded by actually filling above the upper lateral cartilage, that shortens the height of the nasal valve but enlarges the angle (see Chap. 1), and of course this further obstructs the airway [18].

Thinking of a separate internal and external valve is classic two-dimensional compartmentalized thinking. In reality, the nasal inlet (a term first used to describe the unified valve by Shuaib et al. [19] and further analyzed by Tripathi et al. in 2017, [20] is a funnel shaped structure supporting air inlet, that during inspiration begins at the nostril, and tapers internally and gradually toward the internal airway at the bony pyriform aperture. As we discussed in Chap. 2, the turbinate component of the "valve" is actually reactive to nasal underuse and is only a limited obstructive component. It is the *shape* of the funnel shaped nasal inlet that determines form and function. By *shape*, I am referring to the surface area of the nostril opening, the degree of tortuosity or bending of the funnel, and the length of the inlet. The degree of bending of this funnel increases the airflow turbulence, and thus reduces available air to reach the all-important pharynx (see Chap. 4) (Fig. 5.12). In this figure of

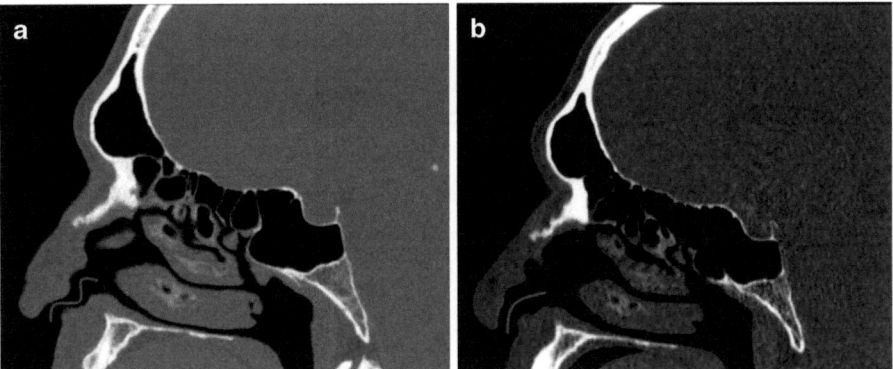

Fig. 5.12 Sagittal CT scans of the nasal inlet. (**a**) Pre-operative, with blue line indicating inlet tortuosity. (**b**). Post-operative, with blue line revealing loss of bending of inlet, suggesting decreased bending and less pressure drop. (Image courtesy of Sage Publication with permission – Naughton et al. [21])

sagittal CT scans from the same patient before and after isolated nasal valve surgery, the nasal inlet is far less bent or tortuous in the postop image. The upper lateral cartilage is largely irrelevant as well, but as we will see shortly, but only appears "collapsed" or narrowed at the "middle third" due to excessive septal length or poor tension on the canopy layer due to lower lateral cartilage droop from its superior attachments to the bony framework layer. Using computational flow dynamics in a patient who underwent isolated nasal inlet surgery, we tested this concept and the effect of changing the shape of the nasal inlet on downstream airflow [21].

As you can see, in Fig. 5.13a, the path from the nasal valve (right) to the pharynx has sharper bends when the patient had a longer and more tortuous nose and nasal valve (pre-op). In Fig. 5.13b, (post-op) the airflow path is shorter, more curved, less sharply bent and thus more efficient at getting air pressure to the nasopharynx (left).

The concept of "pressure drop" is used in physics to denote a differential of pressure between two points in a channel or tube. The nozzle-shaped pipe from the nostril opening to the distal entrance to the nasal cavity can be conceived of as one of these channels which transmits air as its "fluid." The Darcy-Weisbach formula (although designed for non-compressible fluids) predicts that increasing length or degree of bending will result in increasing pressure drop during fluid transmission across the pipe. Thus, in the case of the nasal inlet, a long, overly bent inlet, as in the case of the overly long, nose, as the patient who underwent the computational flow dynamics (CFD) had originally (Fig. 5.12), will cause excessive pressure drop of the inspiratory air column, and will not have sufficient air pressure to stent open the more distal airway from the remainder of the nasal cavity onward. Additionally, if the nozzle is shaped incorrectly, like the reverse of a funnel, with a narrow nostril opening, and then dilated internal nasal cavity, air vortices will form in the dilated cavity, also reducing the pressure-head that finally reaches the distal downstream airway. Experimenting with tidal flow on a beach during a vacation to Amelia island, Florida last year, we can see the same phenomenon, that only inlet dilation

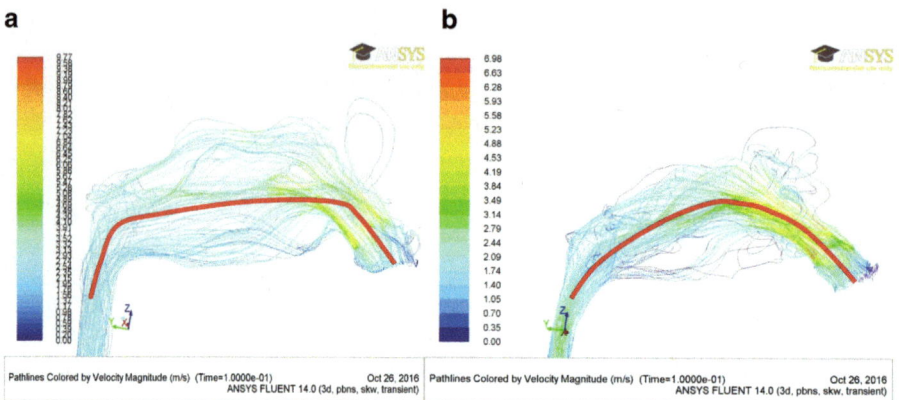

Fig. 5.13 Same patient as Fig. 5.12, with computational flow dynamics showing less acutely bent trend line from pre-operative image (**a**), to post-operative (**b**). (Naughton et al. [21])

(Fig. 5.14a), and NOT dilation along the route of a stream (Fig. 5.14b) will result in improved flow, and any internal dilation will only result in vortices.

In the CFD study discussed above, while the operated upon nasal inlet increased in size in cross-sectional area by between 25% and 45.8% in various sections, downstream, non-operated areas increased by nearly 50%, confirming that improving the shape (and size) of the inlet could result in downstream improvement in airflow, and air passage caliber. As expected, the pressure drop and resistance across the nasal valve from the change in shape improved substantially as well, by over 40%, and airflow increased by similar amounts. We attributed this large improvement to the shortening of the nasal inlet funnel from 24 to 21 mm, and decreasing its degree of tortuosity by shortening the L-strut in this patient to a more favorable length (we will see in the next section how and why shortening works) [21].

So, what does this all show? That it is the *shape* of the whole nasal inlet, not simple attempts to measure caliber of the internal valve that is critical in determining both airflow, resistance, pressure drop, and even down-stream airway size. Thus, the traditional concept of the internal and external separate nasal valves that can be evaluated with internal valve angle or surface area can be considered to be obsolete and replaced with a concept of a cone or funnel shaped nasal inlet that functions better with fewer bends and shorter axis length.

Finally, one can also conclude that attempting to "fix" the downstream airway without addressing a narrow inlet will NOT improve nasal airflow. Instead, as seen in our flow dynamics study, fixing only the nasal cavity will create intra-nasal turbulence that does not contribute to increased flow. A petite inlet and large cavity is a set-up for poor distal airflow, even while the surgeon sees on his endoscope a "large" airway. This is a classic reason why turbinate surgery and limited septal surgery (submucous resection procedures) cannot prevent mouth-breathing and treat sleep disordered breathing (see Chaps. 2 and 3). As we discussed above, this is similar to a narrow but flowing river that at its midpoint experiences a lake-like

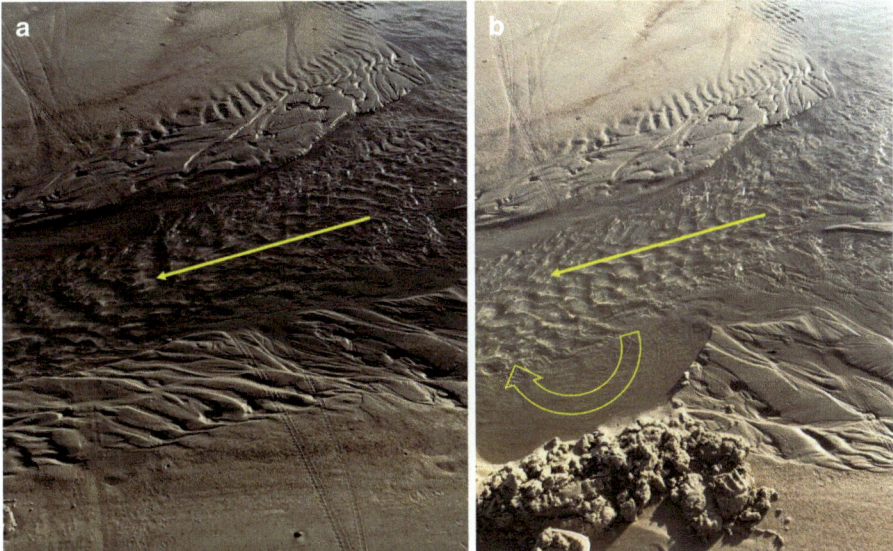

Fig. 5.14 (**a**) Large inlet flowing (yellow arrow), into a stream, (**b**) same inlet, but with downstream dilation does not increase flow, instead creating areas of re-circulation (hollow yellow curved arrow)

dilation (Fig. 5.15). While the lake is large, the increased space actually decreases flow due to circular eddy formation in the lake (Fig. 5.15b). In contrast, when the nasal inlet and nasal cavity together form a funnel shape with minimal bending and length, flow is efficient (Fig. 5.15a). You can use Fig. 5.16a to help visualize our funnel shaped new view of the unified nasal inlet. Figure 5.16b by contrast shows the conventional two-dimensional internal and external nasal valves conceptualized in many texts. Now that we have rethought the nasal inlet concept (think funnel instead of ovoid area of restriction, we can apply this knowledge to our framework model, incorporating both aesthetics (external appearance) and function (nasal inlet shape) simultaneously: This is the subject of the next section.

Putting It All Together: The Framework and Its Relations Using the Dynamic Triangular Prism Model (DTPM), the Nasal Inlet, Aesthetics and Symmetry

Earlier in the chapter, we were introduced to the concept of the DTPM, which includes a foundation or substrate (piriform aperture and septal bones) framework (septum and nasal bones), and canopy (superficial layer of skin and alar cartilages). We discussed how the foundation or substrate is the root cause of most aesthetic and functional problems of the nose. However, it is the framework, or structural layer that is the most important actual determinant of aesthetics and airflow, and even of the form and function of the canopy layer. Into our DTPM, in addition to the all-important framework layer (septal cartilage and nasal bones—Yellow), its underlying foundation of the maxilla and bony septum (Pink), and the superficial

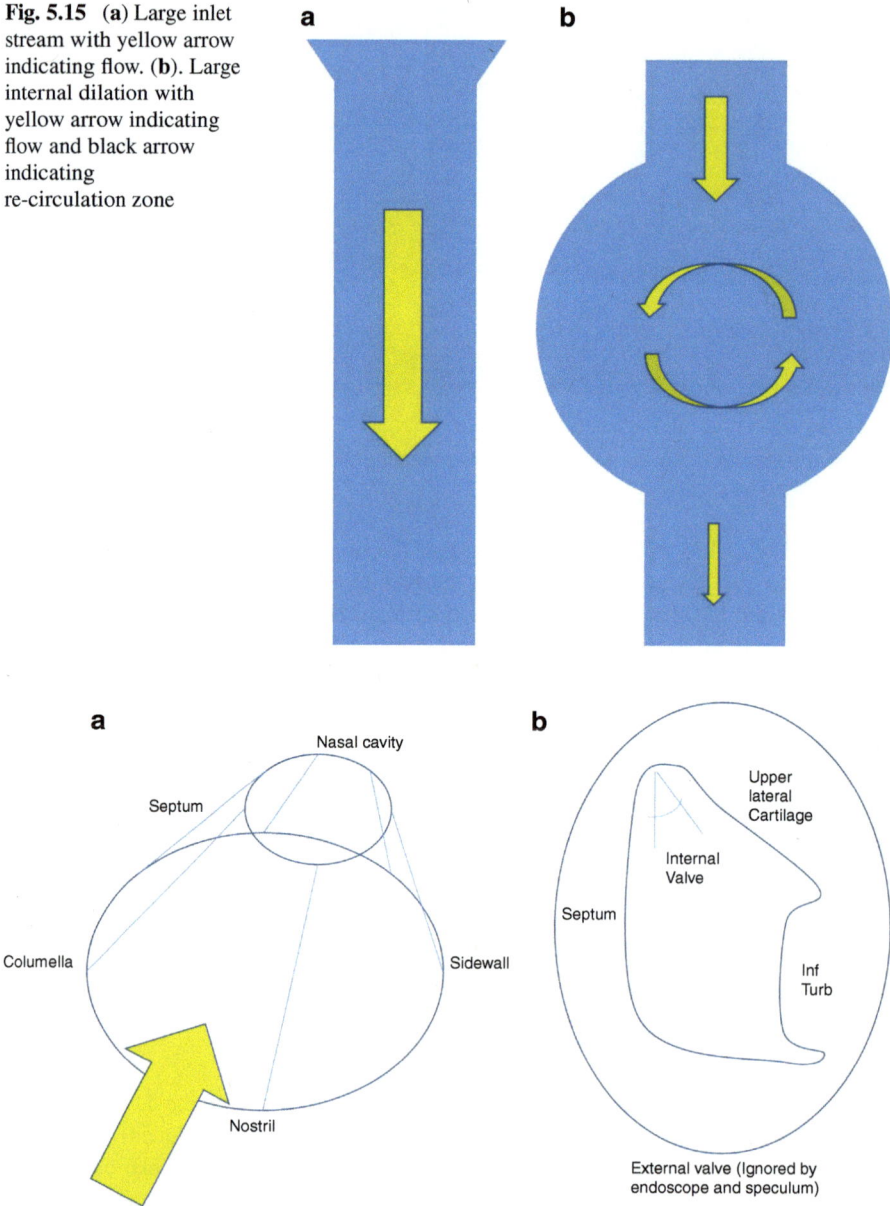

Fig. 5.15 (a) Large inlet stream with yellow arrow indicating flow. (b). Large internal dilation with yellow arrow indicating flow and black arrow indicating re-circulation zone

Fig. 5.16 (a) The three-dimensional nasal inlet is funnel shaped. (b) The conventional internal and external valves represented as overlapping two-dimensional openings

canopy layer (alar cartilages, scroll, and skin envelope—Blue), we will incorporate a three-dimensional cylindrical representation of the new concept of the nasal inlet (transparent grey) (Fig. 5.17). For this advanced model, instead of including an "upper lateral cartilage," we will include the "scroll," the spring-like fibro-cartilaginous soft-tissue layer that connects the dorsal septum to suspend the lateral crura of the alar cartilage (seen here as a black coiled spring embedded in a blue strip). This spring-like structure instead of intrinsic importance serves the role of supporting the lateral crura much like a wing-strut supports the load of a mono-plane wing. Thus, treating this spring does not affect the airway in itself, as being an independent cartilage would infer, but simply is a supportive structure to the alar structure of the canopy. The scroll, functioning as a supportive spring prevents the lateral crura from moving permanently even with force applied, but it also can be stretched or damaged with prolonged force, and with this lost spring elasticity, the lateral crura can become malpositioned.

In contrast, the framework layer, the fusion of the quadrangular cartilage of the nasal bones is so critical to ALL nasal structures, and both functional and aesthetic concerns that I will suggest that the next few paragraphs are the most important part of this book. The significance of this cannot be understated. Most previous models have considered the quadrangular cartilage of the septum to be relatively irrelevant with a small portion removed for deviation, access to the sinuses, or as a supply of grafts. More generous considerations have at best considered the role of the septum to play merely a supporting role, as a "pedestal" in the tripod model, where the tip cartilages are paramount. The septum can also be seen as a nuisance, as in the extracorporeal septoplasty model, where only complete removal and refurbishing on the "back table" can fix the deviation. In contrast, we will describe how the septal framework, largely controls and shapes the canopy or tip cartilage layer, and is

Fig. 5.17 Dynamic triangular prism model (DTPM). Pink indicates the foundation/substrate, golden yellow represents the framework, blue shows the canopy layer, here consisting of the paired medial and lateral crura of the alar cartilage and the spring-like scroll. The grey cylinder represents the nasal inlet, supported by the external nose structures

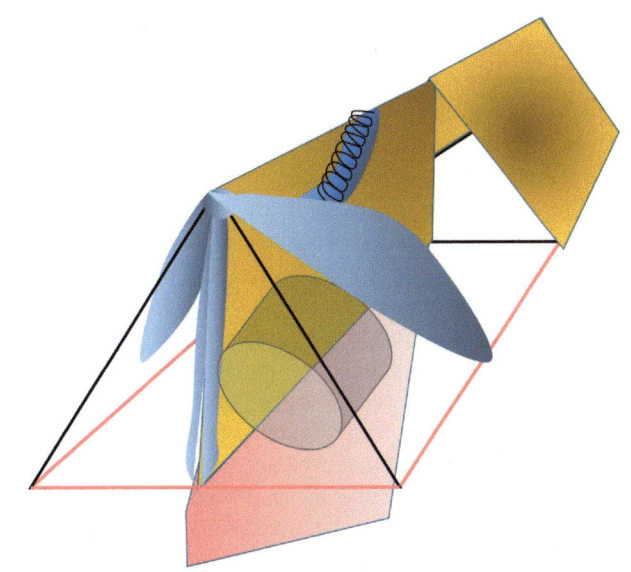

directly or indirectly responsible for almost all-important functional and aesthetic problems, except iatrogenic ones, or those due to misinformation and dated myths propagated by both providers and the internet.

Septal or framework position, as determined by the capacity of the substrate or foundation of the underlying septal bones (see prior sections) determines the aesthetic and functional phenotype of the nose. Like the cardinal points of a compass (north, south, east, and west), there are four distinct septal position extremes that are possible for the *Homo sapiens*. Ideal aesthetics and function lie as some compromise between these various points between over- and under-support of the nose. Between these four pathological states, combinations are possible, like the directional combination of the cardinal points (i.e., south-south-west). And also like a compass, opposites cannot co-exist in the nose, for example, there is no direction that can combine south and north, or east with west, as you cannot have a short and long nose at the same time. The four "cardinal" septal positions are: (1) Superior-inferior extrusion excess (long nose)—called SI+, (2) anterior-posterior extrusion excess (protruding nose) called AP+, (3) superior-inferior deficiency (short nose) called SI–, (4) anterior-posterior deficiency (flat nose) called AP–. When the four extreme conditions are represented graphically as a "Rhinoplasty Compass™" (Fig. 5.18), one can see that the "ideal" nose both functionally and aesthetically can exist at an ill-defined point somewhere in the middle of the compass. In contrast, pathologic, or non-ideal noses can exist as combinations of two cardinal points, for example, a long and protruding nose (AP+, SI+), or a long and flat nose (AP+, SI–). These septal positions also determine the position and shape of the *dependent* canopy layer. For example, a protruding AP+ nose will cause the overlying canopy tip layer to be stretched forward, thus narrowing the sidewalls and creating the illusion that the lateral alar cartilages are collapsed. It is this illusion that permitted the two-dimensional thinking to design batten grafts as a misguided solution to the problem. While the nose appears narrow with this framework, it is narrow because of septal over-projection, not because of alar cartilage problems. In the triangular prism tent, with an oversized framework (support poles too long), the walls of the tent would appear narrow and collapsed. But in reality treating the narrowed walls would be an error. Only shortening the frameworks poles would result in success in un-collapsing the sidewalls. As we will discuss in the next chapter reviewing existing procedures, this is why except in iatrogenic deficiency of alar cartilage, adding material to the sidewall, either cartilage, bone, or in the case of a recently introduced absorbable injectable device, is not only useless, but actually further narrows the airway, although increasing the bulkiness of the sidewalls. And of course, this misunderstanding adds nothing to aesthetics either, but has certainly misled many patients and physicians into believing that a benefit has been added.

By breaking the septal framework position into these four cardinal compass points allows infinite variations by many combinations, accounting for the variability seen among humans. It even accounts for racial differences, or traumatic dislocations of the septum, as one does not need to ascribe a race to a nose, nor a speculation of the degree of trauma, just a positional description. While most texts will refer to different racial sub-types of the nose and rhinoplasty, we will only focus on actual

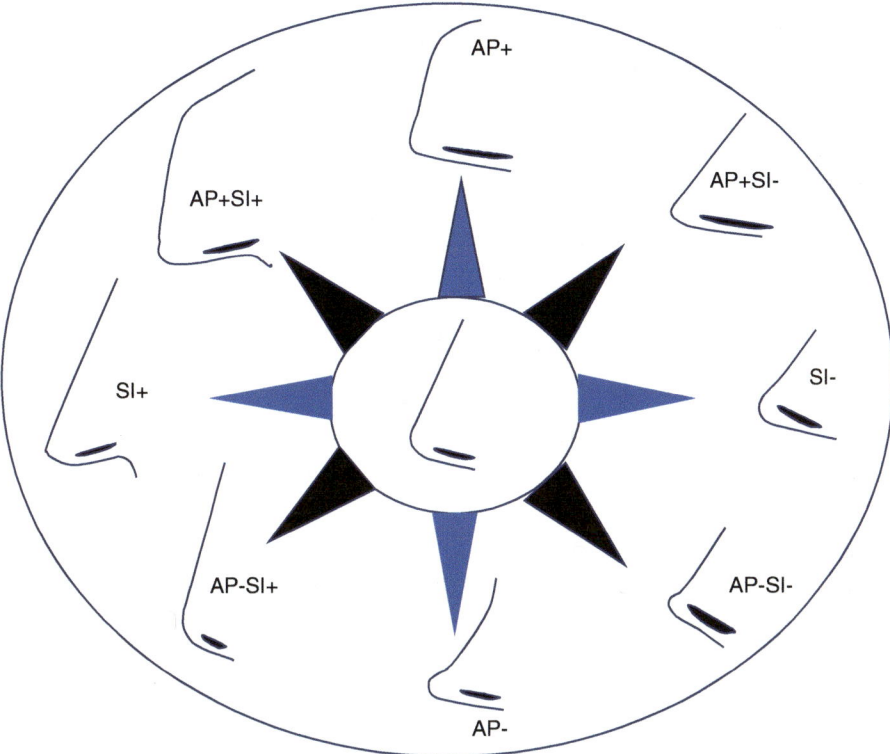

Fig. 5.18 The Rhinoplasty Compass™. The nasal framework has four cardinal points, as in a directional compass, corresponding with north, south, east, and west. The four cardinal points are antero-posterior excess (AP+), antero-posterior deficiency (AP–), supero-inferior excess (SI+), and supero-inferior deficiency (SI–). Combinations of these cardinal points form the rest of the directional structures

description of the framework and septal position, although of course different ethnicities have a tendency toward one framework position or another. By focusing on position only, we can successfully avoid attempting to classify by racial divisions (i.e., Caucasian or Asian rhinoplasty) and simply discuss pathology and treatment by septal framework position, and its relation to the "ideal." As Louis Leakey teaches, all humans have a common origin and most differences between individuals are generally superficial. Of course, there are societo-cultural differences in aesthetics that can be addressed, but this is over a broad continuum and will not be discussed this in this book. Perhaps the "ideal" in the center between these four extreme phenotypes can be fluid and open to individual/cultural interpretation with as much variability as the pathologic extremes. However, I do believe that function and form occupy nearly the same positions on this compass. One could conjecture that this is possibly due to a co-evolution of our aesthetic knowledge as a species and subconscious recording of health with attractiveness by individuals and crowds [22].

By focusing on the four positional extremes, we can see sample noses of these extremes, and also predict the external nose shapes, from a front, side, and base view that go along with these phenotypes. We can also classify noses before surgery into combinations of these extremes and design a more suitable strategy than following a series of steps (see Chap. 7).

First, let's analyze each of the four cardinal compass framework positions one at a time and consider the details of their pathology.

Rhinoplasty Compass Point 1: AP+ (Antero-Posterior Septal Extrustion)

This is one of the most important and common configurations of the septum. Figure 5.19 shows the AP+ profile (Fig. 5.19b) compared with the neutral nose Fig. 5.19a. Now, look at the DTPM (Fig. 5.20) for this configuration. See Figs. 5.21, 5.22, 5.23, 5.24, 5.25, and 5.26 for a sample photographic profile, front, and base view example of this configuration. As you can imagine, this configuration can exist in several variations, but we are presenting a typical version. There can be primarily dorsal "excess" classically manifesting as a dorsal hump and narrow bridge or primarily excess at the tip, causing an over-projected tip and narrow tip. The excess dorsal or inferior septal projection creates the illusion of narrowed sidewalls, just like our example of overly long tent poles. So, you can see that the skin and lateral crura (the canopy layer) assumes a "collapsed" position adjacent to the septum that narrows the nose aesthetically, but also narrows the nasal inlet for airflow. As the septum extrudes dorsally and externally during growth, it also causes the nasal bones to bulge externally, as it is attached at the keystone area, creating a peak at the intersection of cartilage and bone. Thus, these patients frequently have an over-projected pointy tip, and a sharp dorsal hump point, like a hawk's beak.

From a symmetry perspective, if the antero-posterior extrusion is severe enough, over-coming the stretching point of the canopy layer (skin and alar cartilages) in an anterior direction, the septum will tilt as seen on the base view, tilting the whole axis of the nose to one side, sometimes creating an illusion of, or exacerbating pre-existing facial asymmetry. In AP+ (anterior excess), the deviation is most pronounced from the base view, but of course this base deviation will cause the entire A-P axis of the nose to deviate on front view as well, but typically as a complete unit, including nasal bones (see figure). I make this point only in contrast to the SI+ (superior-inferior excess), which tends to form more irregular frontal asymmetries like c- or s-shaped noses as we will discuss shortly. Internally, the septum may actually be straight in the AP+ configuration, with narrowed nostrils, or the internal quadrangular cartilage (posterior portion) can bend in the direction opposite the external septum, taking the septal bones with it, and creating a large "spur" appearing region (see the figure of external effect on internal). Because the septum is protruding anteriorly, it tends to keep the lip under some tension, even if it does not encroach into the lip. These patients can have a shortened, tense lip due to the overly

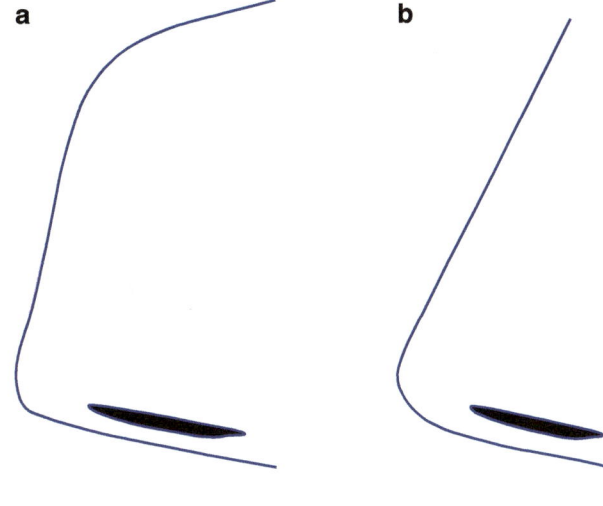

Fig. 5.19 Profile diagram of (**a**) AP+ (excess) SI neutral (0) framework in comparison with (**b**) antero-posterior (AP) supero-inferior (SI) neutral framework (AP 0/SI 0)

a   **b**

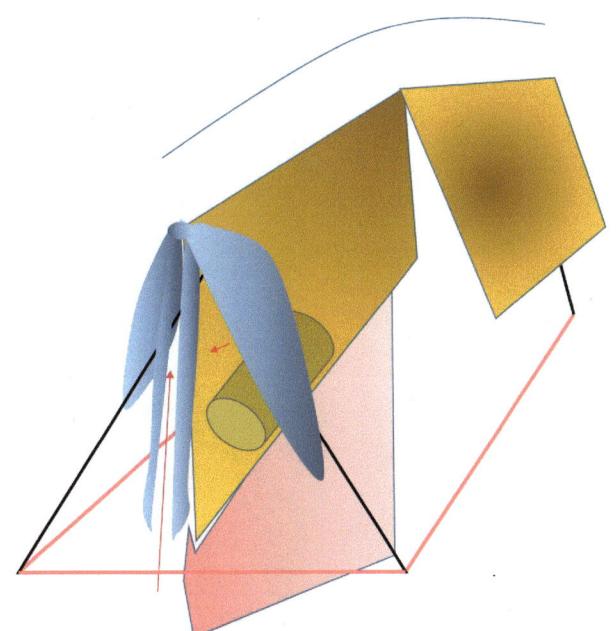

Fig. 5.20 Dynamic triangular prism model (DTPM) of the antero-posterior excess (AP+) framework. Pink indicates the foundation/substrate, golden yellow represents the framework, blue shows the canopy layer, here consisting of the paired medial and lateral crura of the alar cartilage. The grey cylinder represents the narrowed nasal inlet, supported by the stretched external nose structures. Red arrows show the direction of movement

large nose taking up too much skin real-estate for the upper lip to properly close without a lot of effort.

As you are hopefully starting to imagine, treatment strategies will revolve around re-sizing the septum and returning all components back to their midline position independently. (This will be discussed in detail in the next chapters.)

Fig. 5.21 Clinical
photographs of patient
with antero-posterior
excess (AP+). Frontal view

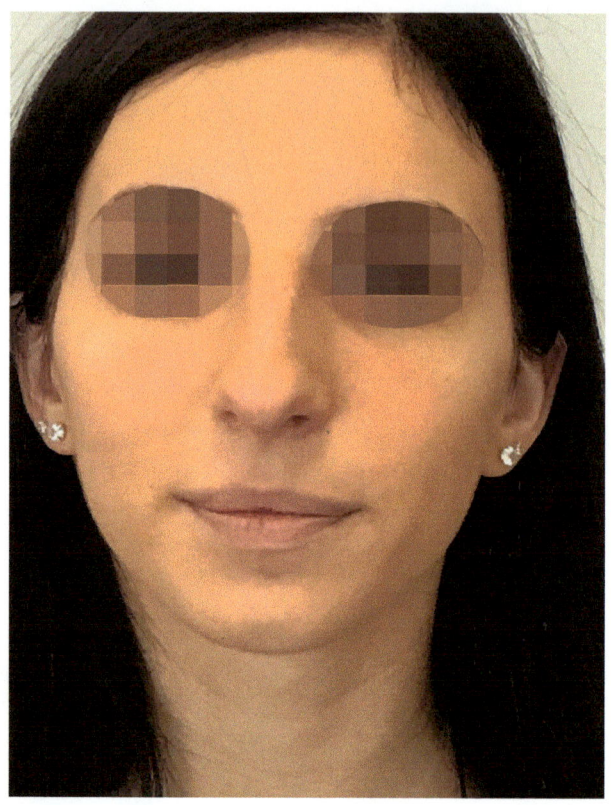

Fig. 5.22 Clinical
photographs of patient
with antero-posterior
excess (AP+). Base view

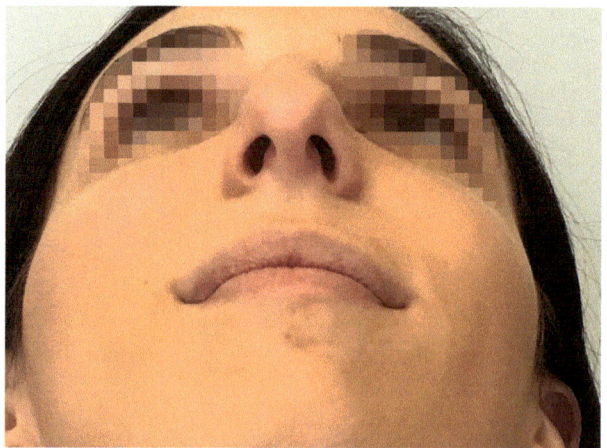

Fig. 5.23 Clinical photographs of patient with antero-posterior excess (AP+). Oblique left view

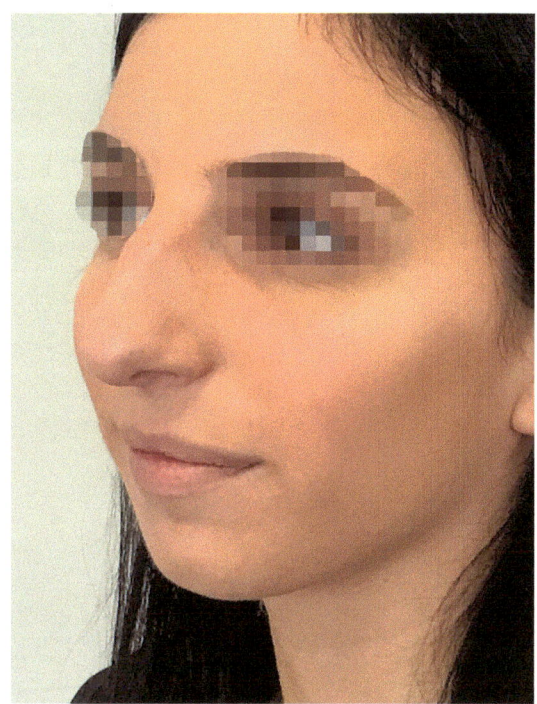

Fig. 5.24 Clinical photographs of patient with antero-posterior excess (AP+). Right profile view

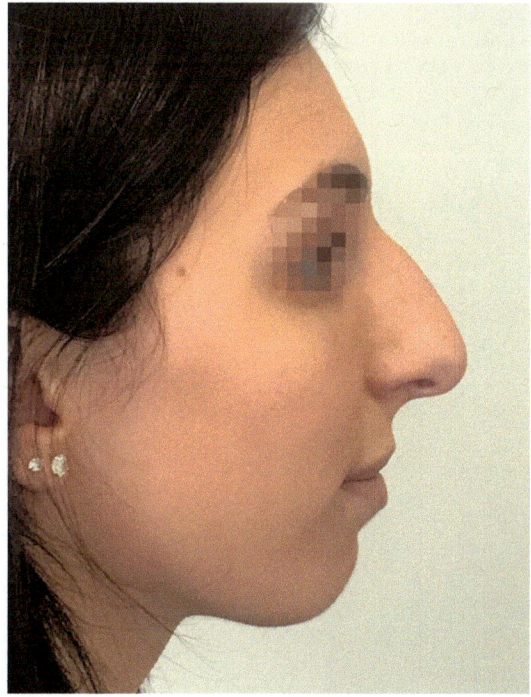

Fig. 5.25 Clinical photographs of patient with antero-posterior excess (AP+). Oblique right view

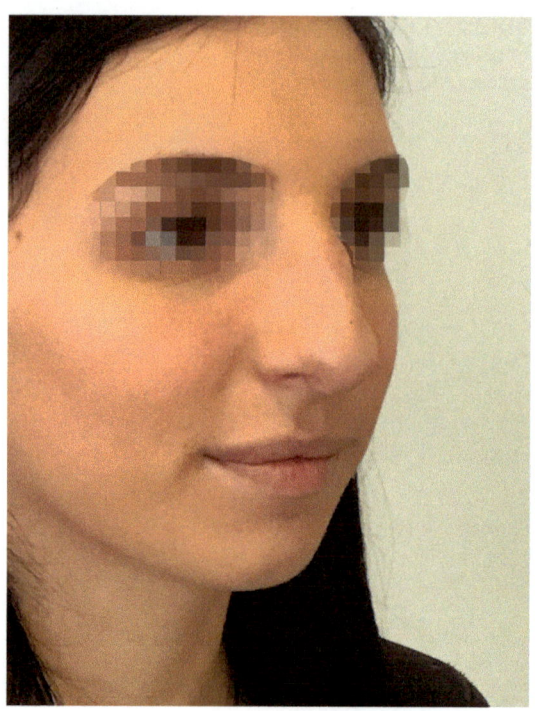

Fig. 5.26 Clinical photographs of patient with antero-posterior excess (AP+). Left profile view

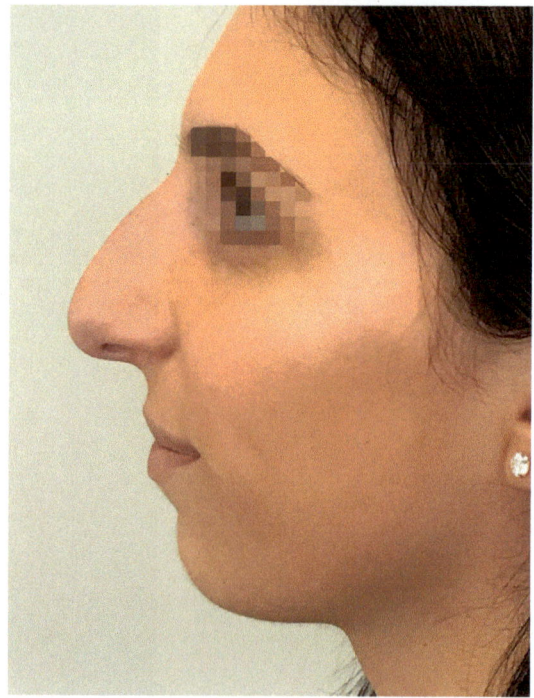

Rhinoplasty Compass Point 2: SI+
(Supero-Inferior Septal Excess)

For reference, see Fig. 5.27a, b, the prototypical SI+ profile compared to neutral (AP/SI neutral) for configuration. For framework, see the SI + DTPM (Fig. 5.28), and for sample photos, see Figs. 5.29, 5.30, and 5.31. While similar in concept as the AP+ septal extrusion that relates to PROJECTION, the superior-inferior extrusion (SI+) relates to nasal LENGTH. In this case, the septum, growing from its ethmoid plate origins, is overly long in superior inferior direction, and protrudes beyond the nasal spine into the lip. The lip will appear shortened substantially not because of tension anteriorly like in the AP+ model, but because the nose is literally occupying the lip. This is most pronounced by smiling and is not due to overactive lip musculature but excessive nasal length. The excessive length of the nose from the frontal view also produces a less attractive, or even prematurely aged view, particularly in a female who are perceived in human esthetics to be more youthful and attractive with a shorter nose relative to the lip and facial height. I do not think numerical measurements as espoused my most authors (while helpful as basic guidelines for students) are as helpful as using one's aesthetic "eye" to determine "proper" nasal length. I believe this sense can be developed by analyzing as many noses as possible and considering whether or not one would consider the person to be attractive, acceptable, or unattractive. (Of course, you do not need to inform the subject or anyone of your conclusions, just form a mental database). The long nose creates an additional frontal view aesthetic problem: narrowing of the middle part of the nose. Now, of course this is referred to as "middle vault collapse" or as the external manifestation of the upper lateral cartilage collapse, but in reality, this problem is usually due to excessive nasal length! How is this possible? By focusing only on the narrow middle "third" of the nose as a static object, a two-dimensional thinker would assume that the narrow middle third is due to collapse of the local walls. In reality, however, if one imagines a nose or septum growing from superior to inferior (toward the lip), one can imagine stretching of the canopy (skin and alar cartilages layer). Thus, in the very short nose of the child, the alar cartilages nearly abut the nasal bones in a superior-inferior direction. When the septum has grown overly long inferiorly, a gap will develop in the middle part of the nose, like the narrowing of an hourglass. Similarly, if one stretches both ends of a rubber tube, they will appreciate narrowing in the central segment. The middle third narrowing can be exacerbated by broad nasal bones, due to a lack of anterior growth in this phenotype, as the nasal bones were never stretched outward like in the AP+ model or the ideal nose. Thus, wide nasal bones will accentuate a "middle third" deficiency in relative terms, particularly with broad alar cartilages. The deviation of the external nose in SI+ patients takes on a distinct "("C")" or even "S" shaped deformity on the frontal view photographs. This is due to a buckling effect of the overly long septum and its effect on the dorsum. If one were to compress a flexible rod, it would take on a similar shape, and would become more complex in more severe compression, thus the "S" shaped deformity in maximal compression. The alar cartilages can appear

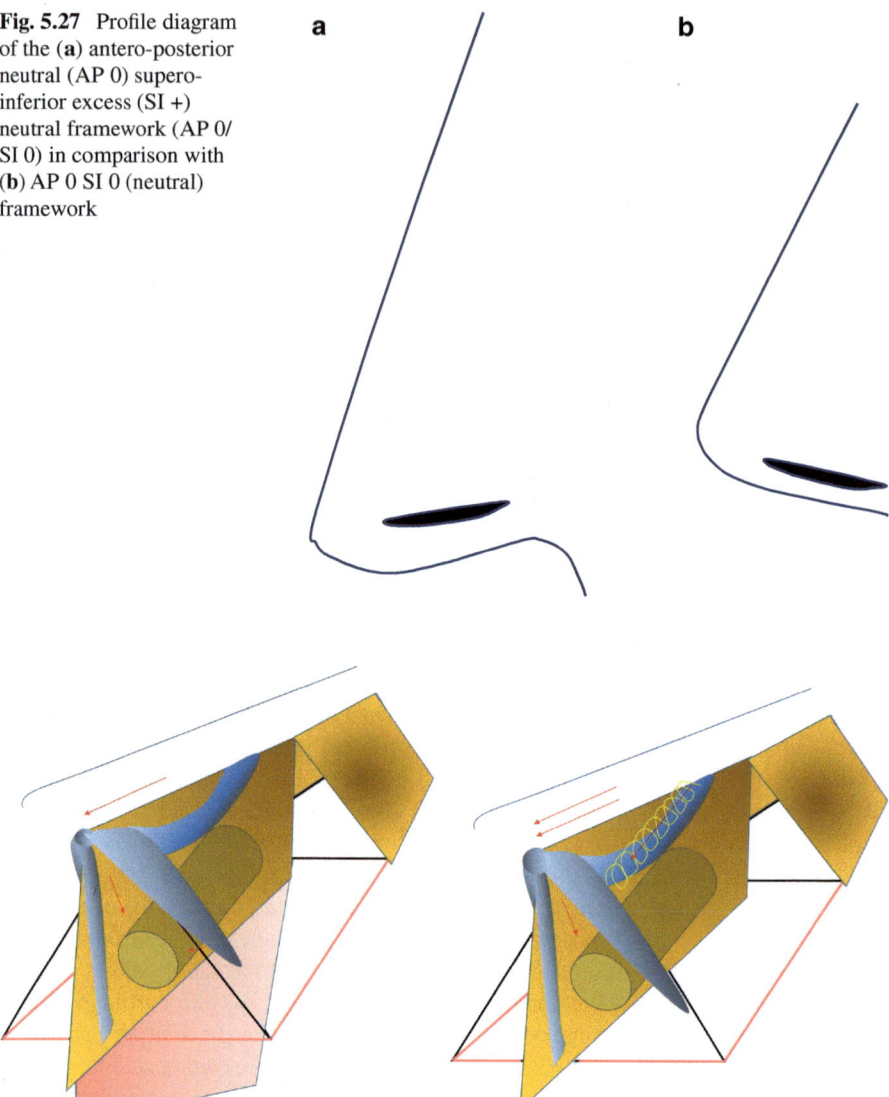

Fig. 5.27 Profile diagram of the (**a**) antero-posterior neutral (AP 0) supero-inferior excess (SI +) neutral framework (AP 0/ SI 0) in comparison with (**b**) AP 0 SI 0 (neutral) framework

Fig. 5.28 Dynamic triangular prism model (DTPM) of the antero-posterior neutral (AP 0), supero-inferior excess (AP+) framework. Pink indicates the foundation/substrate, golden yellow represents the framework, blue shows the canopy layer, here consisting of the paired medial and lateral crura of the alar cartilage. The grey cylinder represents the narrowed nasal inlet, supported by the stretched external nose structures. Red arrows show the direction of movement

ptotic or pointed down, because the anterior septal angle in the SI+ or long nose usually points inferiorly. It is not uncommon to see these "droopy" alar cartilages diagnosed as such primarily, with only treatment of the alar tripod performed, with the septal contribution minimized or ignored. For obvious reasons, treating only the

Fig. 5.29 Clinical photographs of patient with supero-inferior excess (SI+). Frontal view

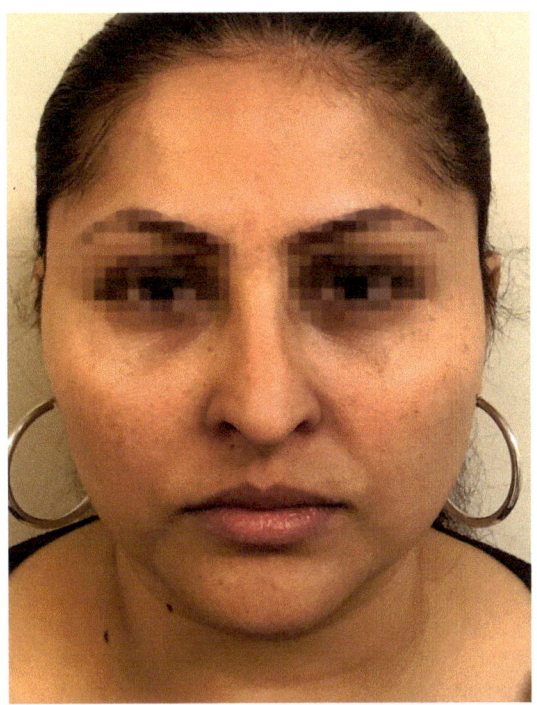

Fig. 5.30 Clinical photographs of patient with supero-inferior excess (SI+). Base view

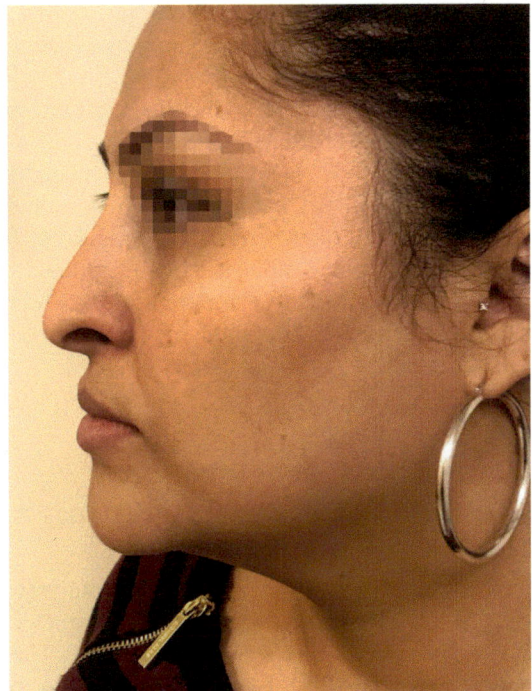

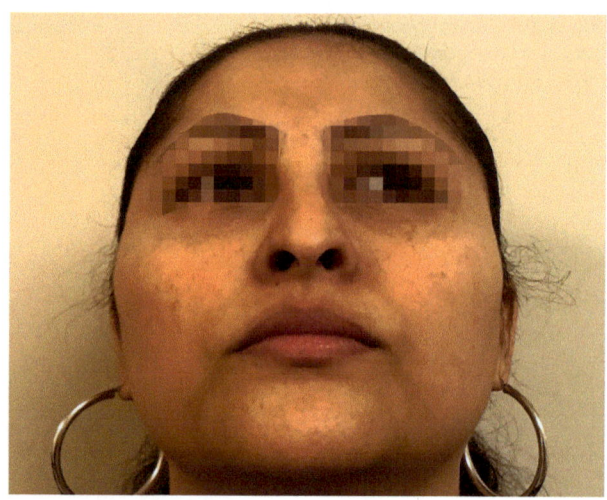

Fig. 5.31 Clinical photographs of patient with supero-inferior excess (SI+). Right side view

alar cartilages, even with extensive grafting and sutures risks failure. On the other hand, the very long SI+ nose, particularly in advanced age, or with a very long nose can result in intrinsically ptotic alar lateral crural cartilages with associated de-rotated tip due to stretching and loss of elasticity of the scroll. Notice in Fig. 5.28 how long the spring-like scroll (blue curve) has become. This supporting fibro-cartilaginous tissue that supports the lateral crura to the framework is stretched over time. Thus, even with shortening of the septum, maneuvers to restore alar cartilage position and rotation can be required such as division and shortening of the scroll and its connection with the lower lateral cartilage.

Finally, the nasal inlet in the SI+ configuration can be long and overly bent with narrowed nostril openings. Thus, even without a septal deviation, true nasal obstruction will exist. The long septum will interfere with the columella, stretching it inferiorly and potentially narrowing the nostril opening. It can also cause deviation of the columella further obstructing the airway. From the resultant ptosis and de-rotation of the alar cartilages from the influence of the long septum, the nasal inlet becomes longer, and is bent more acutely, which as we discussed in the prior chapter results in poor airflow and more loss of pressure supporting the airway (see pressure drop earlier in this chapter).

Rhinoplasty Compass Point 3 (Antero-Posterior Septal Deficiency AP–)

For reference, see Fig. 5.32a, b, the prototypical AP- profile compared to neutral (AP/SI neutral) for configuration. For framework, see the AP—DTPM (Fig. 5.33 and for sample photos Figs. 5.34 and 5.35). Unlike the previous two points (which are due to a growth mismatch of septum to maxilla), the antero-posterior septal

Fig. 5.32 Profile diagram of (**a**) antero-posterior neutral (AP 0) supero-inferior neutral SI 0) neutral framework (AP 0/ SI 0) in comparison with (**b**) AP deficiency (−) SI 0 (neutral) framework (AP–/SI 0)

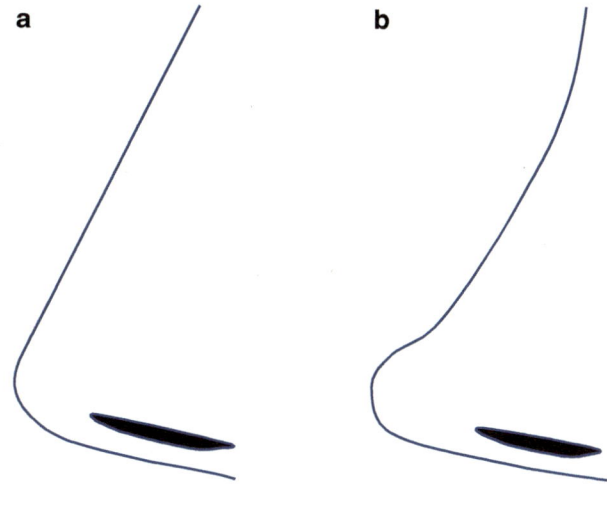

Fig. 5.33 Dynamic triangular prism model (DTPM) of the antero-posterior deficiency (AP–) framework. Pink indicates the foundation/substrate, golden yellow represents the framework, blue shows the canopy layer, here consisting of the paired medial and lateral crura of the alar cartilage. The grey cylinder represents the narrowed nasal inlet, supported by the stretched external nose structures. Red arrows show the direction of movement

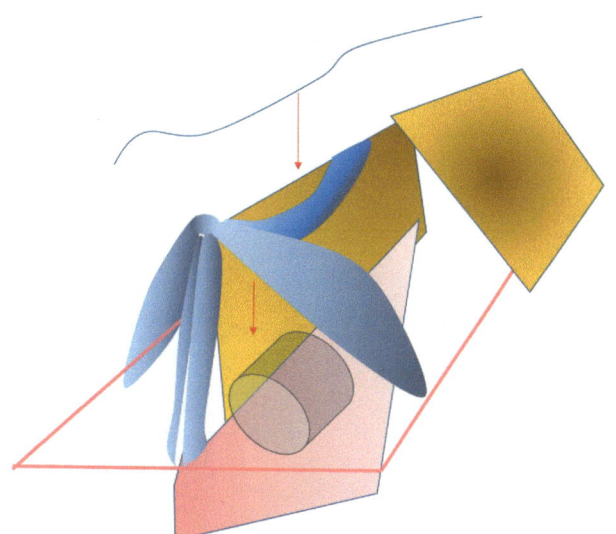

deficiency can be either due to growth disturbance *or* trauma and is commonly known as the "saddle nose deformity" but can be just a "flat" nose if the nasal bones are underprojected as well. In this case, the septum remains excessively inside the nasal cavity and inadequately supports the dorsum, tip, and nostrils. From a frontal view, these patients have a broad nose, sometimes with splayed broad nasal bones, and a wide nasal sill wide-appearing nasal tip cartilages. From a profile perspective,

Fig. 5.34 Clinical photographs of patient with antero-posterior deficiency (AP–). Left lateral view

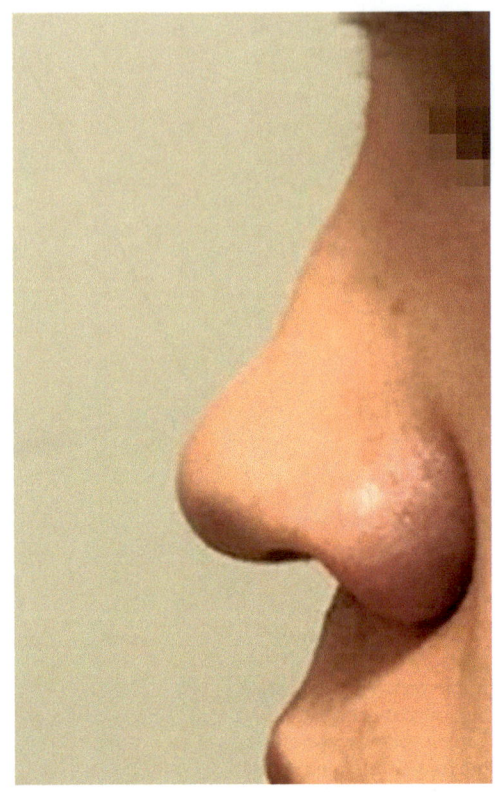

Fig. 5.35 Clinical photographs of patient with antero-posterior deficiency (AP–). Frontal view

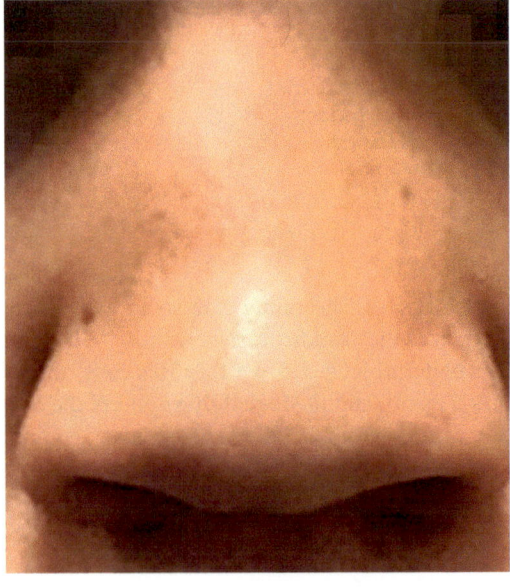

the nose is flattened and inadequately projected. From a base view, the nostrils are flat horizontal ovals that can provide inadequate flow. These patients can have a ptotic tip as well, not from septal overgrowth in an inferior direction pulling the cartilages down, but from failure of the anterior septal angle to support the alar cartilages, thus they fall inferiorly, narrowing the nostrils.

In the case of trauma, particularly a severe head-on trauma, the septum can be telescoped in an interior or posterior direction, and the internal septum can be found to duplicate itself, even appearing as two distinct parallel septums, or frequently with multiple fractures. Because of this, the dorsum can be flat while also deviated. The nasal inlet is narrowed by the flat nostrils and the ptotic tip. Using the classic tripod theory to consider, one viewing the alar cartilages will notice that they look flaccid and ptotic and assume it is due to inadequate cartilage strength, and the nasal tip is broad due to inadequate "definition." In reality, using our DTPM, we can see that the alar cartilages are actually weak due to inadequate framework or septal support. The deviation in these cases will not follow the congenital patterns of bowing seen in the "+" configurations, but will be mostly notable for fractures, telescoping, and apparent duplications. This makes the septal approach portions quite difficult and any surgery prone to risk of flap problems as we will discuss in subsequent chapters.

Rhinoplasty Compass Point 4: (Supero-Inferior Deficiency: SI–)

For reference, see Fig. 5.36a, b, the prototypical SI– profile compared to neutral (AP/SI neutral) for configuration. For framework, see the SI—DTPM (Fig. 5.37 and for sample photos Figs. 5.38 and 5.39). From my experience, this is one of

Fig. 5.36 Profile diagram of (**a**) antero-posterior neutral (AP 0) supero-inferior deficient (SI–) (AP 0/SI–) in comparison with (**b**) AP 0 (neutral) SI 0 (neutral) framework (AP 0/SI 0)

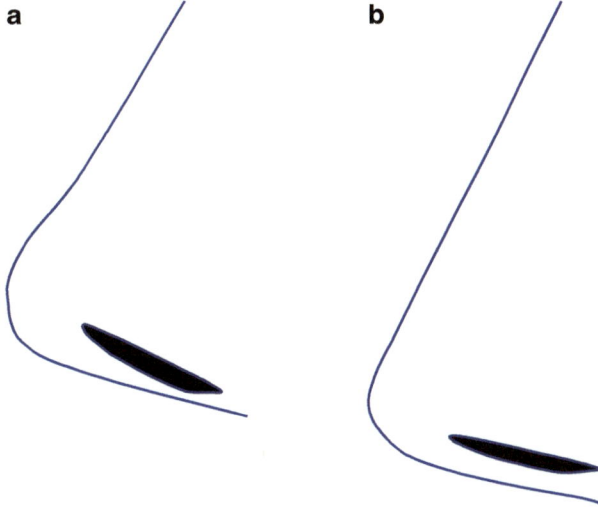

Fig. 5.37 Dynamic triangular prism model (DTPM) of the superoinferior deficiency (SI–) framework. Pink indicates the foundation/substrate, golden yellow represents the framework, blue shows the canopy layer, here consisting of the paired medial and lateral crura of the alar cartilage. The grey cylinder represents the nasal inlet, supported by the external nose structures. Red arrows show the direction of movement

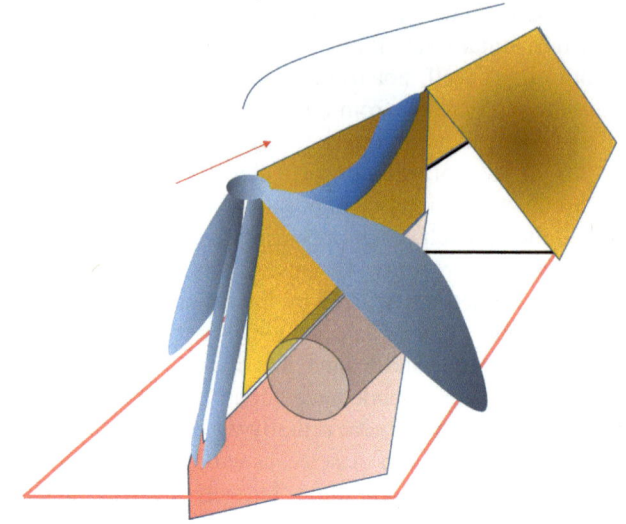

Fig. 5.38 Clinical photographs of patient with supero-inferior deficiency (SI–). Left lateral view

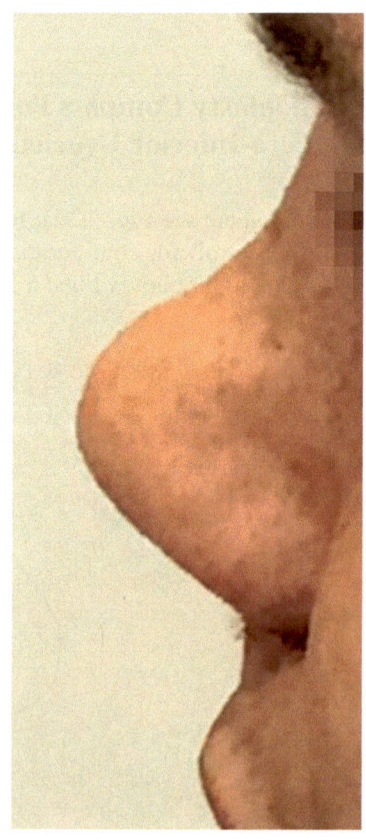

Fig. 5.39 Clinical photographs of patient with supero-inferior deficiency (SI–). Frontal view

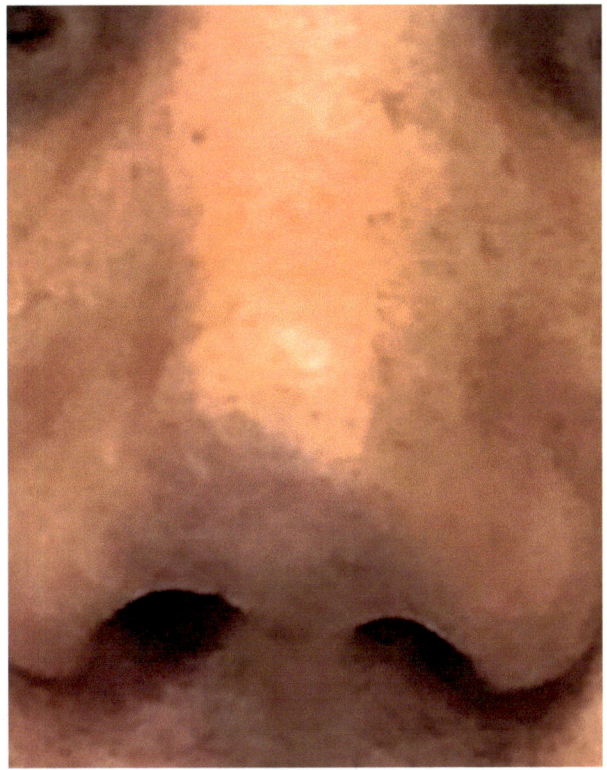

the less common reasons for patients to seek rhinoplasty. These are patients with on overly short nose, which can also be misdiagnosed as an overly "rotated" nose. It is not that these individuals do not have over-rotation of the nasal tip, but that the tip rotation is not the primary problem, requiring tip changes, but is secondary to an overly short septum that provides inadequate inferior or downward directed force. These patients tend to complain of an upturned nose but because their nose differs from the classic rhinoplasty patient, they tend to feel embarrassment about their request and are sometimes unable to adequately verbalize their problem. The empathetic surgeon can help them understand the problem and explain how the structure causes the aesthetic complaint. Deviation is unusual in these cases. Nasal obstruction is also usually more mild than the other configurations and is simply due to columellar retraction due to inadequate septal support compared to the relatively normally positioned nasal sidewalls. This creates an abnormal nasal inlet or nostril and can have columellar thickening or widening due to inadequate septal inferiorly directed force that directs pressure of the midline columella toward the lip. Excessive overhang of the lateral nostril sidewall relative to the columella can cause some obstruction at the nostril or nasal inlet as well due to inadequate funnel opening. The lip can appear overly long in these patients as well.

Combinations

As in the case of the directional compass, all of the cardinal points can be combined with adjacent points, but not opposite points (e.g., while south-west is a possible directional combination, south-north is not, just as AP+, SI– is possible, but AP+, AP– is not). Common combinations for patients seeking rhinoplasty include AP+ combined with SI+ or SI–, while AP–, SI– can be less common from my personal experience, which of course can vary from others. I generally find that the AP + SI+ configuration combination is one of the most common reasons to seek rhinoplasty (Figs. 5.40, 5.41, 5.42, and 5.43 shows photos of an AP + SI+ patient before and after surgical framework re-sizing, Fig. 5.44 shows the AP–SI– and AP + SI+ compass diagrams, while Fig. 5.45 shows the AP + SI—DTMP) and the results can be extremely rewarding to modify (see Chap. 7). Because they have such an oversized framework, the septum and axis of the nose can be severely deviated, and the esthetic problems can be severe as well. In contrast, the AP-SI- is not an uncommon combination, but due to soft-tissue contracture as well as a general lack of a framework, the surgery poses the greatest of challenges to completely re-create the framework.

So, what is the utility of the Rhinoplasty Compass ™ with its cardinal points and combinations? Instead of making disorganized descriptions of various problems during the rhinoplasty consult, for example listing: middle third narrowing, tip ptosis, dorsal hump, caudal deviation, and alar base narrowing, and then having a specific maneuver for each specific problem, one would make a more "global" diagnosis, and then plan a more strategic rhinoplasty that takes into account how the components interact. As we discussed in previous chapters, this is the difference between tactics and strategy to borrow military terms. While it may feel right to plan a series of grafts, sutures, reductions, and removals as four separate maneuvers with four separate goals, it may be more efficient to have a more comprehensive understanding of the nose as a whole, and to set your strategy for that specific nose type (i.e., AP+, SI–) accordingly. Now that we have described the rhinoplasty compass for diagnosis and understanding component interaction with the septal cartilage using the DTPM, we can begin form strategies to assist patients in altering their configuration to be closer to the "neutral" ideal from their directional extremes. But before we discuss specific strategies for each cardinal point (and some combinations), let's consider how the conventional, well-established tactical maneuvers perform using the DTPM. We will estimate the expected functional and aesthetic outcomes, and evaluate these procedures using this model.

Fig. 5.40 Clinical photographs of patient with supero-inferior and antero-posterior excess (AP+/SI+). Frontal view. (**a**) Before surgery and (**b**) after surgery

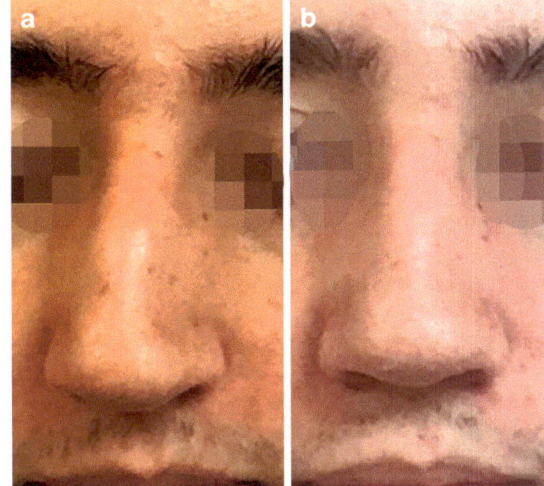

Fig. 5.41 Clinical photographs of patient with supero-inferior and antero-posterior excess (AP+/SI+). Base view. (**a**) Before surgery and (**b**) after surgery

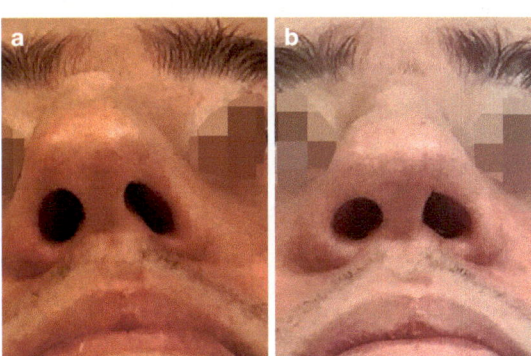

Fig. 5.42 Clinical photographs of patient with supero-inferior and antero-posterior excess (AP+/SI+). Left oblique view. (**a**) Before surgery and (**b**) after surgery

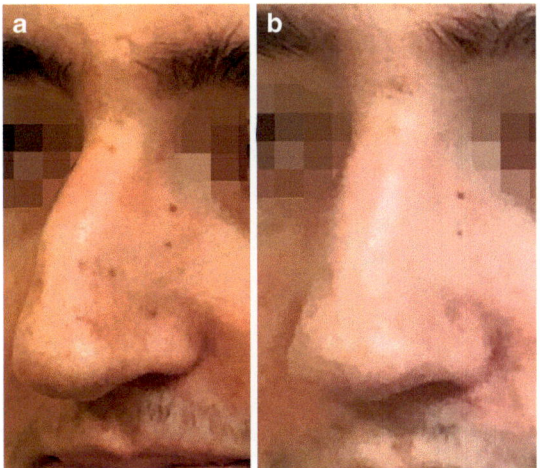

Fig. 5.43 Clinical photographs of patient with supero-inferior and antero-posterior excess (AP+/SI+). Left side view. (**a**) Before surgery and (**b**) after surgery

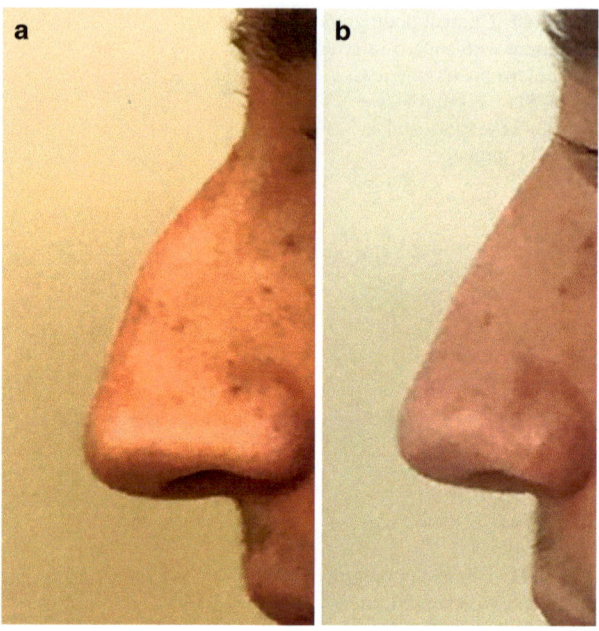

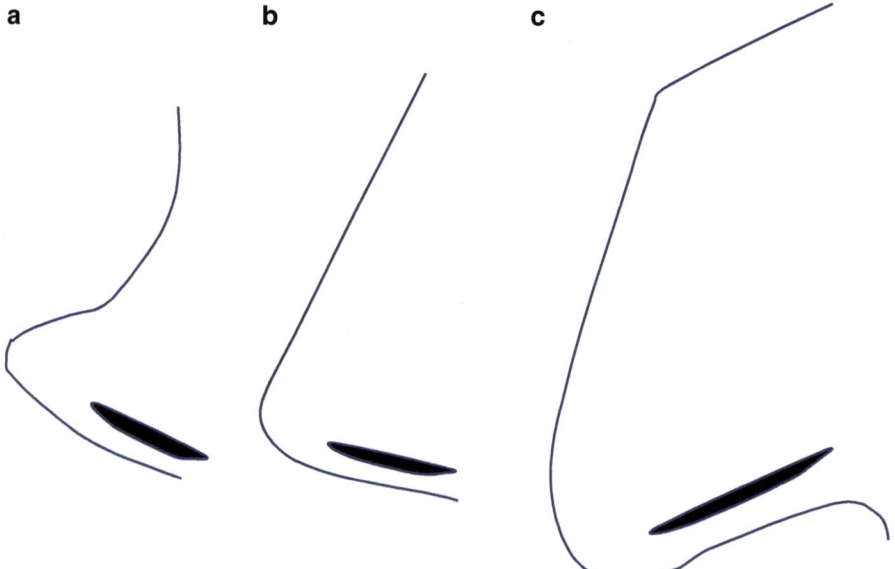

Fig. 5.44 Profile diagram of the (**a**) antero-posterior and supero-inferior deficient (AP–/SI–) in comparison with (**b**) AP 0 (neutral) SI 0 (neutral) framework (AP 0/SI 0) and C) antero-posterior and supero-inferior excess (AP+/SI+)

Fig. 5.45 Dynamic triangular prism model (DTPM) of the supero-inferior and antero-posterior excess (AP + SI+) framework. Pink indicates the foundation/substrate, golden yellow represents the framework, blue shows the canopy layer, here consisting of the paired medial and lateral crura of the alar cartilage. The grey cylinder represents the nasal inlet, supported by the taut external nose structures. Red arrows show the direction of movement

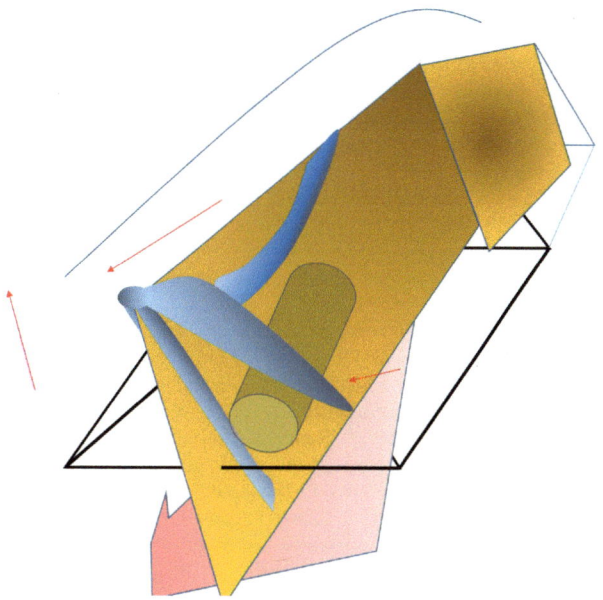

References

1. Kandathil CK, Saltychev M, Moubayed SP, Most SP. Association of dorsal reduction and tip rotation with social perception. JAMA Facial Plast Surg. 2018;20(5):362–6.
2. Johnson CM Jr, Godin MS. The tension nose: open structure rhinoplasty approach. Plast Reconstr Surg. 1995;95:43–51.
3. Lee MR, Geissler P, Cochran S, Gunter JP, Rohrich RJ. Decreasing nasal tip projection in rhinoplasty. Plast Reconstr Surg. 2014;134:41e–9e.
4. Behrbohm H, Tardy E. Essentials of Septorhinoplasty. 2nd ed. Stuttgart, New York: Thieme; 2017.
5. Stupak HD, Weinstock M. Bony/cartilaginous mismatch: a radiologic investigation into the etiology of tension nose deformity. Plast Reconstr Surg. 2018;141(2):312–21.
6. Pernia NE. The dimensions of the nasal septal cartilage: a preliminary study in adult Filipino Malay cadavers. Philipp J Otolaryngol Head Neck Surg. 2011;26:10–2.
7. Miles BA, Petrisor D, Kao H, Finn RA, Throckmorton GS. Anatomical variation of the nasal septum: analysis of 57 cadaver specimens. Otolaryngol Head Neck Surg. 2007;136:362–8.
8. Massie JP, Runyan CM, Stern MJ, et al. Nasal septal anatomy in skeletally mature patients with cleft lip and palate. JAMA Facial Plast Surg. 2016;18:347–53.
9. Dalili Kajan Z, Khademi J, Nemati S, Niksolat E. The effects of septal deviation, concha bullosa, and their combination on the depth of posterior palatal arch in cone-beam computed tomography. J Dent (Shiraz). 2016;17:26–31.

10. Hartman CH. Nasal Septal Deviation and Craniofacial Asymmetries (master of science thesis). Iowa City, Iowa: University of Iowa; 2015. p. 8.
11. Mladina R, Krajina Z. The influence of palato-cranial base (basomaxillary) angle on the length of the caudal process of the nasal septum in man. Rhinology. 1990;28:185–9.
12. Hyman AJ, Fastenberg JH, Stupak HD. Orientation of the premaxilla in the origin of septal deviation. Eur Arch Otorhinolaryngol. 2019;276(11):3147–51.
13. Stupak HD, Park SY. Gravitational forces, negative pressure and facial structure in the genesis of airway dysfunction during sleep: a review of the paradigm. Sleep Med. 2018;51:125–32.
14. Hur MS, Won HS, Kwak DS, Chung IH, Kim IB. Morphological patterns and variations of the nasal septum components and their clinical implications. J Craniofac Surg. 2016;27:2164–7.
15. Mays S. Nasal septal deviation in a mediaeval population. Am J Phys Anthropol. 2012;148:319–26.
16. Trevizan M, Consolaro A. Premaxilla: an independent bone that can base therapeutics for middle third growth! Dental Press J Orthod. 2017;22(2):21–6.
17. Stupak HD. The human external nose and its evolutionary role in the prevention of obstructive sleep apnea. Otolaryngol Head Neck Surg. 2010;142(6):779–82.
18. Bhatia DDS, Palesy T, Ramli R, Barham HP, Christensen JM, Gunaratne DA, et al. Two-dimensional assessment of the nasal valve area cannot predict minimum cross-sectional area or airflow resistance. Am J Rhinol Allergy. 2016;30(3):190–4.
19. Shuaib SW, Undavia S, Lin J, Johnson CM Jr, Stupak HD. Can functional septorhinoplasty independently treat obstructive sleep apnea? Plast Reconstr Surg. 2015;135(6):1554–65.
20. Tripathi PB, Elghobashi S, Wong BJF. The myth of the internal nasal valve. JAMA Facial Plast Surg. 2017;19(4):253–4.
21. Naughton JP, Lee AY, Ramos E, Wootton D, Stupak HD. Effect of nasal valve shape on downstream volume, airflow, and pressure drop: importance of the nasal valve revisited. Ann Otol Rhinol Laryngol. 2018;127(11):745–53.
22. Surowieki J. The wisdom of crowds: why the many are smarter than the few and how collective wisdom shapes business, economies, societies and nations. Doubleday 2004.

Chapter 6
Modeling to Evaluate Conventional Procedures

"The best dividends on the labor invested have invariably come from seeking more knowledge than more power."—Wilbur and Orville Wright, March 12, 1906

As we discussed in the previous chapter, the Dynamic triangular prism model (DTPM) is an excellent way to consider in one place how specific conventional rhinoplasty (tactical) "maneuvers" will affect aesthetics and function by considering the entire dynamic structure of the nose at once, and not just individual sub-regions. In other words, there is but one framework for a structure, not an inside and an outside framework that are treated by conveniently different specialties. By this, we will learn how to avoid the trap of "compartmentalization" that has plagued our treatment paradigms, and then in the subsequent chapter re-think strategies to perform better "big-picture" framework-optimization rhinoplasties that always consider both form and function simultaneously.

An analogy for this type of flawed thinking is found in the story of the quest to design the first aircraft capable of powered flight. At around the turn of the twentieth century, experts throughout the world were competing to fly the first craft capable of sustained, powered flight. Sophisticated engineers like Samuel Langley, head of the Smithsonian Aeronautics division, with prestige, extensive education, funding, and access to resources were the of course the obvious front-runners in this "race." To build his aircraft, Langley configured multiple well-crafted wings, a powerful motor, a stable well-designed fuselage, and contracted an expert pilot. By sourcing the "best" components by the "top" expert in the field, failure seemed to be almost impossible, and the public waited with baited-breath for Langley's inaugural flight, which of course was a complete failure. In contrast, the high-school dropouts from Dayton, Ohio, Orville, and Wilbur Wright tested various simple gliders at the windy coast of North Carolina after studying extensively the flight of birds and the existing field of aviation. By studying and understanding the "big-picture" of flight instead of looking at designing "best" components, they were able to slowly scale-up glider models and eventually achieved a sustained, powered flight in 1903 [1].

© Springer Nature Switzerland AG 2020
H. D. Stupak, *Rethinking Rhinoplasty and Facial Surgery*,
https://doi.org/10.1007/978-3-030-44674-1_6

In the same way, while we focus on expert-named and designed grafts and maneuvers as we perform rhinoplasty, we fail often because we do not consider the big-picture dynamics of the nose and how all the parts interact as a unit. Many of the "experts" I have met casually seemed to be more experts on self-promotion and politics than in in-depth anatomy.

The rhinoplasty compass of the previous chapter is designed to help us think about this dynamic framework structure. Because all of the existing rhinoplasty "components" are so well-established, I feel it is necessary to at least discuss why individually "fixing" these can be less successful than we suspect. Further, before discussing an alternative view-point it is warranted to discuss the flaws and even the occasional benefits of these procedures. We will evaluate these maneuvers by "class," as there are too many variations to consider from implantable devices, to rib grafts. These classes include: Submucous resection septoplasty and L-strut scoring, "Batten" grafts/implants, "Spreader" grafts and implants, Tip suturing techniques, tripod grafts (columellar struts and lateral crural onlay), and finally "Tensioning" techniques of the middle third.

Submucous Resection Septoplasty with/Without Graft Harvesting

One of the most common procedures performed, both independently, and as part of a rhinoplasty, *submucous resection septoplasty* is ubiquitous, and seen as generally benign and helpful to patients. With a simple approach, and a satisfying "ooh" from surgical staff as the cartilage is removed, the procedure is seen as a "classic."

Unfortunately, the procedure is as destructive as helpful. With time-tested adage to *preserve* a 1–2 cm "L"-strut, operators happily overlook and avoid the actual root cause of the deviation, instead, completely avoiding the anterior (dorsal) and inferior (caudal) external portion of the septum, removing only cartilage posteriorly. This cartilage is usually removed at the site of a "spur," or segment of maximal deviation, and after removal, the wound is carefully closed, completing the therapeutic part of the procedure, and the removed cartilage is potentially preserved for grafting usage later in the case.

As we have discussed in previous chapter on the nasal valve and septal oversize, however, avoiding the pathologic septum at the nasal valve but instead solely removing intra-nasal blockages will reduce the visual manifestation of obstruction on endoscopic or speculum exam, but without creating a funnel shaped airway, only intra-nasal vortices will be created, without relieving the negative pressure generated by nasal valve obstruction or mouth-breathing. This is not to say that by removing the peak posterior deformity of cartilage and bone overlap and twisting, airflow cannot be improved. Of course, these maneuvers do increase airflow. However, by only removing a posterior segment of septum, one creates a false sense of security that the septum is "restored," while the septal framework remains unchanged. Worse, if too narrow an L-strut is left, the oversized L-strut will buckle further, even worse with "scoring" or graft reinforcement. Failure to address the actual L-strut, instead only removing less

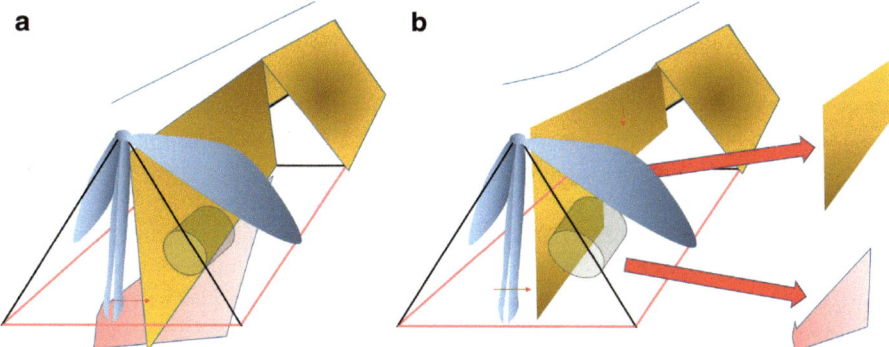

Fig. 6.1 Dynamic triangular prism model (DTPM) of submucous resection for septal deviation. Pink indicates the foundation/substrate, golden yellow represents the framework, blue shows the canopy layer, here consisting of the paired medial and lateral crura of the alar cartilage. The grey cylinder represents the nasal inlet, supported by the external nose structures. (**a**) Indicates a bony and cartilagionous septum deviated from the midline (small red arrows), causing a narrowed nasal airway. (**b**) Represents submucous resection surgery with removal (large red arrows) of maximally deviated cartilaginous and bony components, but the L-strut remains out of position as a component of the nasal valve and can lose some antero-posterior framework support from the resection. Red arrows indicate excision

relevant cartilage behind it is the source of the commonly described "memory" that permits re-deviation and obstruction and causes confusion and discomfort for patients. Further, in planning revision surgery, when re-sizing of the septum would be attempted, due to the narrow L-strut left behind, there is little antero-inferior L-strut that can be safely removed due to the prior resection. See Fig. 6.1, for the DTPM of septal deviation with subsequent submucous resection. There is no change to the nasal inlet (and thus limited airflow improvement), and there is obviously (as is well-known) no aesthetic or structural benefit. Only structural compromise results unfortunately, despite what the "data" shows. What are the positives of submucous resection? During the surgery to reduce, resize, and reposition the entire septum (including the L-strut), there are portions where cartilage and bone overlap, creating the above described spur (see prior chapter). If the deviated or overlapping bony and cartilaginous deviated portions are removed as *part* of repositioning of the entire septum, the relief of obstruction within the depths of the nasal cavity are helpful.

"Batten" Grafts and Implants

In sailing, a batten is a thin piece of wood or plastic that is incorporated into the fabric of the sail to enhance sail stiffness, shape, and wind "lift" efficiency. These devices, while part of efficient sail mechanics, do not provide any actual lift or wind propulsion. Only the interaction of the wind and sail can do this. In rhinoplasty and nasal valve surgery, the "batten" graft or implant is similarly of literally marginal importance. The graft or device is a stiff object inserted into the sidewall of the nose, usually just below the skin or canopy layer, and supposedly "prevents" collapse of the nasal sidewalls. In reality, these objects fill space that otherwise would permit airflow and usually depress the mucosal side of the nasal sidewall further into the airway and actually can worsen collapse as it widens and thickens the nasal sidewall instead of the actual airway. See the attached DTPM of left sided batten grafts placed in the SI+ (overly long nose) and AP+ (overly projected) nose (Figs. 6.2 and 6.3, respectively). Of course, those who promote the continued use of this "easy" procedure will claim that there is a type of "dynamic" collapse that "stiffening" the nasal sidewall will prevent. This is very prevalent in the conventional literature, in web marketing, and even many well-read patients are aware of this and will demonstrate this on consultation. On deep inspiration, these patients can actually close their nostril, and upon inspection, it appears to be "floppiness" or "weakness" of the sidewall. Thus, the batten graft or implant is justified to "stiffen" the nasal sidewall and prevent this "dynamic collapse." What these observers fail to realize is that a baseline narrowed nostril, when substantial negative pressure is applied will be drawn intraluminally, creating the "collapsed" appearance. The correct treatment is to dilate the *nostril* permanently by adjusting the framework size (as we will discuss in the next chapter), not to stiffen the sidewall and worsen actual airflow, despite what we have been told. There is a commercially available version of this device, that is available in an absorbable form, that is supposedly replaced by scar tissue after dissolution.

Will individual physicians continue to use the "batten" class of procedures even as they are eventually discredited? I would imagine so, as because there are few objective measures to determine outcomes beyond "satisfaction," and the procedure requires little skill or forethought, it can generate substantial billing revenue, it may be with us for some time to come.

Fig. 6.2 Dynamic triangular prism model (DTPM) of the use of batten grafts (green) with a supero-inferior excess (SI+) framework. Pink indicates the foundation/substrate, golden yellow represents the framework, blue shows the canopy layer, here consisting of the paired medial and lateral crura of the alar cartilage. The grey cylinder represents the nasal inlet, supported by the external nose structures

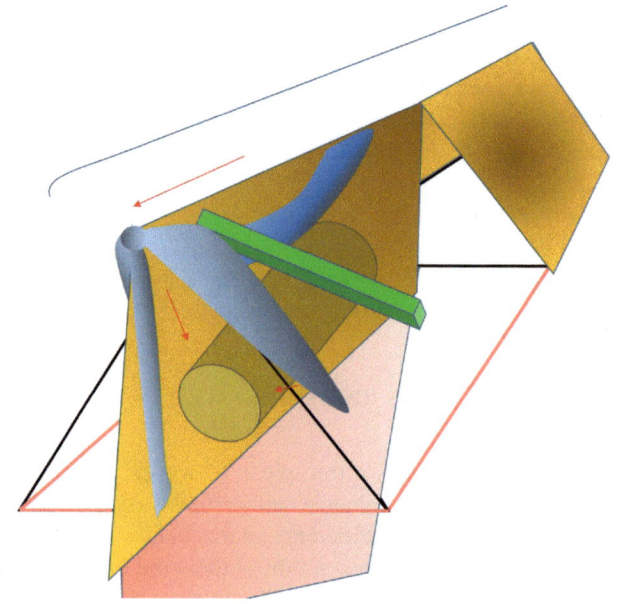

Fig. 6.3 Dynamic triangular prism model (DTPM) of the use of batten grafts (green) with an antero-posterior excess AP+) framework. Pink indicates the foundation/substrate, golden yellow represents the framework, blue shows the canopy layer, here consisting of the paired medial and lateral crura of the alar cartilage. The grey cylinder represents the nasal inlet, supported by the external nose structures

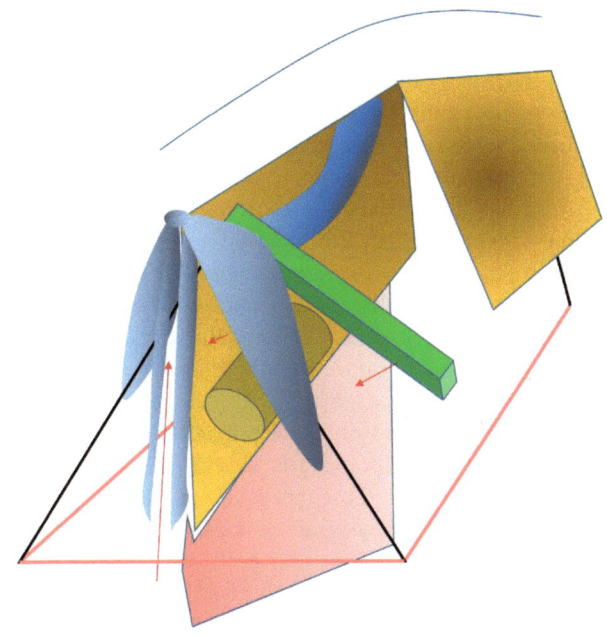

Spreader Grafts (Dorsal Grafts)

No single maneuver has gotten more attention in rhinoplasty than "spreader grafts," with nearly 200 articles in the literature. Spreader grafts reference the placement of a bar of septal or other cartilage in the created space between the dorsal septum and the upper lateral cartilages. Since its description by Sheen in 1978 [2], it has reached mass popularity among surgeons. Mention of the term "spreader grafts" on Pubmed search increases over the 1990s, peaking in 2016, with 20 articles using the term in the abstract or title. Nearly all are confirmatory of the "effectiveness" of the maneuver. More interestingly, as the years progressed, calls for larger, stronger spreader grafts, made of rib [3], or other materials (high density porous polyethylene or Medpor™) [4–6] were made, as though simple septal cartilage grafts we not enough. Like most things in medicine, we double down on failing bets, assuming that more and bigger will solve the problem. This is akin in the above described airplane metaphor to the concept espoused by Langley that only larger or more wings would enhance flight. Of course, in reality, wings optimized for lift and minimized for drag will permit flight with adequate airflow.

At the month of this writing, an article was just published in the (now renamed) Journal of the American Medical Association (JAMA) Facial Plastic Surgery journal which claims that the widening associated with spreader grafts actually is *so* well accepted by patients that aesthetic satisfaction scores actually increased in addition to the ever-present NOSE score improvements, despite the fact that discerning which rhinoplasty maneuver caused aesthetic improvement is impossible due to too many confounders [7]. (I also cannot recall an article in the literature where NOSE scores decreased or stayed the same).

In reality, patients intensely dislike the unnaturally thickened noses created by spreader grafts, and find them frustrating to discuss with surgeons who are unbending advocates for this maneuver. In addition, spreader grafts, like batten grafts take up more airspace than add space for airflow, and are thus obstructive instead of helpful in most cases. They create no inlet dilation, and in many cases make overly long (SI+) septal frameworks even longer! When we analyze spreader grafts on the DTPM, we can see that there is almost no effect besides dorsal widening, and inlet narrowing in the SI+ and AP+ models, (Figs. 6.4 and 6.5 respectively) despite their popularity in the literature for all comers.

When can spreader grafts be helpful? In revision rhinoplasty (mostly SI− or AP−) where the anterior portion of the quadrangular cartilage framework (L-strut using the old-school terminology) is absent, and must be replaced between the "upper lateral cartilages." In these cases, of course it is not a "spreader" graft, but a dorsal framework replacement graft or dorsal onlay graft. (Fig. 6.6) Similarly, in the SI− nose, variations of the spreader graft can theoretically be used to extend the length of the framework if permitted to extend beyond the caudal septum. (Fig. 6.7) In the next section, where we will discuss grafting related to the tripod, we will see using our model that grafts are very effective for *replacement*, and can be helpful for camouflage if repositioning is impossible (rare), but are ineffective for *moving* tissues to a new position, because even the strongest of grafts and implants cannot overwhelm

Fig. 6.4 Dynamic triangular prism model (DTPM) of the use of spreader grafts (green) with a supero-inferior excess (SI+) framework. Pink indicates the foundation/substrate, golden yellow represents the framework, blue shows the canopy layer, here consisting of the paired medial and lateral crura of the alar cartilage. The grey cylinder represents the nasal inlet, supported by the external nose structures

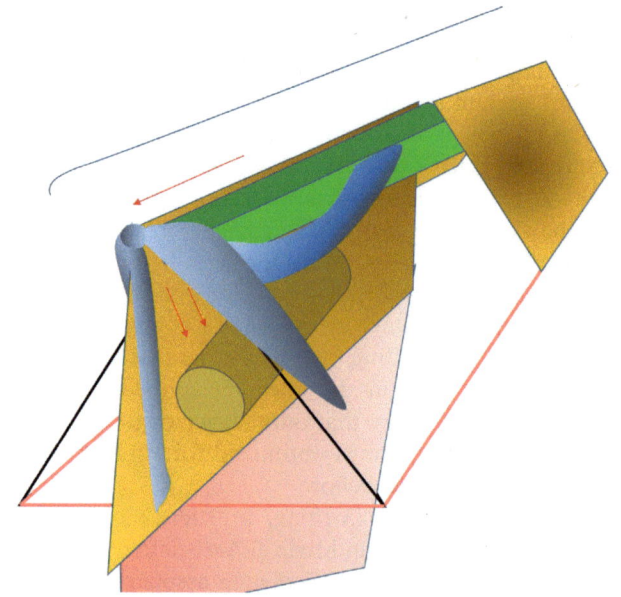

Fig. 6.5 Dynamic
triangular prism model
(DTPM) of the use of
spreader grafts (green)
with an antero-posterior
excess AP+) framework.
Pink indicates the
foundation/substrate,
golden yellow represents
the framework, blue shows
the canopy layer, here
consisting of the paired
medial and lateral crura of
the alar cartilage. The grey
cylinder represents the
nasal inlet, supported by
the external nose structures

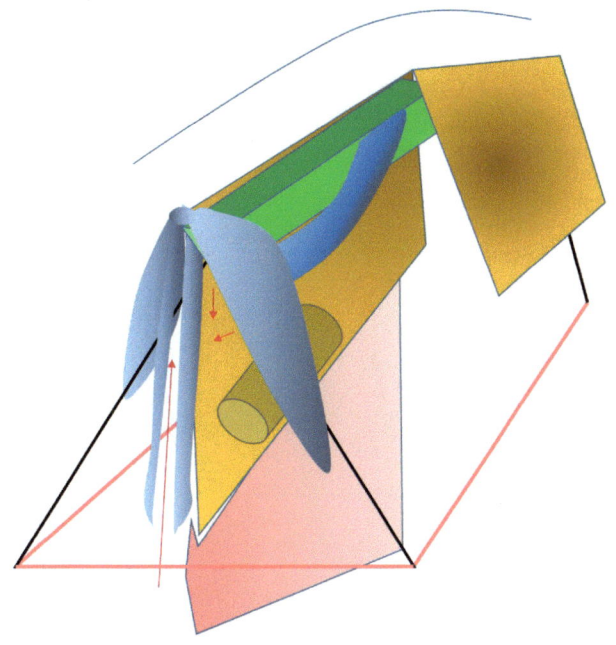

Fig. 6.6 Dynamic
triangular prism model
(DTPM) of the use of
spreader grafts (green)
with an antero-posterior
deficiency AP−)
framework. Pink indicates
the foundation/substrate,
golden yellow represents
the framework, blue shows
the canopy layer, here
consisting of the paired
medial and lateral crura of
the alar cartilage. The grey
cylinder represents the
nasal inlet, supported by
the external nose structures

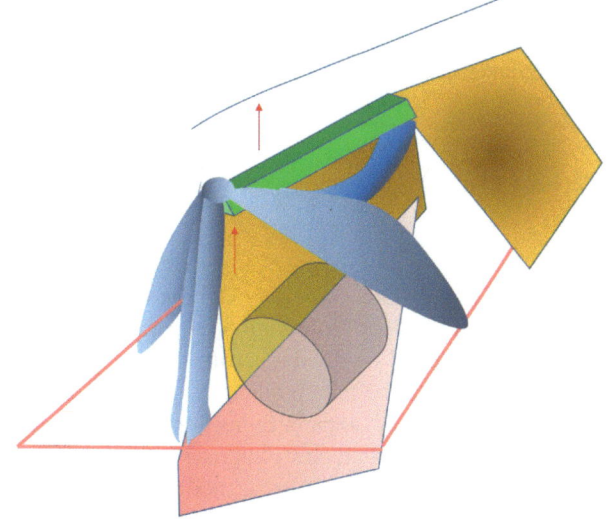

Fig. 6.7 Dynamic
triangular prism model
(DTPM) of the use of
spreader grafts with a
supero-inferior deficiency
(SI–) framework. Pink
indicates the foundation/
substrate, golden yellow
represents the framework,
blue shows the canopy
layer, here consisting of
the paired medial and
lateral crura of the alar
cartilage. The grey cylinder
represents the nasal inlet,
supported by the external
nose structures

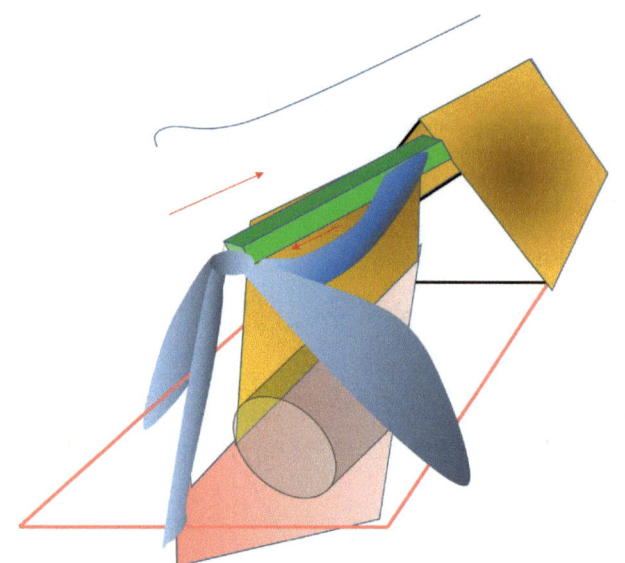

the forces of tension, and certainly cannot efficiently move a misplaced framework simply by their addition. Finally, the "turn-in spreader graft" concept involves no actual grafting. In this scenario, after dorsal cartilage excision, excess nasal side-wall tissue is preserved, which is appropriate. Some use sutures to re-fasten the side-wall to the septum, while others do not. Either way, the maneuver is an exercise in "not excising", and is thus preservative and by "doing nothing" is thus helpful, but of course has nothing to to with the graft concept.

Tripod Grafts and Sutures

One of the most revolutionary events in the history of rhinoplasty was the discovery by Jack Anderson (and eventually Calvin M. Johnson, Jr.) that rhinoplasty could be more than just a reductive operation, where primarily cartilage and bone are simply removed, weakened or divided. Instead, they found that the nose was a dynamic structure that could be manipulated by a variety of interventions by visualizing the nasal tip as a "tripod," apparently as presented at a meeting by Anderson in 1969.

Through the open rhinoplasty approach, a paradigm was established where the nasal cartilages were directly visualized, modified, then strengthened via the addition of a series of grafts primarily created from septal cartilage. Needless to say, the paradigm became broadly accepted following the publication of the text Open Structure Rhinoplasty by Johnson and Toriumi [8]. Framing the alar cartilages this "tripod," the concept consists of imagining the nasal tip structures as a three-legged camera-style tripod, resting on a "pedestal" of the nasal septum. Strength and length of the legs of the tripod determine the orientation (rotation) and projection of the nasal tip relative to the septum. The three legs consist of the two lateral crura and the combined medial crura of the columella being the third leg. Thus, the simplified surgery generally consists of an open approach to the nasal tip after graft harvesting from the septum or ear, L-strut preservation septoplasty (with some dorsal and caudal reduction if necessary). Then, typically a columellar strut is fashioned out of septal cartilage and is placed between the crura to strengthen and rotate the medial leg. Frequently, the domes or lateral crura are divided, then re-attached with sutures, and often with lateral crural onlay grafts added for lateral limb strength. Finally, tip grafts are placed on top of the domes or columella to further enhance projection and definition. Essentially, the tripod is strengthened, projected, and defined as a primary objective relative to the more slightly modified septum.

This has been largely accepted as the most effective way to perform rhinoplasty by most past and current experts. But how will this procedure perform in our DTPM (Dynamic Triangular Prism Model)?

The answer is complicated. In the over-reduced revision rhinoplasty, frequently, SI- or AP-, where the alar cartilages were largely over-excised in prior operations, the procedure performs wonderfully. This over-reduced rhinoplasty appearance was nearly endemic in the 1970s to 1990s, when the open structure rhinoplasty procedure was popularized. Thus, a well-executed tripod grafting procedure was far superior to the severely over-excised rhinoplasty functionally, structurally, and aesthetically (Fig. 6.8). As you can see in the figure, since the tripod was over-weakened, and septum-over reduced in the prior procedure, replacing the missing tissue with grafts to restore tripod strength and projection has excellent results. In addition, using the adage "de-project then re-project," the surgeon can convert and AP+ nose to an AP- nose, then can use the columellar strut to return to AP neutral, (although a better approach could be to go straight from AP+ to AP neutral via framework modification—see the next chapter).

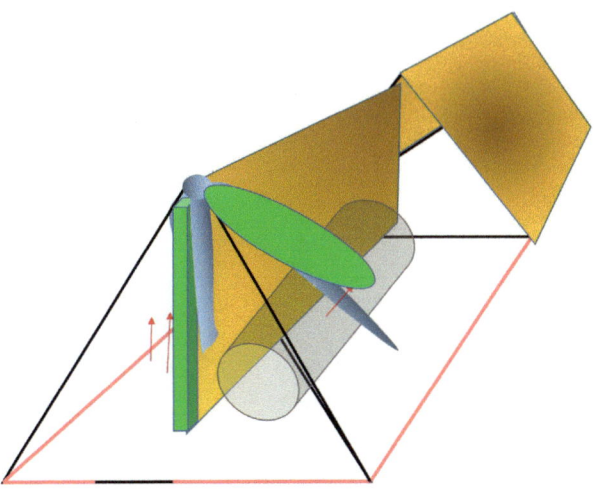

Fig. 6.8 Dynamic triangular prism model (DTPM) of the use of tripod grafts (columellar strut and crural onlay grafts with an antero-posterior and supero-inferior deficiency (AP-SI-) framework and crural over-reduction. Pink indicates the foundation/substrate, golden yellow represents the framework, blue shows the canopy layer, here consisting of the paired medial and lateral crura of the alar cartilage. The grey cylinder represents the nasal inlet, supported by the external nose structures

The problem of course then lay with the *over*-acceptance of this concept, and translation to primary rhinoplasty, particularly the SI+ and AP+ DTPM models. Johnson and Toriumi themselves continued to thoughtfully and carefully analyze on an individual basis the use of the procedure, balancing this procedure with the older reduction rhinoplasty concepts. Others, however promoted a rigid doctrine of complete L-strut preservation, with nearly no modification of septal cartilage beyond scoring, suturing, or treating this all-important structure as a bank for withdrawing grafts. The educational and research establishment, primarily began promoting extensive grafts and sutures to this fixed "tripod model," almost completely failing to look beyond this limited perspective.

In contrast to the revision reductive rhinoplasty DTPM, the primary SI+ or AP+ functional and esthetic rhinoplasty using overly simple tripod grafts is only marginally helpful, existing mostly as a camouflaging operation [9]. One can see in the DTPM for the AP+ or SI+ configurations (Figs. 6.9 and 6.10) that although the sidewalls are narrow, adding cartilage to them, like the batten graft or columellar strut, does almost nothing to reverse the narrowing forces, and may even worsen the problem. Grafts and sutures are also unable to overwhelm the twisted anterior and caudal septum, no matter how thick or strong the material is, but the attempt causes tension, pain, and eventual failure due to what is known as "cartilage memory," or what I call inadequate release of the deviating forces of tension. See Figs. 6.11 and 6.12 as an example of an attempt at camouflage performed at an outside institution that failed to address the framework (A) preoperatively and (B) after framework resizing and graft removal. Along the same lines, in the SI+ nose, where the septum causes the nasal tip to become ptotic, no amount of columellar struts, sutures, or lateral crural onlay grafts will overwhelm this excess septal length until the nasal

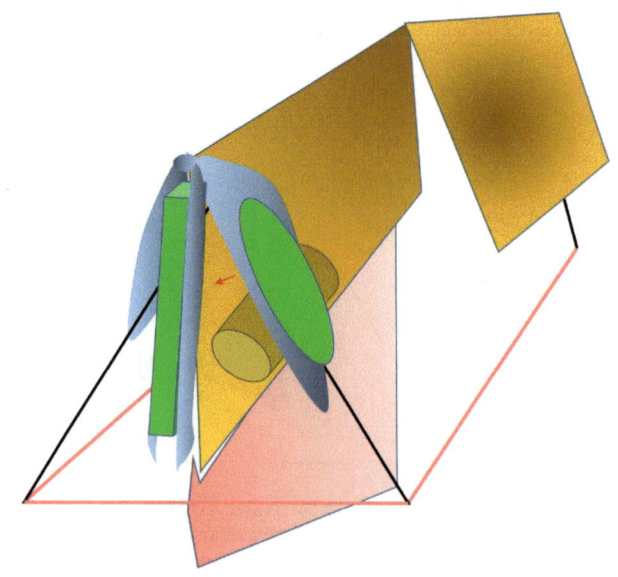

Fig. 6.9 Dynamic triangular prism model (DTPM) of the use of tripod grafts (columellar strut and crural onlay grafts with an antero-posterior excess (AP+) framework and crural over-reduction). Pink indicates the foundation/substrate, golden yellow represents the framework, blue shows the canopy layer, here consisting of the paired medial and lateral crura of the alar cartilage. The grey cylinder represents the nasal inlet, supported by the external nose structures

Fig. 6.10 Dynamic triangular prism model (DTPM) of the use of tripod grafts (columellar strut and crural onlay grafts with a supero-inferior excess (SI+) framework and crural over-reduction. Pink indicates the foundation/substrate, golden yellow represents the framework, blue shows the canopy layer, here consisting of the paired medial and lateral crura of the alar cartilage. The grey cylinder represents the nasal inlet, supported by the external nose structures

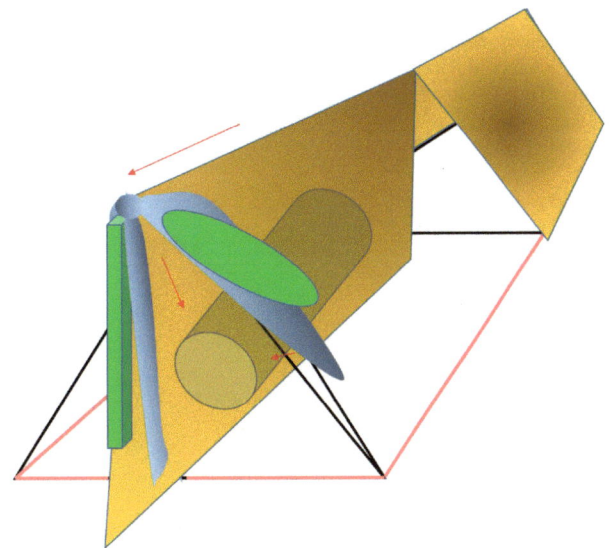

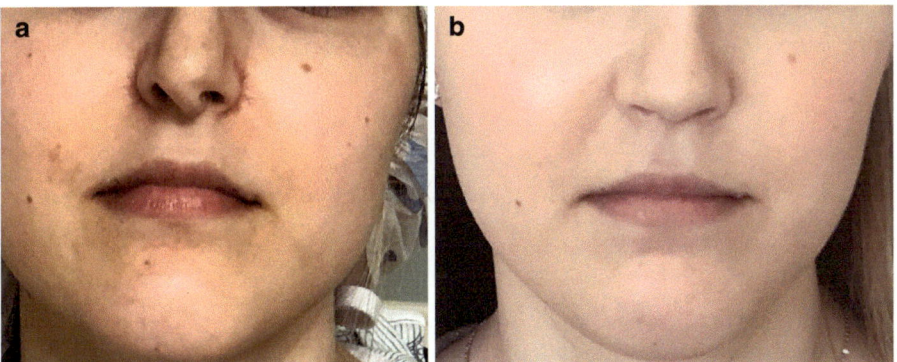

Fig. 6.11 Clinical photographs of patient with attempt at tripod camouflage with supero-inferior and antero-posterior excess (AP+/SI+). Frontal view. (**a**) Before surgery and (**b**) after surgery with antero-posterior and supero-inferior neutral nose (AP 0/ SI 0)

lengthening specific force is reduced (see e.g., Fig. 6.13). Thus, both columellar or alar grafts and sutures are of limited help in the primary SI+ or AP+ models despite their broad current use and large amount of supportive "data" in the literature. That does not mean that columellar and alar grafts are not without any merit. The tripod concept is thoughtfully and effectively presented for more modern usage in a 2004 follow-up book by Johnson and To that discusses nuances of the concept well beyond the scope of this book [10]. Tripod grafts, particularly lateral crural onlay grafts are useful after patients have underdone severe crural reductions as recommended by dated texts (see prior chapter and Fig. 6.14 for DTMP). They are also effective in the AP- and reductive tip rhinoplasty procedures. (Fig. 6.15).

Fig. 6.12 Clinical photographs of patient with attempt at tripod camouflage with supero-inferior and antero-posterior excess (AP+/SI+). Base view. (**a**) Before surgery and (**b**) after surgery with antero-posterior and supero-inferior neutral nose (AP 0/SI 0)

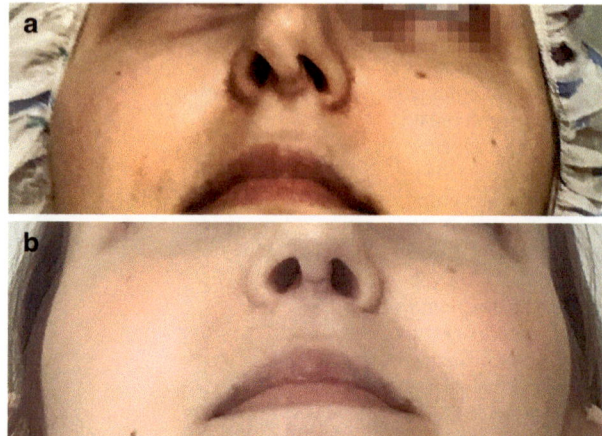

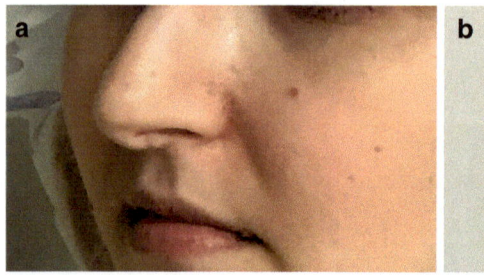
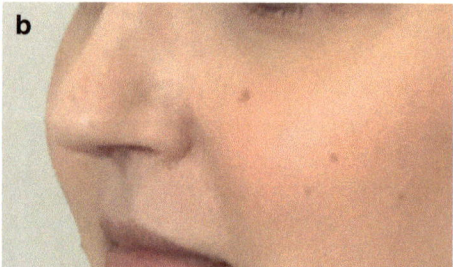

Fig. 6.13 Clinical photographs of patient with attempt at tripod camouflage with supero-inferior and antero-posterior excess (AP+/SI+). Left side view. (**a**) Before surgery and (**b**) after surgery with antero-posterior and supero-inferior neutral nose (AP 0/SI 0)

Fig. 6.14 Dynamic triangular prism model (DTPM) of the use of isolated crural onlay grafts (green) with a neutral framework. Pink indicates the foundation/substrate, golden yellow represents the framework, blue shows the canopy layer, here consisting of the paired medial and lateral crura of the alar cartilage. The grey cylinder represents the nasal inlet, supported by the external nose structures

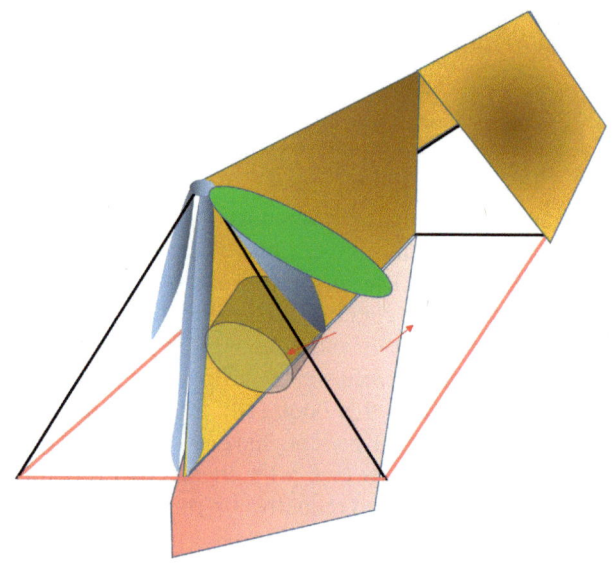

Fig. 6.15 Dynamic triangular prism model (DTPM) of the use of isolated columellar strut (green) with a neutral framework. Pink indicates the foundation/substrate, golden yellow represents the framework, blue shows the canopy layer, here consisting of the paired medial and lateral crura of the alar cartilage. The grey cylinder represents the nasal inlet, supported by the external nose structures

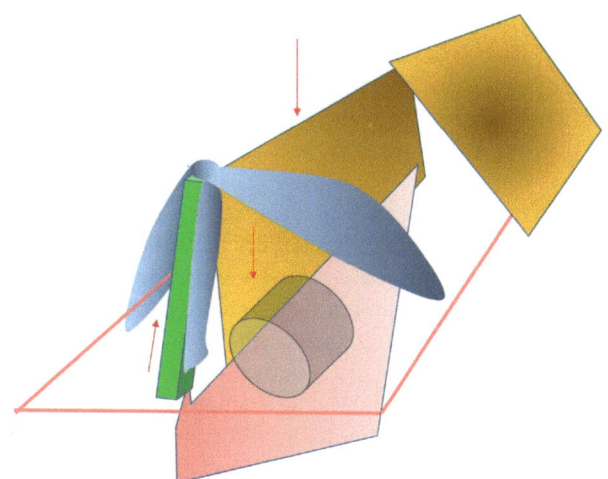

In a final note on the tripod: In the last days before the tripod model became permanently ensconced in stone by the establishment, a series of articles was published by Westreich and Lawson in 2007 and 2008 that respectfully questioned the concept [11, 12]. These two surgeons, with the help of others pointed out essentially that the tripod could not possibly exist in the vacuum that the generally accepted model suggested, and using colorful well-written language, expressed dismay that other forces beyond the tripod were barely considered by most [11–14]. Of particular interest, the authors noted the *extrinsic* spring-like forces that determined tip position outside of the classic model, and the interaction of the tripod with the underlying septum that was well before its time. They even tested the intrinsic spring forces of the individual cartilages removed during rhinoplasty using biomechanical testing of the "modulus of elasticity" of these cartilages. While closer to the framework model we present in this text, the authors remained tripod-centric, but made huge strides by attempting to explain the external forces that act upon the tripod. We will discuss this spring-like concept that they and others of the period described in the next section [12].

Tension-Adjusting Procedures—Scroll and Crural Interaction

The above-mentioned researchers made strides in explaining that the nasal tip "tripod" was subject to *extrinsic forces* (spring-interaction with the surrounding structures) in addition to the commonly described *intrinsic* (strength and length of the cartilaginous tripod legs) forces, attempting to add more value to a limited model of understanding. Further, the researchers described how the spring-like nature of these "cartilages produce elastic potential energy to counteract these external forces and keep its position relatively static." They even went on to discuss the "elastic potential energy" of this spring and described how it can be described in formula form: "Es = 1/2k×2, where k represents the material's stiffness, which for a cantilevered spring can be calculated as follows: K = [3E(Width × Height)3/12)]/Length [3]. Therefore, elastic potential energy in this system can be calculated as: Es = (1/2) [3E(Width × Height)3 /12) ×2]/Length [3]. They went on to calculate the E (modulus of elasticity) for individual cartilage samples removed during rhinoplasty and showed a variable range of elasticity by the cartilage types [12].

While I cannot help but admire the work of these researchers, I believe in some ways they did not venture far enough from convention to describe how the nasal framework interacts with the overlying canopy layer and airway, remaining overly tripod-centric, although they certainly hit upon the key aspects of this viewpoint (in their defense neither did I until more recently). As we presented in the previous chapter using the DTPM, the framework should be viewed (septal cartilage and bones) as the primary structure of the nose. Secondarily, the lower lateral cartilages (canopy layer) are supported medially by the anterior septal angle and suspended laterally by a spring-like structure known as the scroll (traditionally known as the upper lateral cartilage). *The scroll* is the primary structure that provides the spring-like force that gives the tip its dynamic stability, preventing motion in a cephalic (superior) or caudal (inferior) direction due to its spring like shape. This spring itself does not support the airway, but supports the lateral crura via a spring-like septal attachment. Thus, the real foundational errors of the conventional/tripod models are the false primacy of the tip cartilages in structure and as a therapeutic target, but also that the upper lateral cartilage is an independent structure that directly effects structure and airway function. As shown in the DTPM model, the scroll *is* the spring that supports the lower lateral cartilage and the loss of the spring causes airway and structural/aesthetic problems because the lateral crura are not supporting the airway properly, not because of the spring itself blocking the airway. (Fig. 6.16a, b)

Re-analyzing the data from the elasticity study, I calculated the mean E (modulus of elasticity) for the three sample sites from their specimen. The E of the upper lateral cartilage (scroll) is 20.23, the septum is 22.6, while the lateral crura is only 5.9 [12]. This implies that the septum and scroll are the more elastic (spring-like), while the lateral crura is less so. But of course, there are only three specimens for each site, and thus this is not statistically significant, just demonstrating a trend. But, more important than the elasticity of the scroll cartilage, it is the vertical shape of the scroll that gives the scroll the important role as the spring of the tip. When seen in section, it is S-shaped, much like the simplest metal wire springs, which for the same material have much more recoil than a straight wire. One can witness this shape when separating the scroll from its medial attachment during rhinoplasty to view in cross-section, as we will discuss in the next chapter (Fig. 6.17).

So, with this background, we will now discuss a class of procedures that I will refer to as tension-adjusting procedures, that resemble Breathe-right strip (TM) activity, and mostly involve placing the upper lateral cartilage (scroll) under tension to theoretically dilate the nasal airway. The procedures were largely designed to

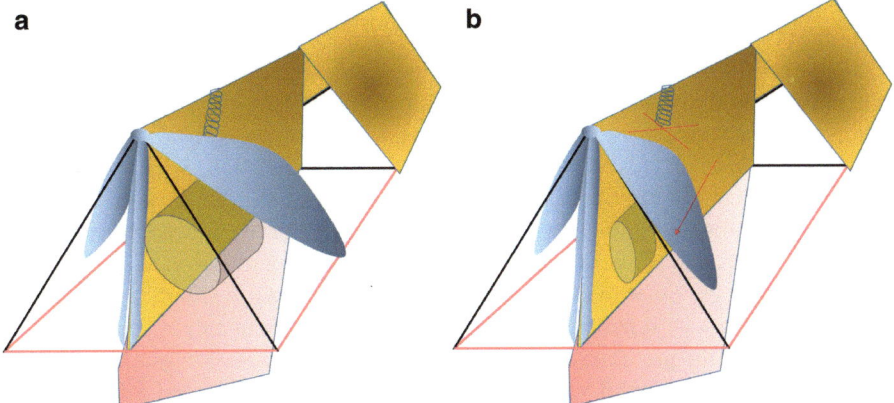

Fig. 6.16 (**a**) Dynamic triangular prism model (DTPM) showing the spring support of the alar cartilage with a neutral (AP 0 SI O) framework. Pink indicates the foundation/substrate, golden yellow represents the framework, blue shows the canopy layer, here consisting of the paired medial and lateral crura of the alar cartilage and spring structure of the scroll. The grey cylinder represents the nasal inlet, supported by the external nose structures. (**b**) DTPM with loss of spring support and resultant malposition of the alar cartilage lateral crus

Fig. 6.17 Intra-operative photograph after separation of the upper lateral cartilage from the septum revealing the S-shape spring-like structure of the scroll

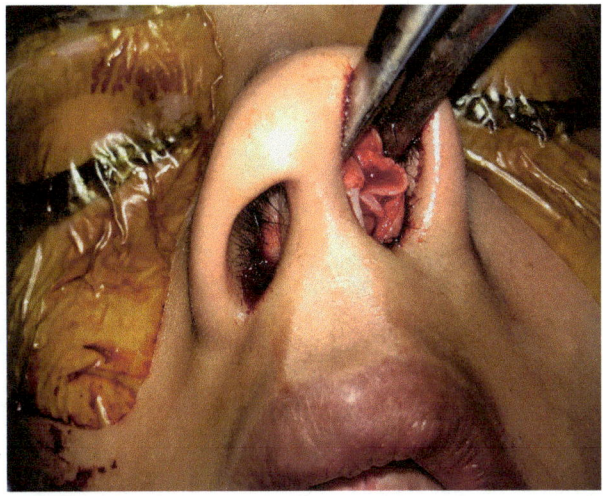

mimic the Cottle maneuver that many patients and physicians believe opens the nasal valve, but of course indirectly the benefit comes from moving the lateral crura laterally. The typical target of these procedures is a "collapsed" or narrow upper lateral cartilage (ULC) or narrowed middle third, a similar target of the "spreader graft." It is believed by most that this cartilage, when over-resected or droopy requires re-tensioning and support in a lateral direction, but of course any benefit is actually due to the restoration of the spring-support function of the lower lateral cartilage (LLC).

One of the most ingenious advancements in this aspect of rhinoplasty was the introduction of the "flaring" suture by Park in 1998 [15]. In general, this procedure involves the suturing of the "upper lateral cartilage" of on side across the dorsal septum to the other side. The suture is placed under tension, which causes the antero-medialization of both cartilages, and thus dilating the "internal nasal valve." This was documented to increase the cross-sectional area in cadavers by about 5% [16] (and was found to work even better in conjunction with spreader grafts). The concept, like many other maneuvers, is both flawed but useful simultaneously, possibly explaining why it has mostly fallen out of popularity in recent years. First, as we discussed in the previous chapter, dilating only the "internal" nasal valve, without modifying the external valve or nostril component of the nasal inlet does not improve airflow, but only makes the nasal airspace seem larger. As we discussed in Chap. 5, in a stream of fluid, only a funnel shaped inlet, with the opening the widest portion will have efficient flow, and a mid-stream dilation (as in this example) will only increase eddys, vortices, and turbulent flow. Using our DTPM (Fig. 6.18) one can see in action, that while the middle of the nose will be temporarily widened, and perhaps an endoscopic exam will reveal a "larger" caliber internal airway, neither aesthetic or functional changes will benefit.

Further, while the device may have performed well in cadavers, as determined by the researchers, even permanent sutures fail over the long run without relief of some tension. While physicians and patients feel a sense of satisfaction at having dilated

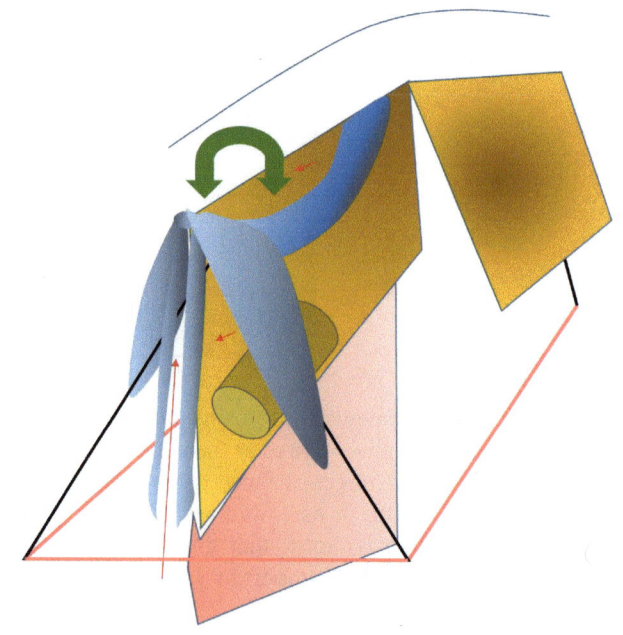

Fig. 6.18 Dynamic triangular prism model (DTPM) of the use of "flaring sutures," which may do little to expand the actual nasal inlet. Pink indicates the foundation/substrate, golden yellow represents the framework, blue shows the canopy layer, here consisting of the paired medial and lateral crura of the alar cartilage. The grey cylinder represents the nasal inlet, supported by the external nose structures

the cartilages, in reality, the suture may eventually either pull through the scroll (AKA upper lateral cartilage), or stretch and release tension. In a real-life analogy, using a nylon string to pull a sapling in a certain direction will likewise fail over time, mostly breaking directly. Only the creation of a raw surface between two tissues will permit long-term healing when combined with a complete release of tension of the structure from opposite directions of motion. In the case of the "flaring suture," tension is not released, and no opposing raw surfaces are placed in contact, thus upon suture failure, surgery may fail. However, if the same concept is applied to the lateral crura of the alar cartilages and the scroll has lost elasticity, cantilevering the lateral crura upon each other (just like Park's flaring suture) can mimic the act of tensioning of the scroll when raw surfaces are opposed and restore alar position (Fig. 6.19).

The "Butterfly graft" procedure popularized in the United States by Ted Cook, but introduced by Hage (1965), uses a conchal cartilage graft in a similar manner to the flaring suture but involves the use of the cartilage tension flaring the middle third of the nose in an anterolateral direction [17]. While the cartilage may create more "airway dilation" than the flaring suture, the same flaws are expected. Of course as

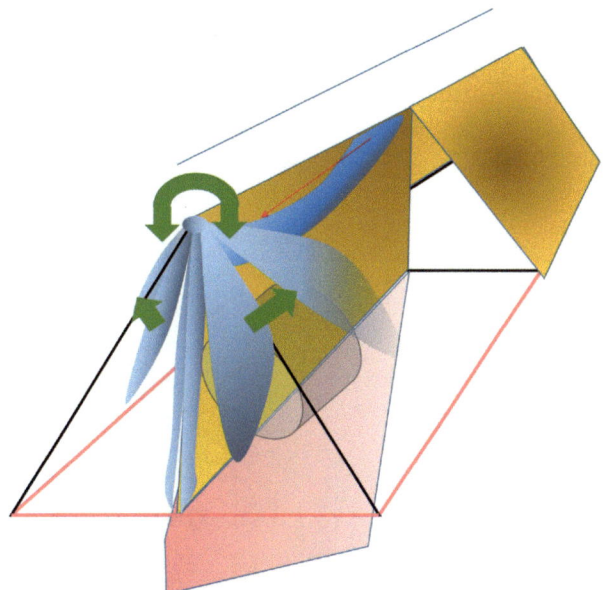

Fig. 6.19 Dynamic triangular prism model (DTPM) of the use of "flaring sutures" specifically of the lateral crus, which simulates re-tensioning of the scroll, by making the alar cartilages mutually dependent. Green arrows indicate direction of motion of the lateral crus, while the green curve represents the direction of lateral crura to lateral crura suture tension. Pink indicates the foundation/substrate, golden yellow represents the framework, blue shows the canopy layer, here consisting of the paired medial and lateral crura of the alar cartilage. The grey cylinder represents the nasal inlet, supported by the external nose structures

recent as 2018, cadaveric studies show improvement in airflow, but I would expect in vivo, only thickening of the middle of the nose results in the long run [18].

I was involved in the development of a procedure that relies on re-tensioning as well, the alar cartilage repositioning procedure, marketed by Medtronic Ear, nose and throat (ENT) as the Alar™ splint procedure. (Disclosure: I do actively receive royalties related to intellectual property for this procedure. I will attempt to be as realistic as possible here, without promoting this device, but of course there is likely inadvertent bias). While the initial description of this technique in the literature mostly invokes tensioning of the ULC, especially in versions that predated my version that uses a splint we have just explained how attempting to move the ULC is largely unproductive, except how it relates to supporting the lateral crura as a scroll component. The residual value of this procedure, unlike that stated incorrectly in my 2011 article, comes not from measurements of the ULC, but from re-positioning the alar cartilages *relative* to the ULC [19, 20].

As we discussed earlier, the upper lateral cartilage, while histologically carti-laginous, serves more as a spring-like-ligament that connects and supports the alar cartilages to the framework (nasal bones and septum via its inclusion in the scroll structure). Thus, when the alar (medial and lateral crural cartilages) structures have descended inferiorly, these ligaments termed the ULC will be stretched inferiorly and appear narrow in the middle third of the nose. This condition is most com-monly due to SI+ noses on the DTPM (Fig. 6.20), where the nasal tip is literally drawn inferiorly by the septum. The aesthetic result is tip ptosis, and the functional problem is due to inadequate nostril support and over-bending of the nasal inlet (see SI+ description in the previous rhinoplasty compass chapter). Shortening of the septum can alleviate the problem, however, there are times when the alar

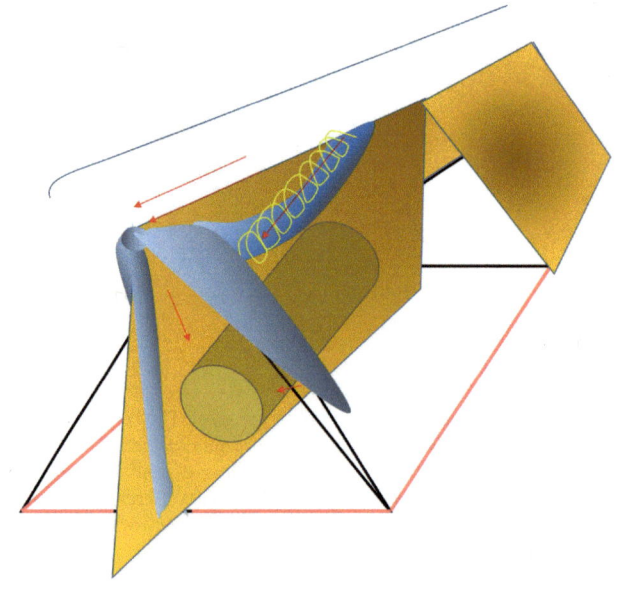

Fig. 6.20 Dynamic triangular prism model (DTPM) of stretched and damaged scroll. Pink indicates the foundation/ substrate, golden yellow represents the framework, blue shows the canopy layer, here consisting of the paired medial and lateral crura of the alar cartilage. The grey cylinder represents the nasal inlet, supported by the external nose structures

cartilages remain ptotic inferiorly even after septal shortening, or even tripod modification. In some variations on nasal aging as well, the alar cartilages can become ptotic even without an SI+ septum, just from loss of ULC ligamentous support, or avulsion in the case of trauma. In these cases, re-tensioning of the ULC ligament, in other words, tightening the VERTICAL support of the alar cartilages or increasing the OVERLAP of the lower lateral cartilage over the ULC ligament aids in shortening the nose and dilating the nostril. There are several caveats, however. First, just as in the other tensioning procedures, if the tension fixing the alar cartilages in their fixed, ptotic inferior position is not corrected, then the procedure will fail regardless of how many splints or sutures are added. In other words, if the SI+ septum is still pulling the tip down, and is not shortened, there may be limited improvement in rotation of the tip. Also, the ligamentous attachments between the ULC and the alar lateral crura serves itself as a spring, retaining memory and the alar in an inferior or caudal position despite attempts to relocate. Only division of the scroll bilaterally (inter-cartilaginous incision) including the midline will allow release of tension to permit re-tensioning of the alar cartilages. This division permits two raw surfaces to heal into the new position, without tension (Fig. 6.21). Thus, the procedure, while reasonable, is only effective in certain conditions, one main one being tip ptosis due to loss of elasticity of the scroll-spring from age. The Alar ™ splint itself is simply a TEMPORARY device used to reinforce the improved tensioning of the alar cartilages with reference to the ULC ligament only after complete scroll release between these two cartilages. Because of the created raw surfaces, the alar cartilage is capable of healing into a new superior position of overlap and tension with reference to the ULC. The sidewalls of the nose are shortened, strengthened, and the nostril is dilated. In my opinion, this procedure is only useful by itself for severe loss of spring function at the scroll from age or trauma,

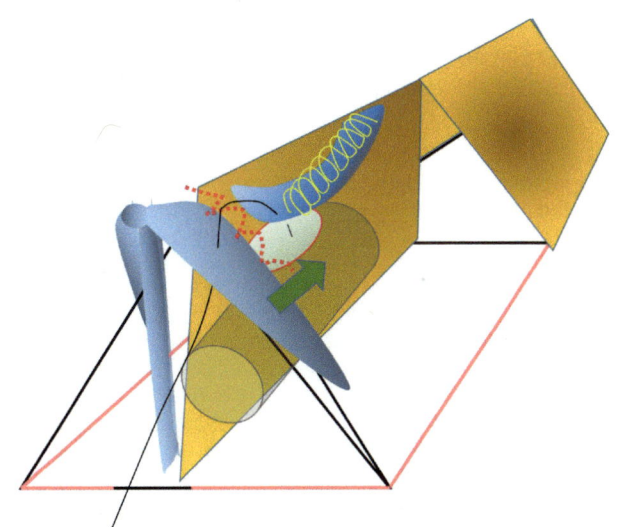

Fig. 6.21 Dynamic triangular prism model (DTPM) of stretched and damaged scroll, now divided and repaired with raw-edge approximation. Pink indicates the foundation/substrate, golden yellow represents the framework, blue shows the canopy layer, here consisting of the paired medial and lateral crura of the alar cartilage. The grey cylinder represents the nasal inlet, supported by the external nose structures

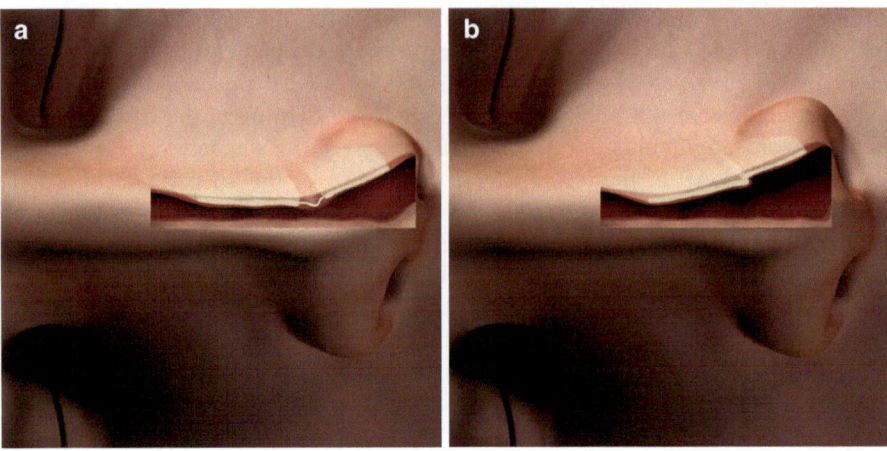

Fig. 6.22 Animation of division of the stretched scroll (a) and (b) re-approximation with improved overlap and spring restoration

but is mostly useful in conjunction with septal shortening of the SI+ nose as we will discuss in the next chapter (Fig. 6.22a, b, Courtesy of Medtronic ENT).

In conclusion, we can see that some traditional procedures can be useful in the right circumstances, while others are less so. Most importantly, though, we can see that grafts are only useful to restore missing or severely damaged structure and serve no purpose for misplaced structures. Similarly, tension restoring procedures are only helpful if tension supporting the alar cartilages to an adequate nasal framework is substantially reduced, and serve no purpose if the framework is damaged or misplaced, or tension is adequate.

References

1. McCullough D. The Wright brothers. New York: Simon and Schuster; 2016.
2. Sheen JH. Spreader graft: a method of reconstructing the roof of the middle nasal vault following rhinoplasty. Plast Reconstr Surg. 1984;73(2):230–9.
3. Fedok FG. Costal cartilage grafts in rhinoplasty. Clin Plast Surg. 2016;43(1):201–12.
4. Gürlek A, Fariz A, Celik M, Ersöz-Oztürk A, Arslan A. Straightening the crooked middle third of the nose: use of high-density porous polyethylene extended spreader grafts. Arch Facial Plast Surg. 2005;7(6):420.
5. Mohammadi S, Mohseni M, Eslami M, Arabzadeh H, Eslami M. Use of porous high-density polyethylene grafts in open rhinoplasty: no infectious complication seen in spreader and dorsal grafts. Head Face Med. 2014;10:52.
6. Kim YH, Kim BJ, Jang TY. Use of porous high-density polyethylene (Medpor) for spreader or extended septal graft in rhinoplasty: aesthetics, functional outcomes, and long-term complications. Ann Plast Surg. 2011;67(5):464–8.
7. Fuller JC, Levesque PA, Lindsay RW. Analysis of patient-perceived nasal appearance evaluations following functional septorhinoplasty with spreader graft placement. JAMA Facial Plast Surg. 2019;21(4):305–11.

8. Toriumi D, Johnson CM. Open structure rhinoplasty. Philadelphia: Saunders; 1990.
9. Seneldir S, Nacar A, Kayabasoglu G. A novel method for smooth contouring of nasal tip: camouflaging alar tip graft. J Craniofac Surg. 2015;26(7):2171–3.
10. Johnson, C., To, W. A case structure approach to open rhinoplasty. Philadelphia: Saunders; 2004
11. Westreich RW, Lawson W. The tripod theory of nasal tip support revisited: the cantilevered spring model. Arch Facial Plast Surg. 2008;10(3):170–9.
12. Westreich RW, Courtland H, Nasser P, et al. Defining nasal cartilage elasticity biomechanical testing of the tripod theory based on a cantilevered model. Arch Facial Plast Surg. 2007;9(4):264–70.
13. Adams WP, Rohrich R, Jollier L, et al. Anatomic basis and clinical implications for nasal tip support in open versus closed rhinoplasty. Plast Reconstr Surg. 1999;103(1):255–61.
14. Adamson PA, Litner J, Dahiya R. The M-arch model: a new concept of nasal tip dynamics. Arch Facial Plast Surg. 2006;8(1):16–25.
15. Park SS. The flaring suture to augment the repair of the dysfunctional nasal valve. Plast Reconstr Surg. 1998;101(4):1120–2.
16. Schlosser RJ, Park SS. Surgery for the dysfunctional nasal valve. Cadaveric analysis and clinical outcomes. Arch Facial Plast Surg. 1999;1(2):105–10.
17. Hage J. Collapsed AL/E strengthened by Conchal cartilage (the butterfly cartilage graft). Br J Plast Surg. 1965;18:92–6.
18. Brandon BM, Austin GK, Fleischman G, Basu S, Kimbell JS, Shockley WW, Clark JM. Comparison of airflow between spreader grafts and butterfly grafts using computational flow dynamics in a cadaveric model. JAMA Facial Plastic Surg. 2017;20(3):215–21.
19. Cárdenas JC, Carvajal J, Ruiz A. Securing nasal tip rotation through suspension suture technique. Plast Reconstr Surg. 2006;117:1750–5.
20. Stupak HD. Endonasal repositioning of the upper lateral cartilage and the internal nasal valve. Ann Otol Rhinol Laryngol. 2011;120(2):88–94.

Chapter 7
Rhinoplasty Strategy and Tactics Using the Rhinoplasty Compass™

He pointed out to him the bearings of the coast, explained to him the variations of the compass, and taught him to read in that vast book opened over our heads which they call heaven, and where God writes in azure with letters of diamonds.—Alexandre Dumas, The Count of Monte Cristo

A healthy young woman, of unclear age, hailing from the Mediterranean part of the world enters your office for a rhinoplasty consultation. She has occasional nighttime mouth-breathing and nasal blockage, but most importantly, wishes she had a nose that fit her face better. After extensive discussion, exam and analysis, you notice that while she has no dorsal hump, nasal narrowing or droopy tip to fix with grafts, or sutures, you instead consult your handy Rhinoplasty Compass™, and realize that she is has an SI+, and slightly AP+ nose, and you decide that this framework problem is the root of her aesthetic and breathing problems. Her family insists that she is fine and is concerned that she is seeking rhinoplasty, while her friends confirm that she has a "classic" nose and don't recommend surgery. After you explain your analysis to her, and monitor her expectations carefully, you present to her a computer simulation, and when she seems pleased with the result, you begin to plan framework surgery strategy (Fig. 7.1).

Finally, we have reached the point in this text where we have discussed enough background, physics, and physiology to describe a general plan to treat most nasal deformities. Unlike most texts, here we will not attempt to convince you that if you follow the exact steps that we take, that you will be successful. In contrast, we are simply trying to change how you think about the structures of the nose and face so better for you to formulate effective strategies for each patient. Thus far, we have established and explained the Dynamic Triangular Prism (tent-shaped) Model (DTPM) and used this to discuss phenotypes of nasal deformity in previous chapters. We have also used the DTPM to discuss and analyze currently available conventional procedures, and their true weaknesses and strengths with an understanding of how they are affected by the forces or physics instead of a regurgitation what is reported by esteemed experts. Now, using the septal/nasal phenotypes located on the eight point Rhinoplasty Compass™ (Chap. 5), we will describe a plan of attack

© Springer Nature Switzerland AG 2020
H. D. Stupak, *Rethinking Rhinoplasty and Facial Surgery*,
https://doi.org/10.1007/978-3-030-44674-1_7

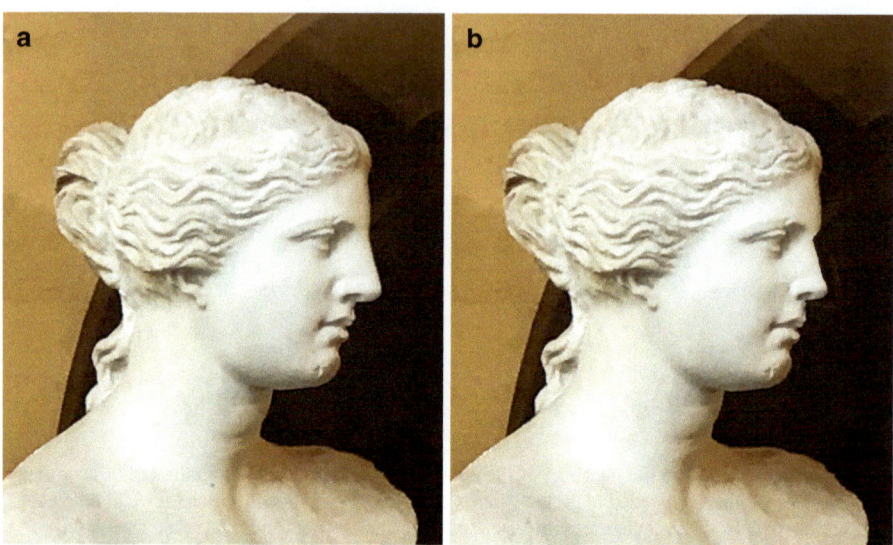

Fig. 7.1 (**a**) Lateral view of 2000 year old sculpture Venus de Milo taken at the Louvre Museum, Paris. (**b**) Computer simulation of framework reduction for same photograph made on Adobe Photoshop Essentials™

for appropriate surgical management for these variations, although of course many more variations exist! We will however, use these cardinal phenotype points as a frame of reference. Instead of the simplified and often two dimensional "procedure" tactical descriptions, we will break down the strategic surgical plan into six stages: plan, approach, release, re-size, reposition, and reinforce. Once we have discussed and mastered these principles pertaining to the nasal framework (septum and nasal bones), we will discuss complementary maneuvers to this basic plan, including dealing with severe deviation of bones and cartilage and canopy surgery (alar cartilage and skin).

Overall Strategy (The Plan)

Of course the key to any endeavor, whether surgical or otherwise, is first a careful analysis of the situation. Only by understanding the root cause of a problem can an efficient, and reasonable solution be found, and this can be tailored to any individual, based on anatomic variation. The Rhinoplasty Compass™ was designed to assist the surgeon in classifying the root framework problem. In this section, we will assume that the patient's framework has been correctly classified to a specific point (or at worst between two points) on the Rhinoplasty Compass. This classification will allow us to plan a specific corresponding procedure that essentially reverses the pathologic framework phenotype of that specific rhinoplasty point and permits the nasal structure to be shifted toward to ideal center of the rhinoplasty chart. The center of the chart essentially consists of a framework neutral nasal length (SI neutral {0}) and neutral nasal projection (AP neutral {0}). So, our global rhinoplasty strategy is: Once a patient's framework is determined to have a SI or AP surplus (+) or deficiency (−), or combination thereof, the essential goal of surgery is to reverse these surpluses and deficiencies not to extremes, but to neutral position (AP 0, SI 0). AP and SI neutral positions may not even be a fixed state, but could vary between surgeons, time periods, and cultures. But, by understanding that there is an AP and SI neutral framework ideal, the surgeon can plan surgery more readily.

Only *after* this "neutralization" of the framework size has been achieved, and after release of retaining forces, can the framework be restored/mobilized to the midline (deviation repair). Subsequently, the canopy layer (alar/tip cartilages and skin), can be modified to match the neutralized framework. While this overall strategy may differ substantially than the listed steps found in most rhinoplasty texts, and can be confusing or even pointless at first, I ask that you the reader be briefly patient and permit me to explain the phases of this strategy. We will discuss the five phases at length, and then discuss how to apply this to each point of the compass, then finally we will address how best to utilize specific additional maneuvers to achieve the overall mission of a well-structured, attractive, and functionally adequate nose.

The Approach

Surgeons love to talk about their *favorite* approaches to different surgical procedures. Many discussions around rhinoplasty, both with patients and surgeons at conferences revolve around the open rhinoplasty approach versus the "endonasal" approach, called the "closed" approach by disparaging open rhinoplasty surgeons. It becomes an animated controversy at rhinoplasty conferences, and for patients seeking multiple opinions prior to surgery, it can become a focal point of fixation. Frequently, the patient or physician become so focused on the approach phase, on the incision planning and decisions around this, that they forget that there is absolutely zero therapeutic value in the approach. The approach is simply an avenue to access the target framework. The more efficient the approach is, there will be less collateral damage to tissue from the surgery, shorter surgery duration, and a less disrupted blood supply. In contrast to this, many rhinoplasty surgeons pride themselves on an extensive approach, usually "open" rhinoplasty, which they justify with "excellent visualization," permitting intra-operative diagnosis, and "great exposure" to place much-needed grafts. Some surgeons pride themselves and spend hours upon hours on a single rhinoplasty procedure, maximizing exposure, and maximizing "attention to detail" to perfect the location and precision of the approach, grafts, and sutures, and they always imply that this extra effort yields good long-term outcomes. Unfortunately, while this "detailed" approach sounds appealing to some patients and surgeons, the situation is a perfect example of the use of tactics over

Table 7.1 Fallacies of approach

Open rhinoplasty is better for visualization and education.
Visualization of cartilages is important to make diagnosis.
Never make a full transfixion—tip will collapse.
A separate approach is required beyond the transfixion incision to approach the nasal dorsum.
Visualization is superior to feel in surgery.
The most anterior/inferior part of the septum is not worth approaching as this "L-strut" is "untouchable."

strategy. These discussions are all about details that sound perhaps high-tech, or even scientific, but almost completely fail to explain *how* the technique will yield structural change beyond what the weak literature (usually generated by these same individuals) promises as we discussed in the prior chapter. There is little reasoning applied that considers the root cause of the deformity in this approach, and once considered, there are rarely thoughts on reversing this root cause.

So, what is the alternative to picking a "favorite" approach and then sticking to it? The flexible, rationale, and efficient approach. This means that instead of participating in the ongoing and possibly irrational discussion about which approach is best, consider what the target tissue you need to get to, and what is the quickest, most direct way to get there that causes the least collateral damage. In reality, a master rhinoplasty surgeon is familiar and even facile with ALL approaches, and can create hybrid approaches with only a little forethought, and can use whichever of the existing approaches best serves their present need. I have listed some of the classically taught myths about rhinoplasty approaches below (Table 7.1). I point these out because we will be referencing these oft-quoted fallacies as we discuss a simplified approach. These fallacies include: (1) open rhinoplasty is better for visualization and education; (2) direct visualization of cartilage is important to make diagnosis; (3) a full transfixion incision (separating the columella from the caudal septum completely) will somehow cause "tip collapse" because this connection is part of tip support; (4) approaching the dorsum of the nose is a separate approach than septoplasty requiring a separate incision; and (5) the most anterior/inferior part of the septum is not worth approaching as this "L-strut" is "untouchable."

As we will discuss below, most of these adages are complete nonsense, and must have arose during an era of confusion about cause and effect in nasal restructuring, as many mythic medical adages have. Despite the broad expansion of evidence based medicine, most of these have never been properly tested or questioned, but are swallowed and accepted by trainees for time.

If our overall strategy is to first and foremost improve the framework of the nose by re-sizing this structure to achieving a SI and AP neutral (0) nose from a nose with superfluous or deficient framework, then the goal of our approach phase is to access the septal and bony framework while causing the least collateral soft-tissue damage and risk to blood supply and taking the least time. In my opinion, the open rhinoplasty approach is overly destructive of tissue and blood supply despite the extensive visualization it permits, and in actuality it provides poor visualization of the caudal septum without extensive dissection (destruction) of the alar cartilage attachments. While most would say that this is the ONLY procedure to access the septal and bony framework while also accessing the tip cartilages, I will attempt to describe a simpler, less invasive approach that can possibly get a more easily accessible view of the septum.

Transfixion Approach to the Entire "L"-Strut—Exposure and Access

Most surgeons who operate on the nose are capable of finding the caudal-most portion of the nasal septum where it contacts the columella. The septum is loosely attached to the columella mucosa and skin, so that once pressure is applied between these two structures with a nasal speculum the sharp edge of the caudal external septum becomes very prominent. This places the mucosa over this sharp edge under tension, which allows a stable incision, as well as temporary hemostasis from pressure on the adjacent mucosa. A curved incision is made on either side of the septal mucosa, but of course one can start with a hemi (one sided) transfixion incision, and move toward the second side later in cases where the caudal septum is so deviated that the sharp edge is only visible on one side or the other. Once the incision has been completed from the anterior to posterior septal angle and nasal floor, flaps are raised broadly as possible, from upper lateral cartilage to piriform aperture (Fig. 7.2). The two hemi-transfixion incisions are then connected in a complete fashion (Fig. 7.3). When I mean complete, I mean the columella must be completely disconnected from the caudal septum as much as possible, otherwise later in the

Fig. 7.2 Intra-operative photo of transfixion incision along the full length of caudal septum

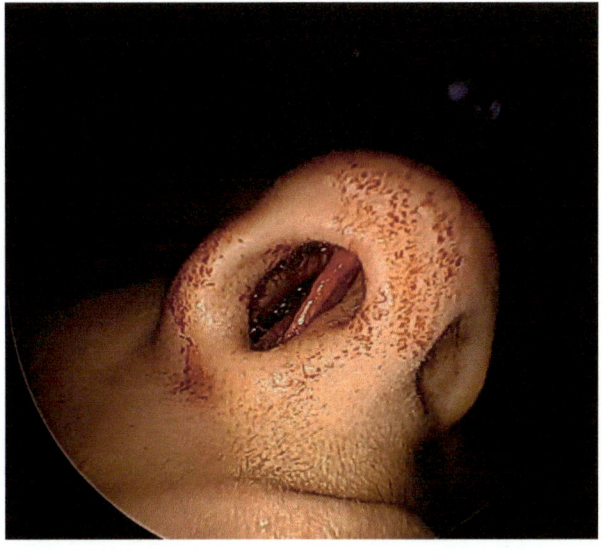

Fig. 7.3 Intra-operative
photo of the completion
and release of the full
transfixion incision

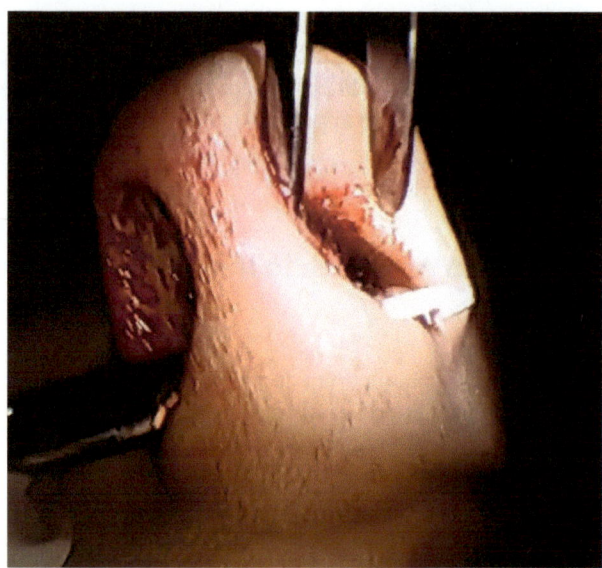

Fig. 7.4 Intra-operative
photo of the released
caudal septum during
left-sided flap elevation

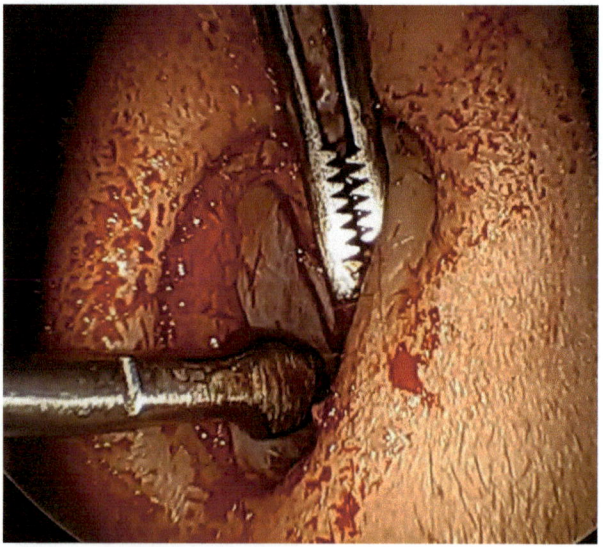

procedure, one will not realize why the view is restricted (Fig. 7.4). In the severe
AP+/SI+ septum, the antero-inferior septum will be cup-shaped with a concave and
convex sides. This is because it is buckled in a supero-inferior fashion and antero-
superior fashion (Fig. 7.5). Fibrous webs, even in the non-traumatized primary rhinoplasty will accentuate the concavity, and make flap elevation on the concave side
of the septum very difficult until these fibrous bands are released, which may not be
possible until after maximal completion of the full transfixion incision (Fig. 7.6).

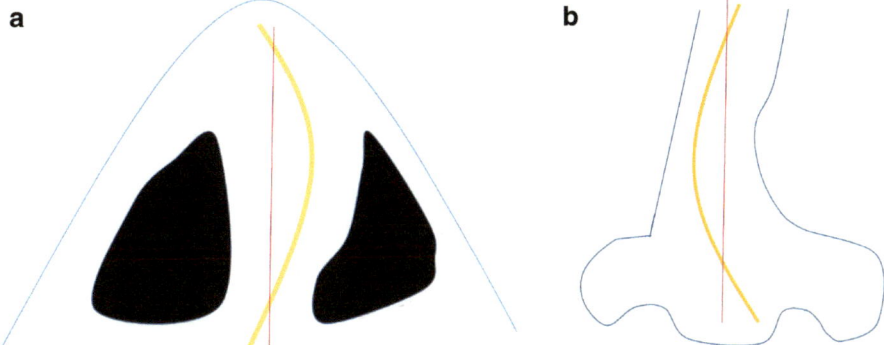

Fig. 7.5 Diagram demonstrating (**a**) antero-posterior septal buckling (yellow indicates buckled, red indicates normal). (**b**) supero-inferior buckling (yellow indicates buckled, red indicates normal)

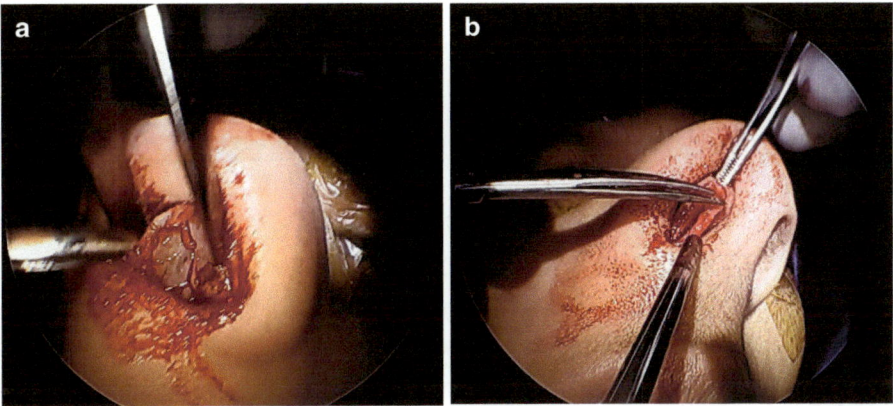

Fig. 7.6 Intra-operative photograph of (**a**) exposure of the curled anterior septal angle and (**b**) release of bands after exposure

The convex side of the septum can be equally challenging, because the peak of the convexity can about the bony pyriform aperture making passage of the speculum and even elevator difficult (Fig. 7.7a–g). It is easy for a novice surgeon to be frustrated and intimidated in these circumstances, especially when one can become disoriented by the severe contouring of the septum. Again, while conventional wisdom dictates that the surgeon should abort this portion of the surgery and move on to a camouflage stage, or proceed to "tip-work" via the much easier "open rhinoplasty" approach, I suggest a different strategy. Slow it down, and take a step back. Try to see in your mind's eye the contours of this bent, contoured, buckled structure, and use FEEL to mentally visualize the structure. Then, find a place on the septum where you are sure of your orientation, and start to elevate again slowly. Don't quit until you need to, but keep trying until you have skeletonized the septum and preserved the flaps to the degree possible. Then, once the most buckled parts of the septum are improved, the flaps will be under less tension and will be less likely to develop perforation even if one flap has a sizeable hole (Fig. 7.8a, b). In the words of Hannibal, "If I can't find a way, I will make a way." Get the job done, but of course don't recklessly create perforations.

Then, once you have achieved extensive flap elevation, you are ready to approach the dorsum. The transfixion incision you have already made and released from the septum and columella is more than adequate to reach the cartilaginous AND the bony dorsum, if you follow this next part of the approach phase. A nasal speculum is placed to straddle the anterior septal angle, with each tine stretching its respective flap. The mucosa over the inferior most part of the dorsal septum will be seen to be under tension as it is stretched by the speculum. Then, a single tine of a curved scissors is inserted into the space created by speculum, its opposite tine on the dorsal surface of the mucosa (Fig. 7.9). Once the scissors are in this position, a cut is made and then duplicated on the other side of the septum. A further series of cuts are continued between the elevated septal flap and the medial border of the upper lateral

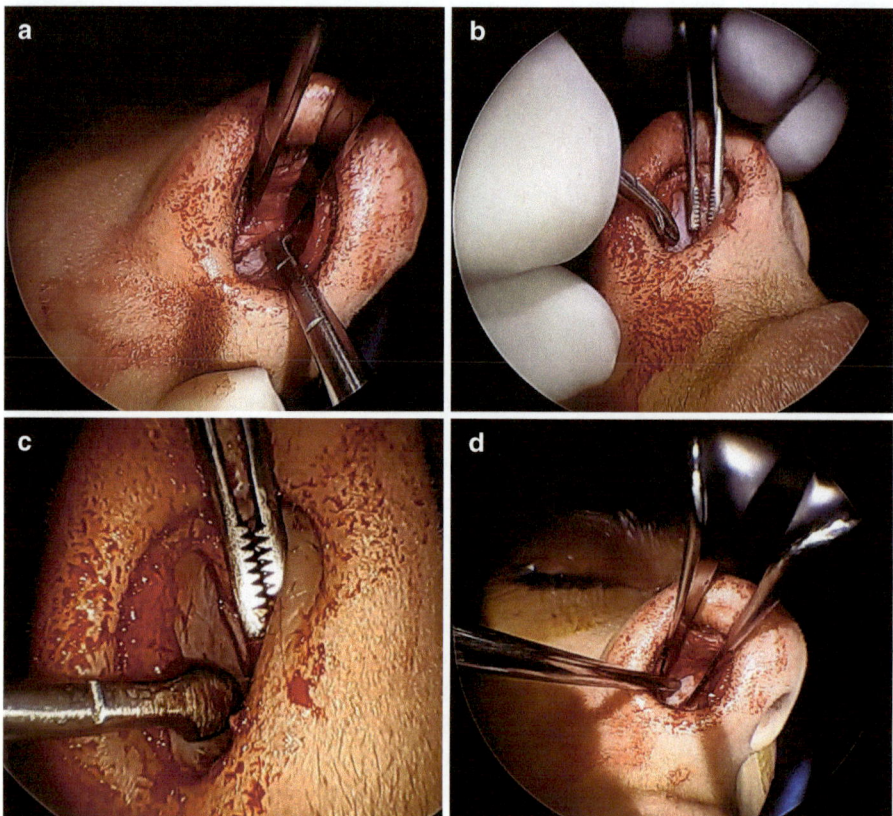

Fig. 7.7 Intra-operative photographs of the anterior septal angle, flap elevation at various states (**a–g**)

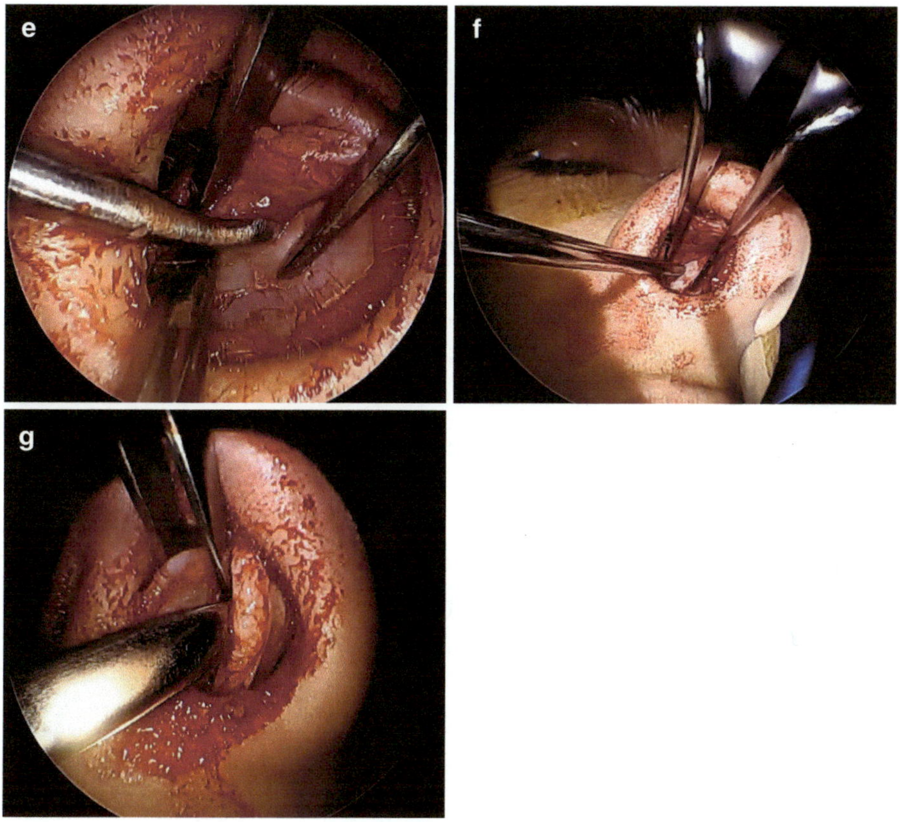

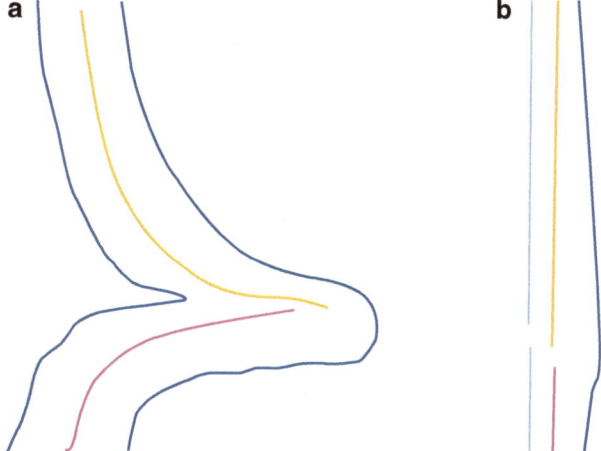

Fig. 7.7 (continued)

Fig. 7.8 Schematic of coronal view of (**a**) the severe septal spur at junction of maxillary crest (purple) and quadrangular cartilage (yellow), with flaps in grey. (**b**) After correction of the deviation, even with a damaged flap, the lack of tension from the spur allows natural flap re-approximation especially with splint use and repair, mostly without perforation

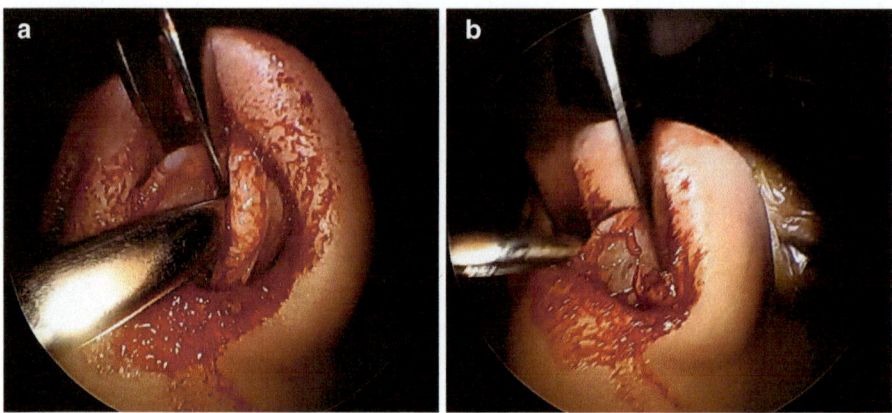

Fig. 7.9 Intra-operative photograph of nasal speculum "stradling" the septum, with concurrent cephalic pressure to begin exposure of the dorsum. (**a**) Left-sided and (**b**) right sided

Fig. 7.10 Intra-operative photograph of dorsal elevation via transfixion with scissors cuts continued between the elevated septal flap and the medial border of the upper lateral cartilage, thus isolating the dorsal (anterior) septum from its lateral attachments. The curvature of the dorsal septum is visualized

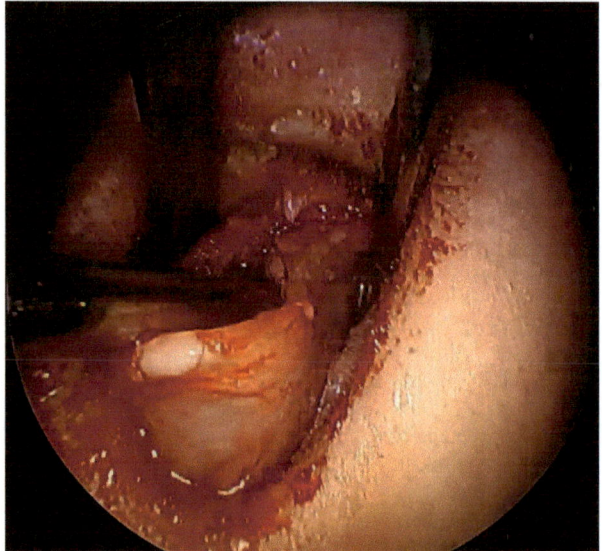

cartilage, thus isolating the dorsal (anterior) septum from its lateral attachments (Fig. 7.10). Technically, as we will discuss in the Release section, this exposure of the dorsal and caudal septum is the earliest stage of the freeing of the septal structure from its surroundings, not only providing visual exposure, but also the earliest steps in permitting mobility.

Once the septal transfixion incision has thus been extended for several millimeters medially by the speculum and scissors, the speculum is traded for an Aufricht, or preferably a Converse dorsal retractor. This device stretches the remaining dorsal mucosa anteriorly, permitting the scissors to dissect in a dorsal plane that is not

Fig. 7.11 Intra-operative photograph of extensive dorsal elevation via the transfixion incision with separation of the upper lateral cartilages from the septum complete

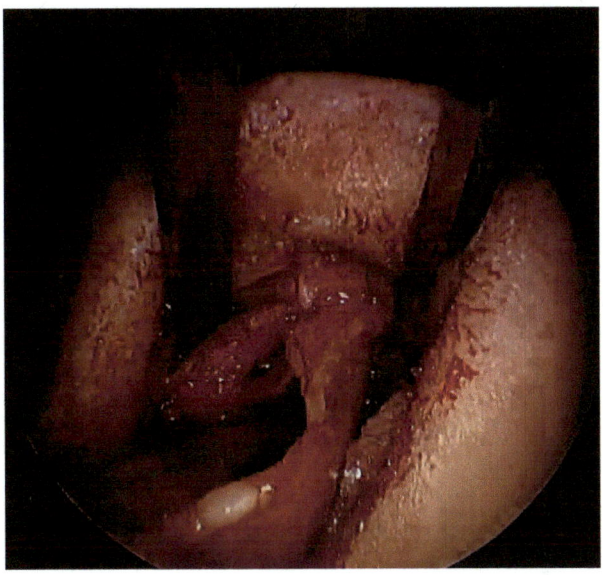

dissimilar to raising a septal flap. The dissection continues along the dorsum with a scraping, snipping action, advancing the dorsal retractor superiorly with all progress (Fig. 7.11). The transition from cartilaginous dorsum to bony dorsum frequently does not go smoothly, because of a change in plane from a sub-perichondrial to a subperiosteal plane. This is particularly challenging in an AP+ nose, as there is little room to work between the bony dorsum and the skin envelope. Enough room must be created to fit the dorsal retractor all the way to the top of the bony dorsum.

Finally, to confirm adequate exposure of the anterior septum, be sure that the cartilaginous dorsal and caudal septum are fully freed from the columella and dorsal skin in continuity, permitting full view of the anterior septal angle, and the contours of the entire anterior septum (Fig. 7.12).

The Release

Possibly one of the most critical aspects in the re-engineering of the nose is the release phase. Unlike in the open rhinoplasty "camouflage" operation, where exposure permits only the addition or subtraction of tissue, in this reconstruction, a full release of the quadrangular cartilage from its anterior inferior and posterior attachments is essential. Full release is the ONLY way to permit the re-sizing and repositioning stages of the operation that are the actually therapeutic portions, otherwise the residual tension WILL cause the structures you plan to mobilize to eventually revert to their original position despite the extensive grafts, sutures, splints, or even hardware you place! (Fig. 7.13). The septum is now completely released from the

Fig. 7.12 Confirmation of the full skeletonization of the dorsal and caudal septum with good visualization of buckling forces

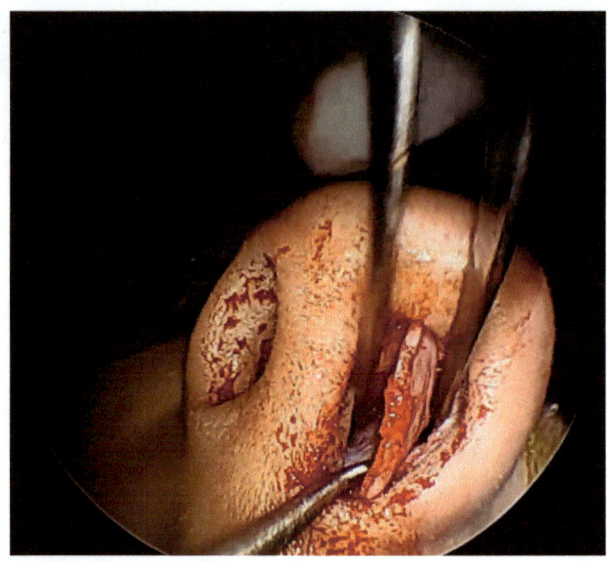

Fig. 7.13 Diagram of sagittal view of septal components. The septum is now completely released posteriorly from the maxillary crest, spine, and vomer as it was already released from the skin or canopy layer at the columella and dorsum and all the tissue in between (red line). However, it is critical to maintain at least one centimeter of attachment at the fusion of the ethmoid, and the septum just inside the keystone area (purple circle), or the procedure becomes an "extra-corporeal" septoplasty

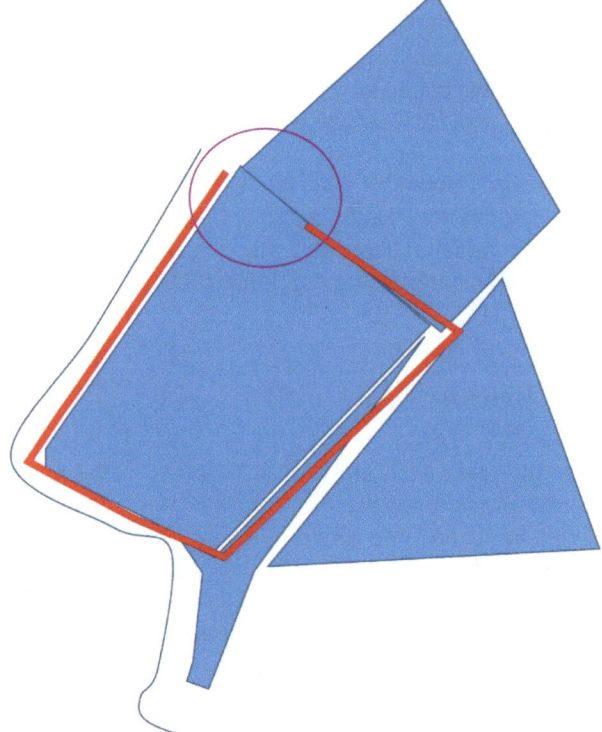

Fig. 7.14 Intra-operative photograph of releasing the septum from the upper lip and nasal spine

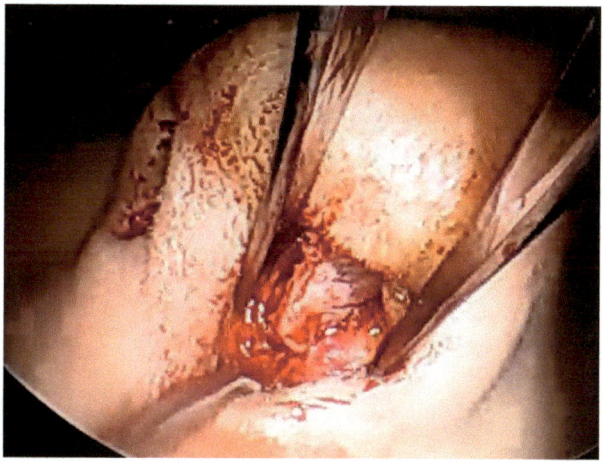

columella and dorsum and all the tissue in between (red line). However, it is critical to maintain at least a cm of attachment at the fusion of the ethmoid, and the septum just inside the keystone area (purple circle), or the procedure becomes an "extracorporeal" septoplasty that has a much less structurally predictable outcome due to mobility of the septum.

As we transition from the approach to the release phase, additional bands connecting the columella to the bony nasal spine at the posterior-most aspect of the transfixion incision are released first. This will permit better access to the posterior septum (foundational release, not just spur removal), but more importantly will permit access to the upper lip (Fig. 7.14). In the common SI+ nose, the caudal septum literally grows into the space normally occupied by the upper lip. (In Fig. 7.15, see an AP+SI+ patient with a shortened upper lip pre-operatively and the appearance of a longer lip after on the right). As discussed in the previous chapter on the SI+ nose, these individuals appear to have a shortened upper lip, and the long septum can even interfere with upper lip closure. During smiling, the shortened lip appears excessively short, with excessive gingival show, and making the nose appear excessively long. Most of the literature mistakenly attributes this problem to an overactive depressor septi muscle with the articles believe pulls the nasal tip inferiorly. While there is upper lip muscular contracture during smiling and the tip appears to descend, in reality, it is the lip shortening, not the nose moving at all [1].

This illusion is similar to a prank played on the audience by Mel Brooks in the 1982 film "To be or not to be." In this scene, an actor peering out the window of a train notices that the station outside the train is slowly beginning to move, and he of course assumes that this signifies the motion of the train itself. In reality, as the camera's vantage point switches to an external shot, the audience is shocked to see that instead a group of soldiers has literally begun to move the station itself, while the train remains stationary.

So, a depressor septi muscle that pulls the nose inferiorly need not be divided. Even in the 2014 objective study, the lip is actually found to shorten MORE on

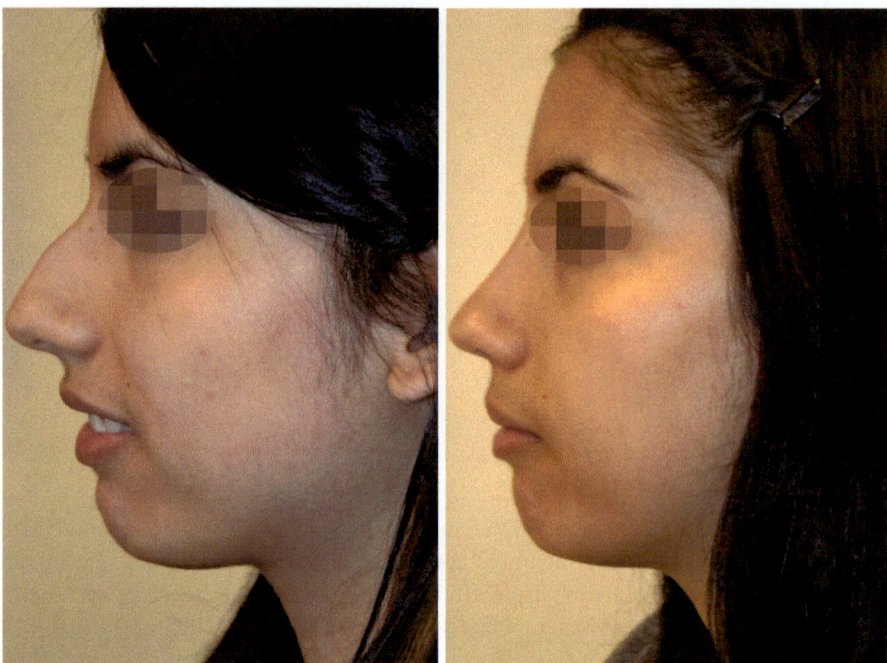

Fig. 7.15 Lateral view of patient with AP+SI+ framework (**a**) Before and (**b**) after re-sizing and release procedure, that permits re-draping and improved function of the upper lip. The pre-operative view was taken at rest. (Image reprinted with courtesy of Wolters-Kluwer). Shuaib et al. [9]

average, by a tiny amount, displaying a minimal amount at best of efficacy [1]. Instead, this "maneuver" should be abandoned and replaced with a complete release of the upper lip from the prominent nasal spine and caudal septum as part of the release of the columella from the septum. The operator will find that with firm colu-mellar retraction during surgery, an easy to reach, although sometimes vascular plane over the bony premaxilla can be dissected with just a few snips of a scissors. In the SI+ nose, this exposes the nasal spine for later removal (see re-sizing phase), but more importantly, permits separation of the upper lip from its pre-maxillary attach-ments that encourage its shortened position in addition to the overly inferior septum making the lip appear short. As seen in Fig. 7.15, release of these attachments allows better lip draping over the teeth, and substantial lengthening of the upper lip for bet-ter mouth-closure (see chapter on mouth-breathing), and for lip to nose relationship aesthetics. A side effect, however, of this quick dissection is that patients will notice temporary (a week or so) edema of the upper lip during the immediate post-operative period. This nuisance can be minimized by explaining how critical lengthening of the upper lip relative to the nose is, particularly in the SI+ nose.

Once the transfixion, dorsum, caudal septum, and lip have been successfully released from the septum, (revealing the entire midline framework of the nose from nasion [top of the nasal bones] to the pre-maxillary alveolar ridge inferior to the nasal spline), release of the intranasal septal cartilages and bone is now facilitated. The sub-perichondrial plane already dissected over the surface of the quadrangular cartilage is now extended over the bony maxillary crest, from nasal spine anteriorly, to vomer posteriorly, and up to the bony nasal floor and sill (Figs. 7.13, 7.16, and 7.17). Once this is completed bilaterally, the interaction of the inferior quadrangular

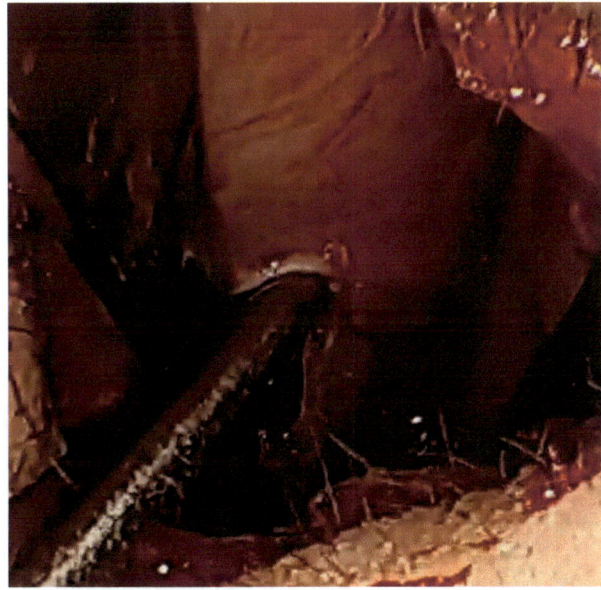

Fig. 7.16 Intra-operative photograph of blunt separation of the quadrangular cartilage from its posterior bony attachments

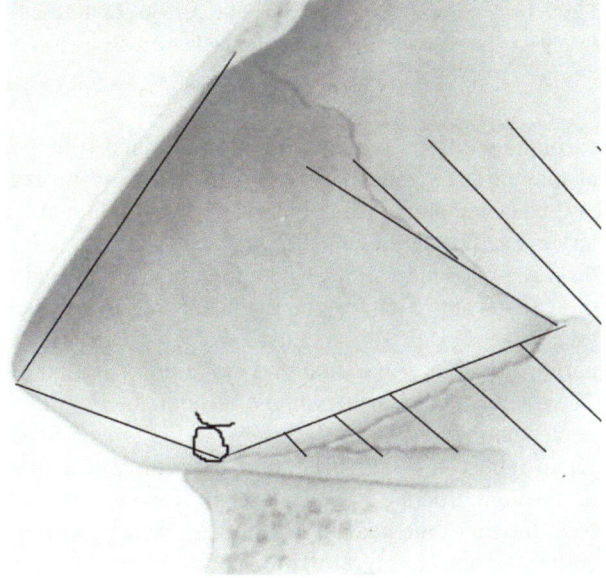

Fig. 7.17 Diagram of area of separation of septal cartilage from its bony attachments (covered by diagonal lines). The "suture" loop indicates eventual re-attachment of the septal structure to the midline. (Image reprinted with courtesy of Wolters-Kluwer). Shuaib et al. [9]

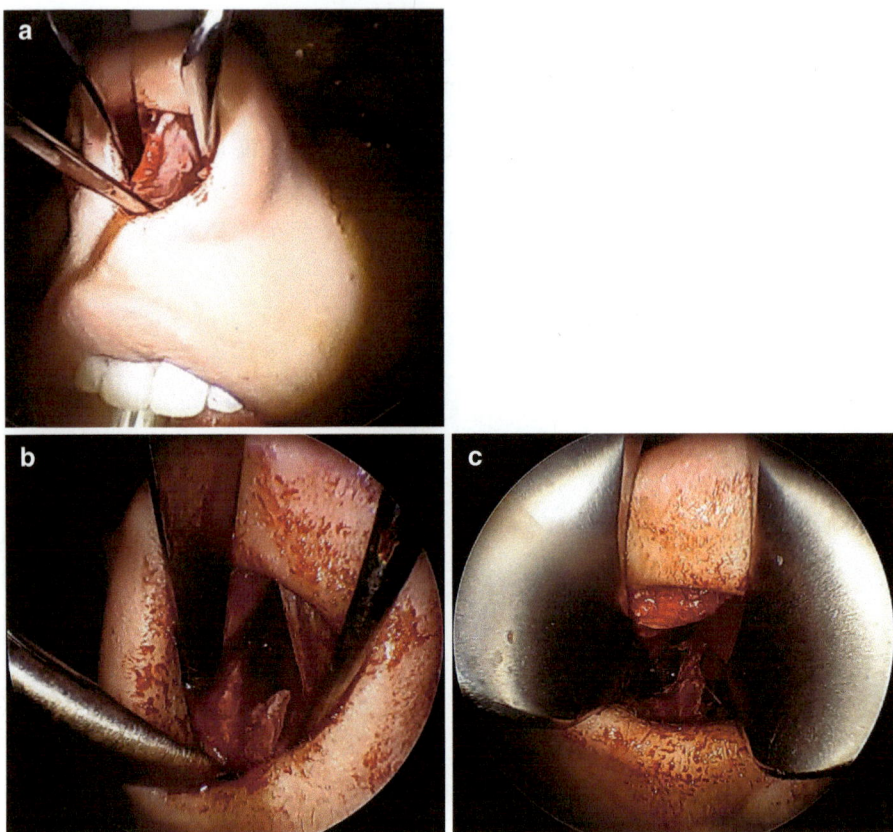

Fig. 7.18 Intra-operative photograph of separation of the caudal quadrangular cartilage from the maxillary crest. (**a**) External view. (**b**) Maxillary crest isolated internally after separation of cartilage. (**c**) Maxillary crest remnant

cartilage with the maxillary crest is revealed (Fig. 7.18). As we discussed in the chapter on the pathogenesis of septal deviation and extrusion, the severely extruded or deviated septum will exhibit severe crumpling at its connection with the maxillary crest. The cartilage and bony crest, like tectonic plates that have collided will display peaks and valleys where they have competed for space, giving the illusion of a "septal spur," but in actuality is the apex of the buckling of these structures. The great view afforded by extensive release, even in severely deviated septums will permit the blunt separation and isolation of the bony and cartilaginous structure. The quadrangular cartilage must be completely released from the crest, spine, and vomer until the entire free inferior edge is free-floating, from vomer to anterior septal angle. This is not dissimilar, but is more extensive than the "tongue in groove" or "swinging-door" procedure of the caudal septum [2], except that this extends from the tip of the nose to the most posterior portion of the septum, freeing up the entire L-strut and septum from its inferior attachments, and is not just a limited caudal procedure. Finally, once freed inferiorly, the septum is separated from the ethmoid plate from posteriorly, from its intersection with the vomer to approximately 1 cm from the keystone area of the dorsum (Fig. 7.17), preserving this attachment at all costs, otherwise the operation becomes the much less predictable "extra-corporeal septoplasty" procedure that relies on having the entire septum become a graft [3].

Note: There is some obvious overlap between the approach and release phase. The surgeon must not be so rigid to be unable to rapidly switch back and forth between these two stages. For example, frequently, release of the septum extensively from the columella will assist in more exposure of the posterior endonasal septum and dorsal septum, even though technically the approach precedes the release. This release of the transfixion incision is thus both part of approach exposure and is therapeutic in that it releases this structure from the pull of the columella attachments eventually permitting repositioning in a later stage.

The Re-sizing/Repositioning Phases

Goal

"War is peace. Freedom is slavery. Ignorance is strength." Nineteen Eighty-Four by George Orwell (Copyright © George Orwell, 1949) Reproduced by kind permission of Bill Hamilton as the Literary Executor of the Estate of Sonia Brownell.

In the book "1984," Orwell [4] uses the above counter-intuitive, paradoxical state mottos to describe how the totalitarian political party dominated the minds of its subjects. Similarly, we have recently been conditioned that the only way to treat any functional or aesthetic deficiencies in rhinoplasty is to ADD grafts. Modern textbooks and the literature are simply full of references where the very concept of "all deficiencies need added material" predominates. As one 2018 entire abstract informs us: "With the adoption of open structure techniques, rhinoplasty has become more reliant on the use of structural grafts to resist change that occurs over time owing to both gravity and the aging process. As surgical procedures have become more technically complex, the type of grafts use for both primary and secondary rhinoplasty have undergone significant evolution" [5].

Because this concept is so pervasive, it becomes challenging to question or unlearn, because it is so simple, and makes so much sense. The problem, unfortunately, is that in rhinoplasty, strength does not come from adding material, but in most cases (counter-intuitively) in *subtraction*. So, we will introduce the concept of "Strengthen nasal support via removal, not addition." Many of you will scoff at this concept, having been exposed for so long to the seemingly obvious "Only grafts = strength" model," but I ask that you keep reading, and hear the compelling argument of why "Septal re-sizing and strategic reduction results in increased strength."

As we learned in earlier chapters, the majority of primary nasal deviation and deformity is due not to overgrowth or under-growth of nasal cartilage, and deficiency of materials, but due to a mismatch of septal cartilage with its bony structure causing the appearance of extrusion or deficiency externally, or buckling of this structure. We went on to describe a "Rhinoplasty Compass™," where we diagnose the specific malposition of this structure as either extruding or deficient in a superior-inferior direction (SI+ or −), or extruding of deficient in an anterior-posterior direction (AP+ or −). Only once we have clearly and consistently made our appropriate diagnosis using the Rhinoplasty Compass (AP_, SI_) can we determine what needs to be done during the re-sizing, repositioning stage.

No matter what the AP/SI compass diagnosis is, though, a thorough release must be completed first, of nearly the entire septal cartilage save the keystone area that attaches the septum framework to the nasal bones.

SI+

In the SI+ noses, the septal cartilage and bony maxillary crest are competing for space in the midline, causing the septum to extrude externally and buckle. So, the first step, after skeletonizing the maxillary crest that is frequently very deviated, is to excise the majority of this structure, (Fig. 7.18a) especially the parts that are intrinsically bent. This deviated or overly prominent maxillary crest, as in a typical septoplasty is removed piecemeal with an open-Jansen-Middleton when deviated, or even when competing with the quadrangular cartilage for midline space, as is the vomer. Frequently, we are tempted to ignore the maxillary crest, as it is difficult to elevate flaps over, and can be a frequent source of septal perforation when flaps are too damaged. However, this structure cannot be ignored or the septum will never reach the midline.

Once the crest is no longer an obstacle (Fig. 7.18b), shortening of the septum can proceed, in order to allow the entire structure to find the midline. The septum is shortened from the anterior septal angle beyond the point of overlap over the maxillary crest, nasal spine and nasal floor to the point where the septum contacts the vomer. This does of course not need to be removed at once, but is safer to do piecemeal, especially when new to this procedure, to avoid taking too much. In stark contrast to the adages about never removing part of the L-strut, this cartilage is removed directly from the inferior limb of the L-strut (Fig. 7.19). As you can see in Fig. 7.20, by not removing the submucous resection posterior box, there is a brand-new L-strut inferior limb just behind the old one that will take its place. Essentially, the cartilage removed and preserved is the *exact opposite* of the classic submucous resection with or without cartilage graft harvest! Care must be taken of HOW to shorten the external caudal septum—it is not just an all or nothing problem. The *angle* of the cuts determines the rotation of the nasal tip (Fig. 7.21). Rotation of the tip of course differs from shortening, in that shortening reduces the overall length of the nose, while rotation of the tip is the angle of the columella relative to the lip. So,

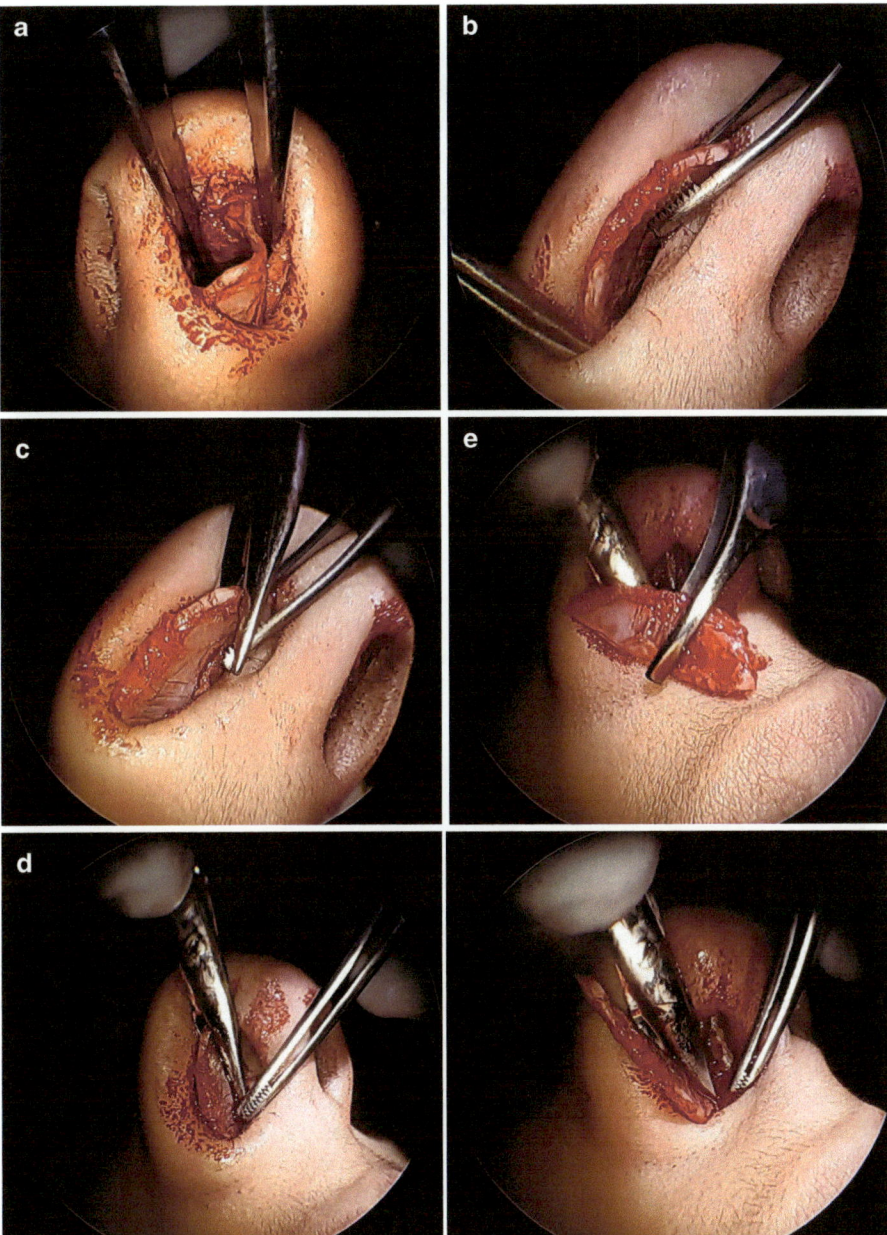

Fig. 7.19 Intra-operative photographs in sequence of shortening of the caudal portion of the L-strut (**a–e**)

Fig. 7.20 Sagittal CT scan of AP+SI+ framework (also called-tension nose) with a diagram of the excised excess L-strut (red lines) and the preserved quadrangular cartilage. (Image reprinted with courtesy of Wolters-Klewer). Stupak and Weinstock [10]

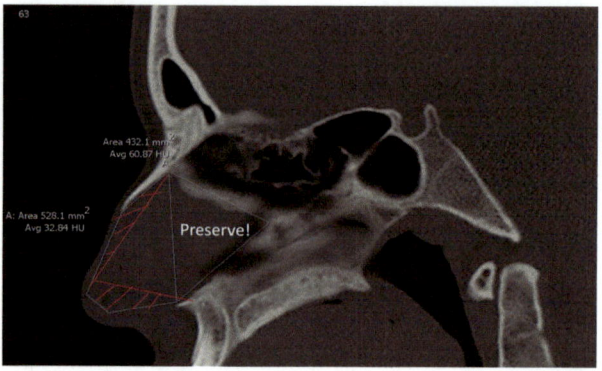

Fig. 7.21 Diagram of the sagittal or lateral view of the septum (yellow), with varied pitch of the caudal incision and resultant nasal profile (left)

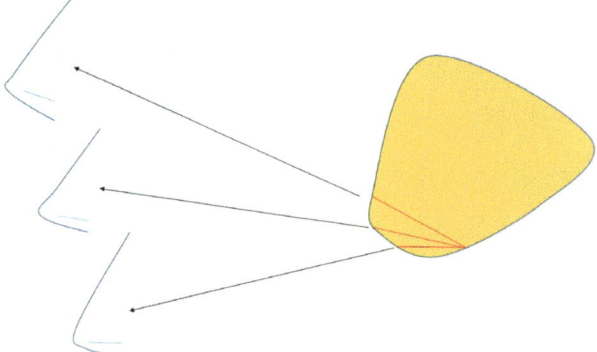

the angle of the caudal septum relative to the lip will determine the rotation of the nose. By shortening the caudal septum with a cut parallel to the previous caudal septum, rotation will stay the same. By changing this angle, rotation, or de-rotation can be achieved, by increasing or decreasing the pitch of the caudal shortening incision respectively. To use yet another aviation analogy, pitch of an airplane is analogous to rotation, while the altitude of the airplane is analogous to nasal length.

As the maxillary crest is reduced, and caudal and inferior (internal) septum are trimmed from below, the naturally elastic septum will now literally spring toward the midline (Fig. 7.22). In other words, you do *not* need to push this structure, it will literally rebound to a straighter structure. But not completely straight yet. Now that you have shortened the entire inferior L-strut limb, it will be less buckled, but in the substantially deviated nose, can still be off midline (see Fig. 7.23 showing the difference between buckling and deviation.)

Even though the septum is still on a deviated trajectory at this stage, it is still much better than buckled and deviated in a superior inferior fashion. The septum (and nose) is still deviated because of the dorsal attachment of the septal cartilage at the keystone area of the nasal bones. If the axis of the nasal bones remains even slightly deviated, the entire shortened septum will follow, and be off axis,

Fig. 7.22 Dorsal view of the nasal septum after caudal excision of excess septum, the entire dorsal septum now approaches the midline due to elasticity with no sutures required to move

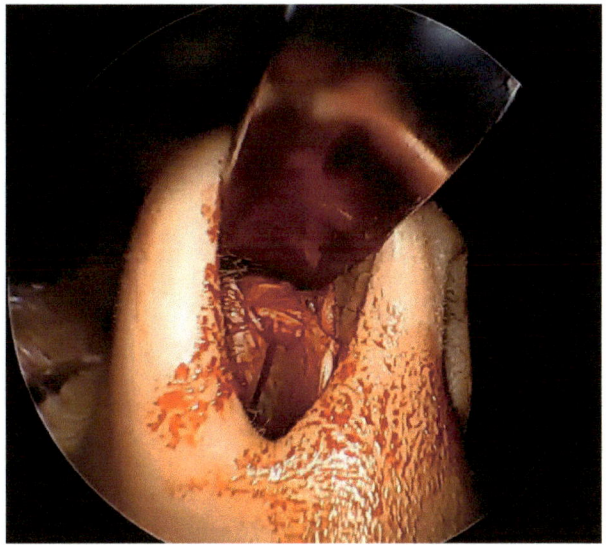

Fig. 7.23 Coronal (frontal) diagram of the SI+ septum with buckling. Despite straightening of the septum after removal of excess caudal septum, the septum is no longer deviated, but is still off axis as it is attached to the nasal bones superiorly, which themselves are still off axis. Only lateral osteotomy and straightening of these bones as a unit now that the septum is shortened will permit midline mobilization

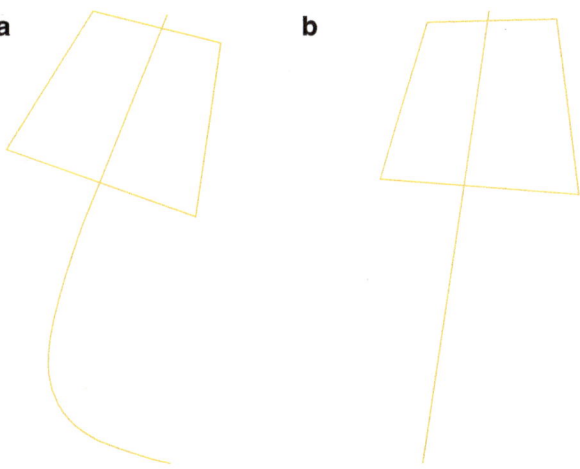

sometimes worse than pre-surgical, because the inferior attachments that kept the septum and nose "C"-shaped have now been released to give the nose a "/"—shape. Only complete lateral osteotomies (technically part of the release and reposition phases) will fix this problem, but ONLY after the inferior/caudal septum has been released and shortened, as otherwise, osteotomies in isolation will just rebound back to their original deviated position (traditionally called "memory") by those who camouflage.

The nasal bones are thus repositioned only after the release and re-size of the connected septal framework. A separate pyriform aperture stab incision is made, with periosteum elevated bluntly along the line of the osteotomy. A straight

Fig. 7.24 Skull model and diagram of osteotomy path. Yellow line is the trajectory of the path of lateral osteotome, separating nasal bones from maxilla at the naso-maxillary groove. The red line is the direction of fracture after the osteotome is rotated, thus in-fracturing the remainder of the cephalic bone

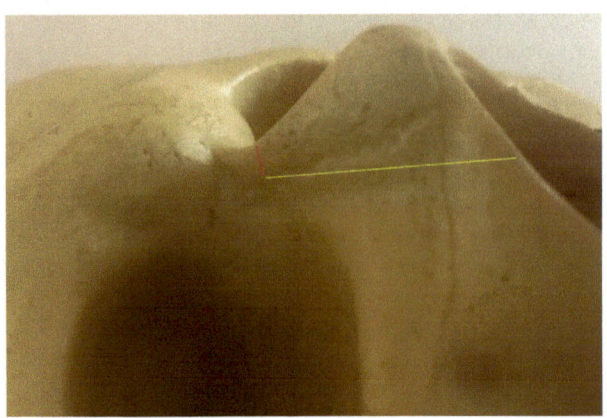

guarded osteotome is used to chisel a straight line through intersection of the nasal bones and the maxilla from their inferior extent to the level of the medial canthus, or top of the nasal bones. Once at its apex, the osteotome is twisted to medialize (or in-fracture) the bone (Fig. 7.24). Learning to perform osteotomies is mostly a "feel" process, so do not be discouraged if you cannot fully visualize this concept before you have done this yourself. The lateral osteotomy is performed on the side the nose is deviated AWAY from, in order to release a space between the maxilla and nasal bones for the opposite osteotomy to close. The contralateral osteotomy will straighten the entire nasal structure if the septum has been shortened and released appropriately, and very little resistance will be felt. Because of the release, these complete and straight osteotomies do not require external splints because the memory that causes the nasal bones to require additional manipulation and support should have been removed. If the axis of the nose is still deviated at this point, you may not have done enough shortening or release of the septum, or your osteotomies were incomplete. The majority of severely deviated noses are SI+, so the above is a good plan to re-size and reposition the common SI+ framework.

The final caveat with the SI+ nose is that even after shortening substantially the septum in individuals with the extremely long nose, or elderly individuals who have lost elasticity [6–8], the nasal tip will remain droopy and the tip will remain long. So, in addition to converting the septal height to SI neutral, the alar cartilages must be re-tensioned to a more superior position. This occurs in the elderly or in noses that have lost elasticity due to stretching of the spring-like ligaments (the scroll) that supported the alar cartilages to the pyriform aperture and septum. In a way, the "upper lateral cartilage" IS the suspensory spring ligament of the alar cartilages that gets stretched. So, using the endonasal alar re-tensioning technique described in the previous chapter, or using open rhinoplasty to reposition or shorten the alar cartilages can be a useful adjunct. The medial-most aspect of the residual upper lateral cartilage and even its attached mucosa can be shortened with great care in the extremely long SI++ nose to ensure adequate shortening.

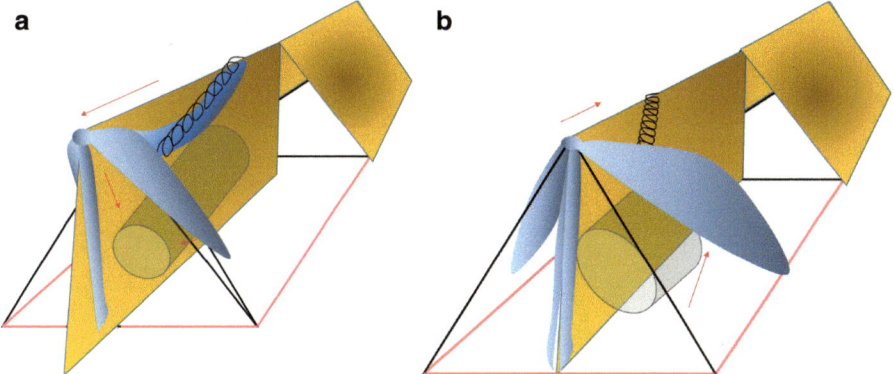

Fig. 7.25 Dynamic triangular prism model (DTPM) showing the (**a**) *stretched* spring support of the alar cartilage due to a supero-inferior excess (AP 0 SI+) framework. Pink indicates the foundation/substrate, golden yellow represents the framework, blue shows the canopy layer, here consisting of the paired medial and lateral crura of the alar cartilage and spring structure of the scroll. The grey cylinder represents the nasal inlet, supported by the external nose structures. (**b**) DTPM with natural recovery of spring support after shortening of the SI+ framework to SI 0 neutral framework. In this case, the spring is stretched, but has not lost its elastic rebound

Usually, however, especially with youth, lack of severe trauma, and moderate nasal length, as we can see from our DTPM, (Fig. 7.25a, b) shortening of the extruded SI+ caudal septum, will cause the alar cartilages to relax to a less inferiorly directed due to the intact and narrow position to a more superior position with airway widening, even with no further direct treatment.

SI−

But, what about SI− (overly short noses) septums? These can be more complex and challenging, but fortunately is an increasingly rare indication for rhinoplasty. First of all, because the septums are short in these individuals relative to the height of the pyriform aperture, there is usually little deviation to correct, and thus limited "crooked nose" or airway symptoms. Second, many females in particular desire a shorter nose in general so have fewer complaints than their longer-nosed peers. But, what about "over-rotation" and "decreased columellar show"?

First, as discussed above, rotation of the tip MUST be distinguished from shortening. Patients and physicians alike confuse over-rotation with shortening. Again, rotation is the angle of the columella relative to the lip that approaches 90° in males, and ideally 100° in females.

The SI− nose may have normal tip rotation, or tip over-rotation (turned-up), which can be dealt with, but should not be confused with nasal length. Decreased columellar show, or columellar retraction can be another sign of the SI− nose needing surgery. When the lateral alar rims descend below the columella, this is the condition that ensues and it can appear unattractive. It can also cause airway

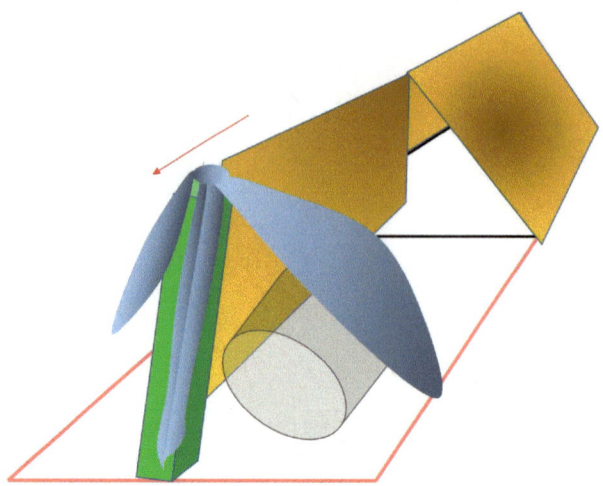

Fig. 7.26 Dynamic triangular prism model (DTPM) of the supero-inferior deficiency (AP 0 SI−) framework. Pink indicates the foundation/substrate, golden yellow represents the framework, blue shows the the canopy layer, here consisting of the paired medial and lateral crura of the alar cartilage and spring structure of the scroll. The grey cylinder represents the nasal inlet, supported by the external nose structures. The green structure is a caudal extension graft

obstruction because the funnel of the nasal inlet is not properly supported, and the columellar tissue collapses into the medial part of the nostril creating obstruction.

The good news, however, is that in most PRIMARY rhinoplasties, even the SI− nose can be improved via re-sizing and repositioning but not how you might imagine. The instinct of the rhinoplasty surgeon when confronted with the SI− nose is to use the commonly discussed "septal extension graft." This of course consists of another piece of cartilage or other material that overlaps the caudal part of the septum, fixated into position and then re-constituted to the columella (Fig. 7.26). I would imagine that these grafts are most useful in revision rhinoplasty or other conditions where the caudal septum is deficient from removal or complete destruction. I find them to be cumbersome, and despite their reputation, unpredictable and prone to shifting over time due to soft-tissue contracture.

In contrast, in most cases of SI− noses seeking primary rhinoplasty, the cause of the SI− deficiency is *displacement* not *absence* of the caudal septum. The caudal septum can be displaced inside the nose, as may be expected with a frontal-directed trauma that pushed the septum inward (or posteriorly). It can be displaced from its appropriate position interacting with the columella due to buckling internally, where the caudal septum is so displaced in its intranasal component (C or S shaped deformity), that the superior inferior height of the septum appears to be shortened caudally. Finally, in the most paradoxical displacement, in the severe AP+/SI− nose, a severe AP over-projection can draw the nasal tissues so far anteriorly that tension appears to shorten the nose, lifting the columella up against the caudal septum (Fig. 7.27). The treatment for all of SI− due to displacement? Release, re-size, and

Fig. 7.27 Lateral view of
the AP+ nose that
paradoxically gives almost
an SI– appearance

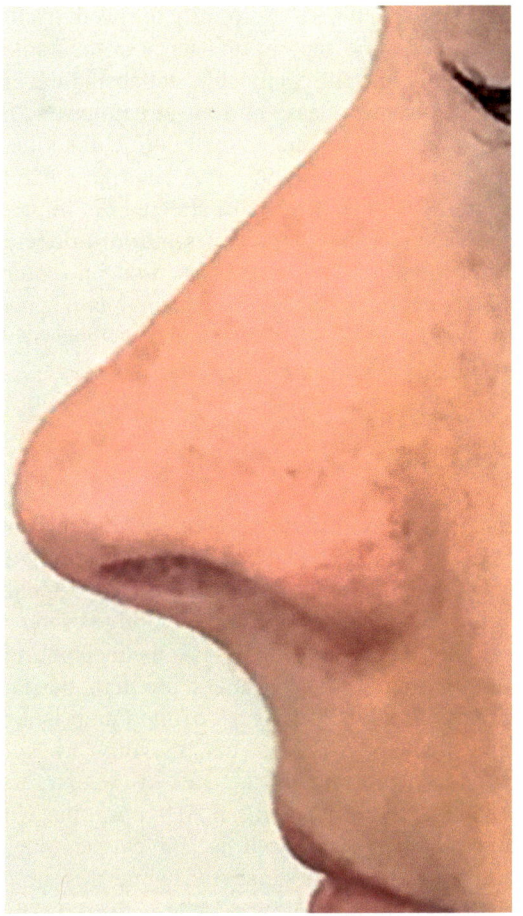

reposition. As expected, the septum that is vertically buckled and appearing short
due to inadequate pyriform aperture height can be lengthened to an SI (0) or neutral
position by correcting the buckling simply with release of the inferior septum and
removal of the maxillary crest and nasal spine that caused the septum to buckle.
Then, the inferior septum, if released from its restraining attachments to the upper
lateral cartilages and ethmoid (as described above in approach and release sections)
will mobilize due to its inherent elasticity to the midline and will appear longer as
it's no longer buckled.

In the AP+/SI– deformity, where the nose is so far over-projected that the nose
appears short and over-rotated, the simple treatment after release is to correct the
AP+ excess septum, which will not only make the septum appear longer relative to
its projection, it actually will lengthen to SI (0) neutral position because the tension that pulled the nasal tissues and columella anteriorly and superiorly will relax,
and the columella will take a more appropriate more inferior position relative to
the lip.

Finally, in the SI− deformity to severe frontal trauma, (typically a AP−/SI− configuration), the septum and nasal bone framework are displaced posteriorly and internally into the cavity, thus collapsing the entire external nasal framework. Only with extensive release of these structures and manual repositioning can the nose be restored in an AP and SI direction. Unlike the elasticity that allows a buckled septum to find the midline after appropriate release, the AP−/SI− traumatic nose requires manual externally directed dis-impaction, as it was internal impaction of the septum that caused the framework deficiency. Frequently, as the force of the impact was high, the dis-impaction can require an equal and opposite force, only once released. One must always maintain concern for excess traction on the septum to avoid avulsion of the septum or worse avulsion of the ethmoid cribiform with resultant cerebra-spinal-fluid leak.

AP+

There is no more classic patient seeking rhinoplasty maneuver than the one with the AP+ septum, frequently the AP+/SI+ configuration. This, perhaps, is one of the most common reasons for patients in the United States to seek rhinoplasty, mostly referring to their "bump" on the bridge of the nose.

The "bump," however, is just the metaphorical "tip of the iceberg" and is actually not the source of the aesthetic problem, despite what most believe. Thus, the commonly discussed "shaving" of the bump is a completely unsatisfactory procedure and should be avoided. This "shaving" procedure, while quite simple and effective sounding, just reduces the apex of the extruded septum and nasal bones, and after healing, the nose is still an AP+ nose, but with a chunk missing, that looks very operated appearing and is the classic "bad rhinoplasty" performed by well-intentioned practitioners. And while this simple procedure appeals to patients as well until they see the results, it is the duty of the operating surgeon to explain the lack of utility of the maneuver and to refuse to do it. Reducing the AP+ septum, however, to an AP (0) neutral septal position/size of course utilizes a different strategy than "shaving the bump," but is similar in limitedness of invasiveness and risk but more appropriately creates an aesthetic and functional solution.

Just as in the SI+ variation, exposure of the dorsal septum from caudal septum to anterior septal angle including the entire midline nasal bones must be completed as described in the approach and release phase. This is done via the full transfixion incision and includes complete sharp separation of the dorsal septum from the restraining upper lateral cartilages. Then, once the entire midline framework is visualized in a three-dimensional fashion from the anterior and posterior septal angles to the top of the nasal bones, the reduction can be completed. In the SI+/AP+ nose, the AP excess can be performed after the septum has already been shortened, and the anterior and posterior septal angle has essentially been mobilized superiorly. Now, the entire anterior (vertical) limb of the L-shaped strut (of course this is not shaped like an L because no posterior septum has been removed) is sharply reduced including in many cases the anterior septal angle (Fig. 7.28). This cut is carried up

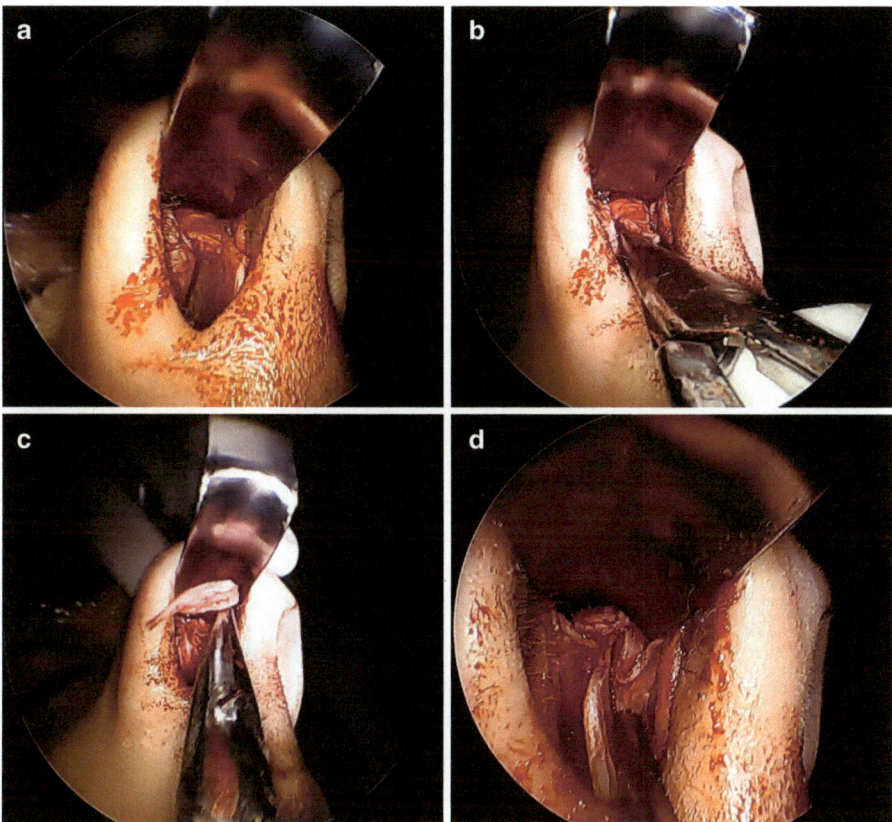

Fig. 7.28 Intra-operative view of the nasal dorsum (**a**) after caudal reduction but before dorsal reduction, with skin/canopy layer protected by Aufricht retractor and (**b**) during sharp scissors dorsal reduction, with skin/canopy layer protected by Aufricht retractor. (**c**) After dorsal reduction, showing V-shaped cartilaginous dorsal fragment. (**d**) Revealing reduced dorsum

to the nasal bones, where scissors and scalpel will no longer be useful due to the bony hardness. The removal can be as little as a single millimeter in mild cases, to over 5 mm of removal, depending on the degree of AP+ over-projection. Typically, the direction of this cut parallels the desired AP(0) neutral dorsum that is desired. At the nasal bones, despite prior adages that this is the true cause of the aesthetic deformity, the amount of reduction is only performed to match the parallel amount of cartilaginous septum removed. This transition area must be handled carefully either with conservative Ruben-style osteotome reduction or with substantial rasping (Fig. 7.29).

The AP+ nasal configuration is associated with a basal view deviation, in contrast to the SI+ front view deviation. This is because as the septum is overly extruded anteriorly, it is buckled in an AP direction. This is corrected with release, re-sizing, and repositioning of the entire septal/bony framework as discussed previously.

Fig. 7.29 Intra-operative view of the nasal dorsum after cartilaginous dorsal and caudal reduction, now engaging the midline nasal bones for bony dorsal reduction to match new cartilage projection using a 1 cm wide straight unguarded osteotome with skin/canopy layer protected by an Aufricht retractor

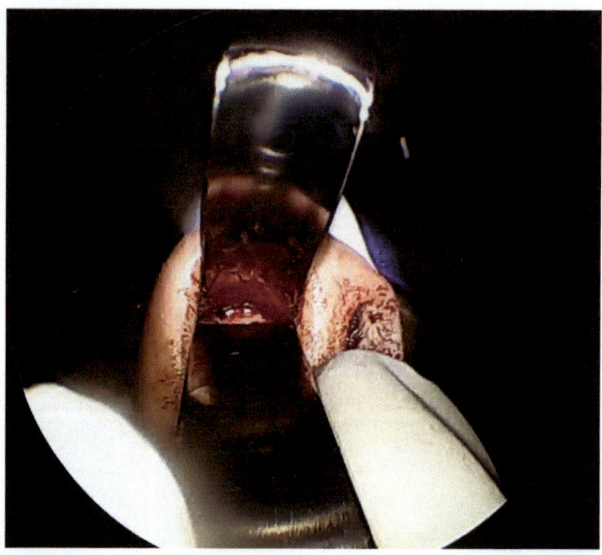

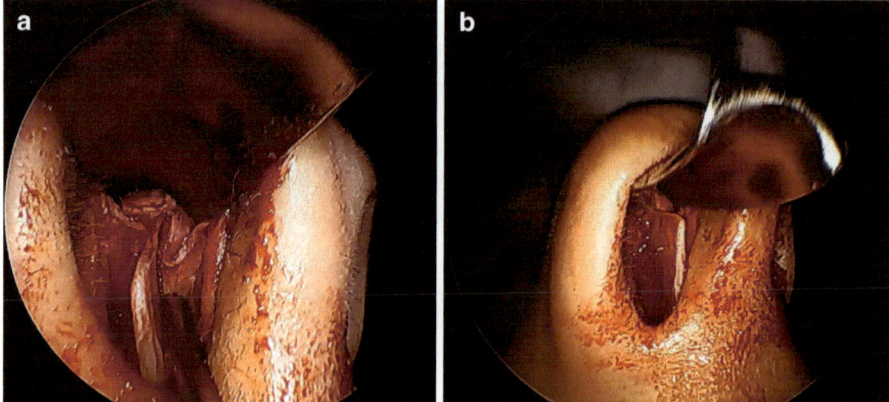

Fig. 7.30 Intra-operative view of the now antero-posterior supero-inferior neutral framework (AP 0 SI 0) revealing a (**a**) straight dorsum with no more buckling but still providing adequate support and (**b**) straight anterior septal angle

As with the SI+ nose, reduction of the AP+ nose to an AP(0) neutral position will as shown in our DTPM cause a relaxation of the tense alar cartilages and permit dilation of the nasal inlet simply by reducing the tension on the sidewalls. This is similar to the sidewall relaxation expected if a tent with overly long poles and narrowed walls had the pole framework replaced with appropriate size poles. Thus, as the profile of the nose and nasal framework is re-balanced with the underlying face and substrate, both aesthetics and function are corrected.

Before surgery is complete, the framework should be checked for straightness without tension (Fig. 7.30), that matches the external view of symmetry as well. The AP+/SI+ patient for whom the intra-operative pictures were generated is pictured pre- and post-operatively in Fig. 7.31. During the surgery, as I learned from my

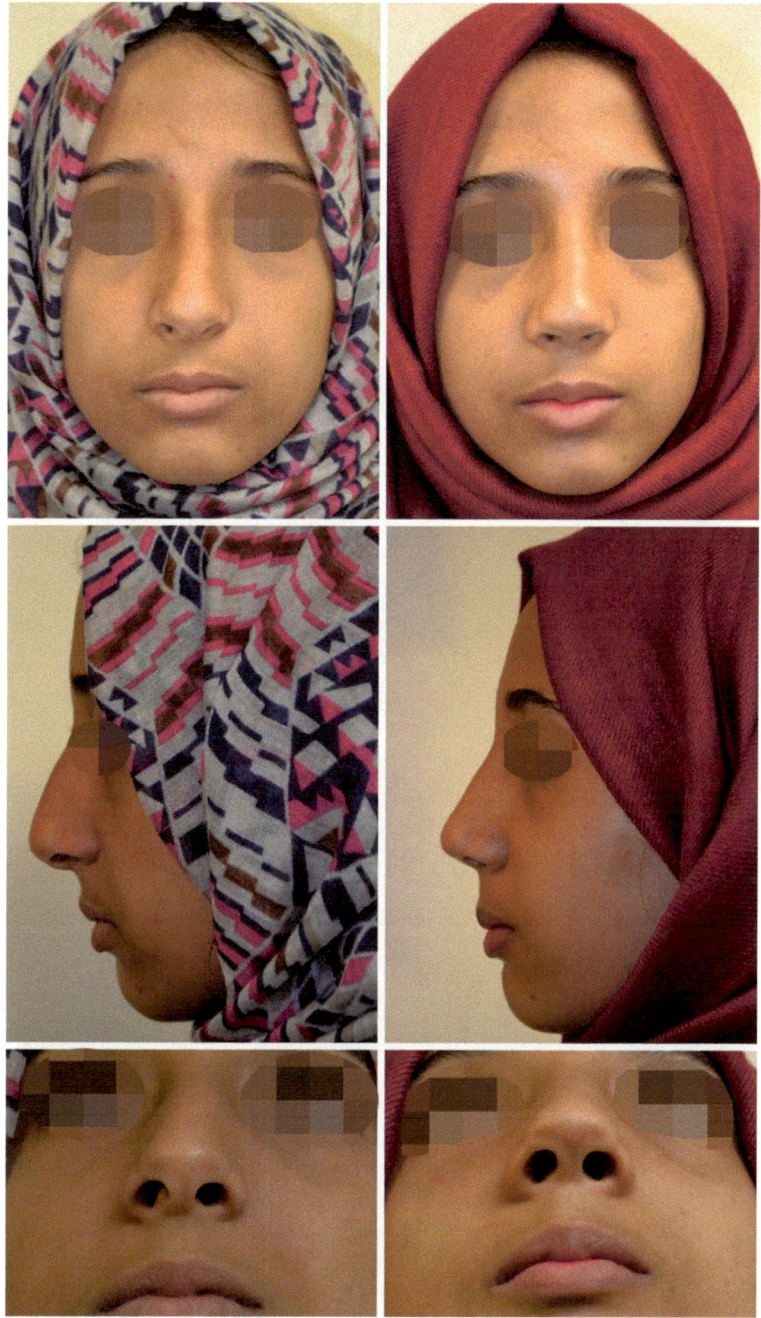

Fig. 7.31 Pre- (right side) and post-operative (left side) photographs of the patient pictured in the intra-operative photographs seen in this chapter. The top set is the frontal view, the middle the left lateral view, while the bottom is the base view. Notice the framework size reduction, improvement in lip-draping, and the size increase of the nasal inlet or nostril. (Photographs courtesy of Wolters-Kluwer). Stupak and Weinstock [10]

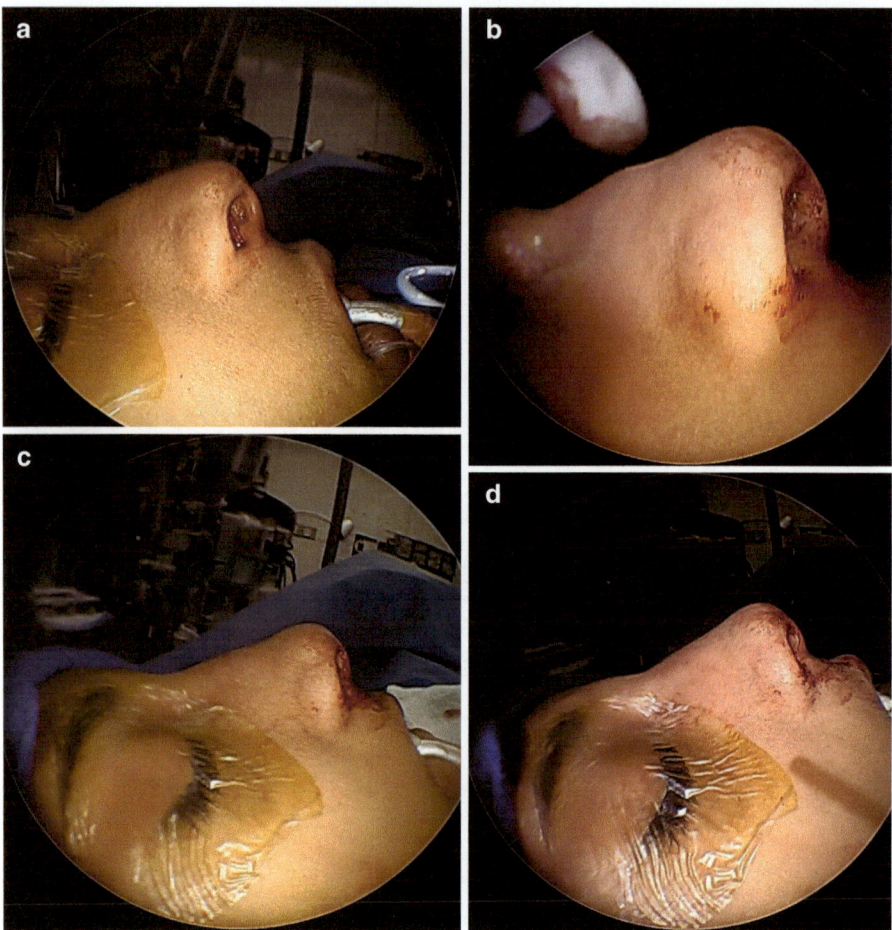

Fig. 7.32 Intra-operative photograph of various stages of the nasal dorsum during surgery. (**a**) The patient is pictured after prior to re-sizing and (**b**) the cartilaginous dorsum has been reduced, revealing a "saddle" relative to the bony dorsum. (**c**) After osteotome bony reduction where the bony dorsum is evened with the cartilaginous one and (**d**) after smoothing of the dorsum with the rasp and final caudal reduction

mentor Calvin M. Johnson, Jr., MD, the profile must be checked and rechecked as the procedure unfolds to confirm accuracy. In Fig. 7.32a, the patient is pictured after prior to re-sizing. In Fig. 7.32b, the cartilaginous dorsum has been reduced, revealing a "saddle" relative to the bony dorsum. This is reduced before Fig. 7.32c, where the bony dorsum is evened with the cartilaginous one, and finally, in 32D, the rasp has been used to smooth the remaining bony dorsum and to finalize septal shortening of the caudal septum.

AP−

Like the SI− phenotype, the AP− phenotype is a little more complicated in patients seeking primary rhinoplasty. Like our discussion of the SI− phenotype, the strategy for treatment can be counter-intuitive, even backward to what one might expect from the conventional world. Many patients who have a mild SI− deformity do not seek rhinoplasty unless the septum is substantially inadequate in supporting the bridge and nostril size (via support of the domal apex). Some configurations of the nose have an effective SI neutral position that is functionally and esthetically normal but would be considered SI− (negative) in patients of different geographic heritages. Thus, the SI neutral position is not a fixed one-size-fits-all for all-comers, but can vary both temporally and based on age, sex, and geographic heritage. The rhinoplasty surgeon must be a student of human aesthetics and desires and should have frank discussions with their patients about their beauty ideals. The description by the conventional literature of the "saddle nose deformity" is a classic SI− phenotype that is correctable without requiring addition of material as most authors imply.

The "saddle nose deformity" is characterized by a saddle shaped appearance of the middle third of the nose, where it is depressed relative to a prominent tip and bony dorsum. While most authors of course recommend augmenting this middle third deficit, there are much more thoughtful and less invasive alternatives present, as implants and grafts are much more prone to shifting, external extrusion and unnatural appearance over the long-term than most authors are willing to admit. Because of restrictions of the soft-tissue envelope of the middle third, simpler is better. The simplest way to restore the SI− nose, via the same approach we previously discussed is to release, re-size, and reposition the septum to its proper position, combined with a RELATIVE reduction in the bony dorsum to match the desired new cartilaginous dorsal position. The same strategy has both aesthetic and functional benefits simultaneously.

Like the other Compass configurations, the AP− (saddle) nose is usually not due to a completely missing or intrinsically absent septum, but a malpositioned one. Obviously, there are many exceptions to this including the total perforation cocaine nose or the over-reduction revision rhinoplasty nose. But, the traumatized and developmentally AP− nose usually have an inwardly displaced septum or L-strut, frequently buckled from its cramped position contained inside the bony nasal cavity and forced to compete with space with the bony septum. Once the septum adequately released from these bony attachments and the upper lateral cartilages, the septum can be rotated and reposition (if no remaining tension) to its more favorable external position. Sometimes this requires medial osteotomies to release the inwardly displaced bony keystone area from its impacted environment. Once at its new position, the cartilaginous septum can be palpable from the dorsal side and as an increasing support of the tip. Sometimes, the new position of the septum will manifest as well as SI+, interfering with the nasal spine, and either this spine can be removed, or the septum shortened and permitting full externalization of the anterior septum. The AP– configuration is always a challenge for me, and I find it far easier to perform AP+ maneuvers. This being said, there is little to lose in the attempt to reposition the AP– septum even if you have every intention of applying a graft to the dorsum or tip. The indirect approach described here has less complexity that can fail in the future.

Infinite Combinations to Tailor to Your Patients

Any combination of the above procedures can be imagined and performed to any degree. It all depends on first making the right diagnosis using the Rhinoplasty Compass (AP_SI_), then adequately approaching, releasing, re-sizing, and repositioning. As expected, the chiefly therapeutic phases of this surgery are the re-sizing and the repositioning phases. This is in stark contrast to the frequently discussed camouflage procedure of open rhinoplasty (approach) with grafts (reinforcement), both non-therapeutic phases. We will spend just a few moments on the reinforcement, as contrary to popular belief, it is rather irrelevant. But first, here are a few other samples of framework re-structuring rhinoplasty, as seen in Figs. 7.33, 7.34, 7.35, and 7.36.

Reinforcement

While many of us are taught the adage during residency that "the only thing the patient sees is the dressing," implying that this is the most important, I find that the opposite is true. I have seen many surgeons pride themselves on their cast-molding or precision taping technique but never achieving consistent results. This is because if tension is not released and structures not re-sized, no amount of pressure at the end of surgery will create any lasting effects, and of course the phenomenon known as "memory" will overwhelm and splint positioning during the course of time. So, in order not to excessively rely on external splints, I tend not to use them, as I must rely on the previous surgical phases to achieve any improvement. Besides, I have seen reactive or burned dorsal skin as a result of the splint.

While packing is never necessary, (better to let some bleeding egress externally) I do use Doyle splints to prevent synechia, re-approximate septal flaps, and to maintain a nasal airway. I think they also help stabilize the repositioned septum. Finally, we do use absorbable sutures to gently re-approximate the columella and caudal septum, to reinstate the transfixion incision. For me, less suturing is preferable, as it causes less soft-tissue trauma and diminishment of blood supply. In the severely shortened AP+ or SI+ noses, sometime the septal flaps need to be shortened to accommodate the shorter septum.

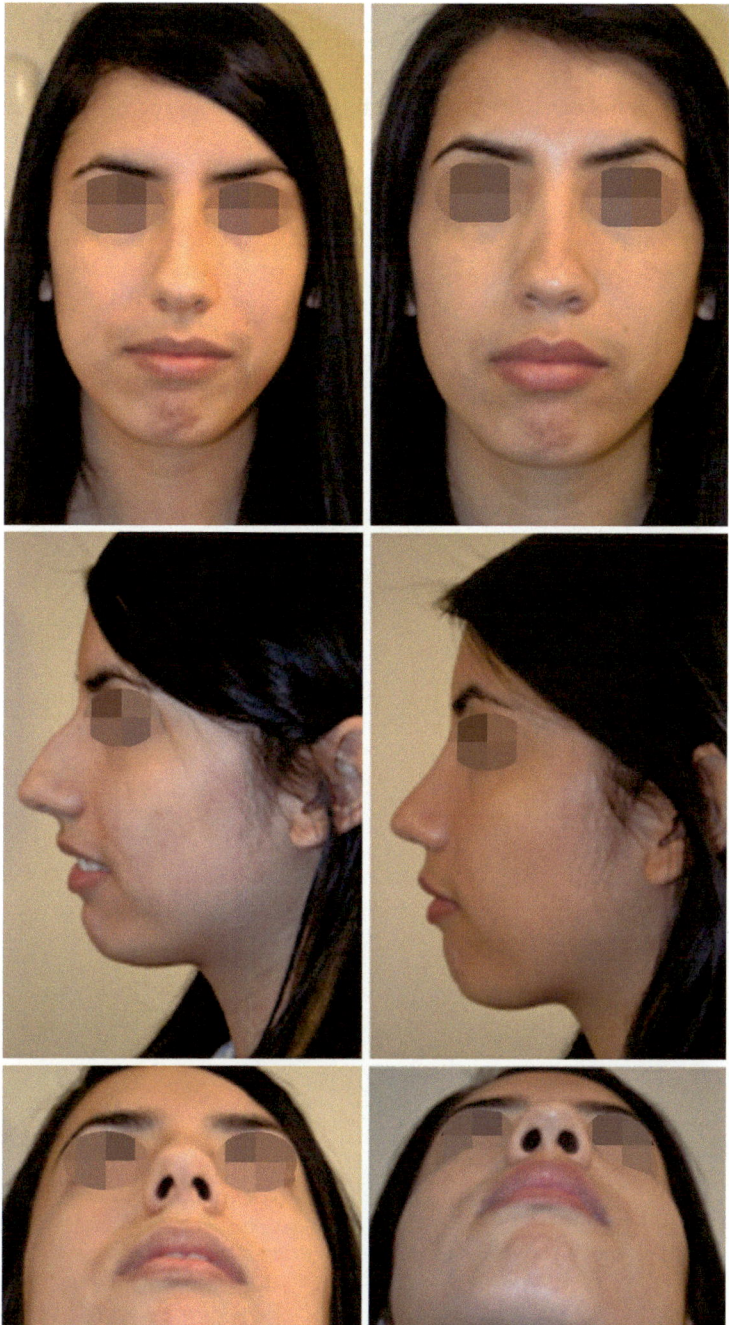

Fig. 7.33 Pre- (right side) and post-operative (left side) photographs of an AP+ SI+ (antero-posterior and superior excess patient). Left photographs are before surgery, right is after surgery. The top photographs show the frontal view. In the middle, the photographs show the left lateral view, while the bottom photographs represent the base view. Notice the framework size reduction and the size increase of the nasal inlet or nostril. (Photographs courtesy of Wolters-Kluwer). Shuaib et al. [9]

Finally, I do tape the dorsum theoretically to maintain the skin in approximation to the framework. In essence, the reinforcement phase is the least critical phase, and from my perspective should be the shortest phase, the surgeon doing as little as possible to maintain the extensive repositioning from the prior therapeutic phases.

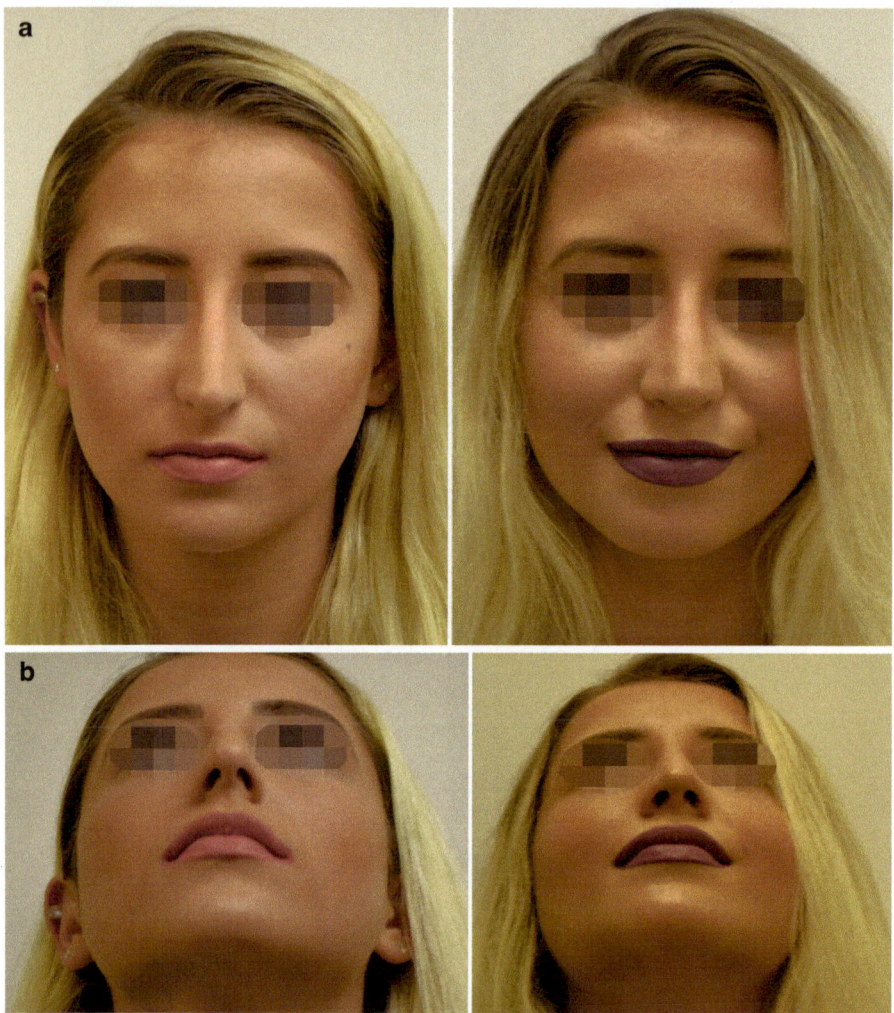

Fig. 7.34 Pre- (right side) and post-operative (left side) photographs of an AP+ SI 0 (antero-posterior excess supero-inferior neutral patient). (**a**) Frontal view, (**b**) base view, and (**c**) the right lateral view. Notice the framework size reduction, improvement in lip-draping, and the size increase of the nasal inlet or nostril

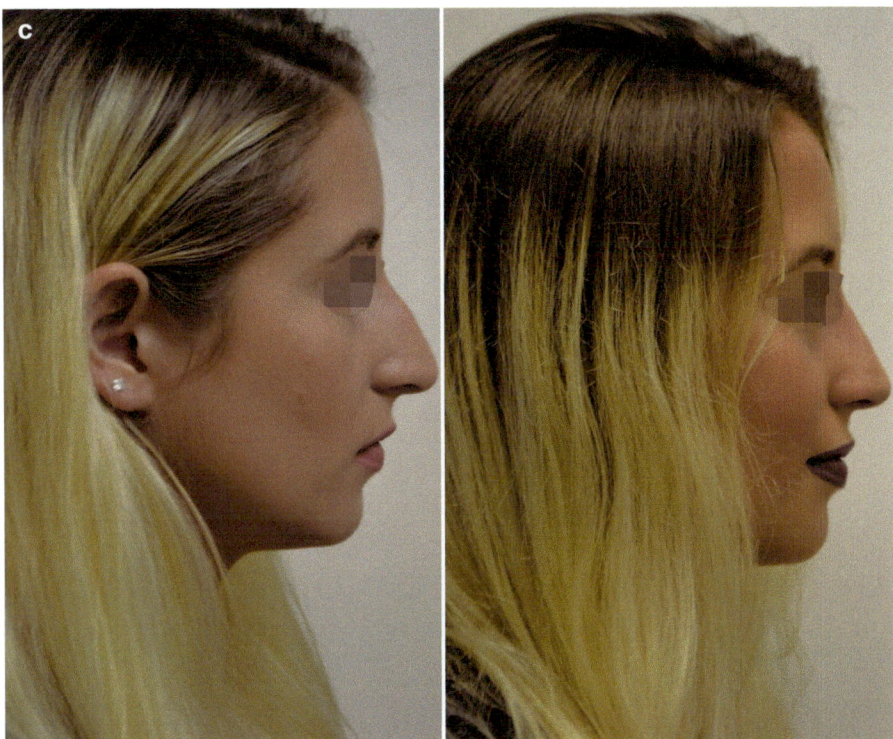

Fig. 7.34 (continued)

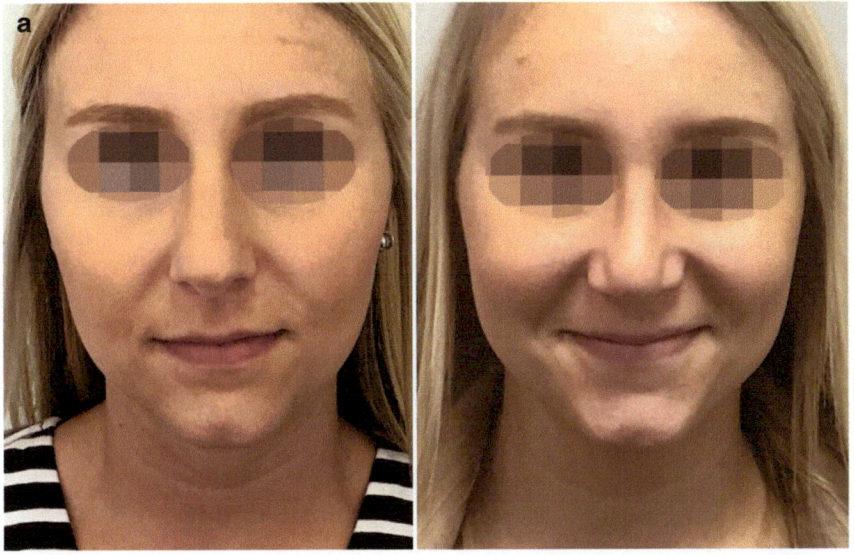

Fig. 7.35 Pre- (right side) and post-operative (left side) photographs of an AP+ SI 0 (antero-posterior excess supero-inferior neutral patient). (**a**) Frontal view, (**b**) base view, and (**c**) the right lateral view. Notice the framework size reduction, improvement in lip-draping, and the size increase of the nasal inlet or nostril. (Photographs courtesy of Springer). Hyman et al. [11]

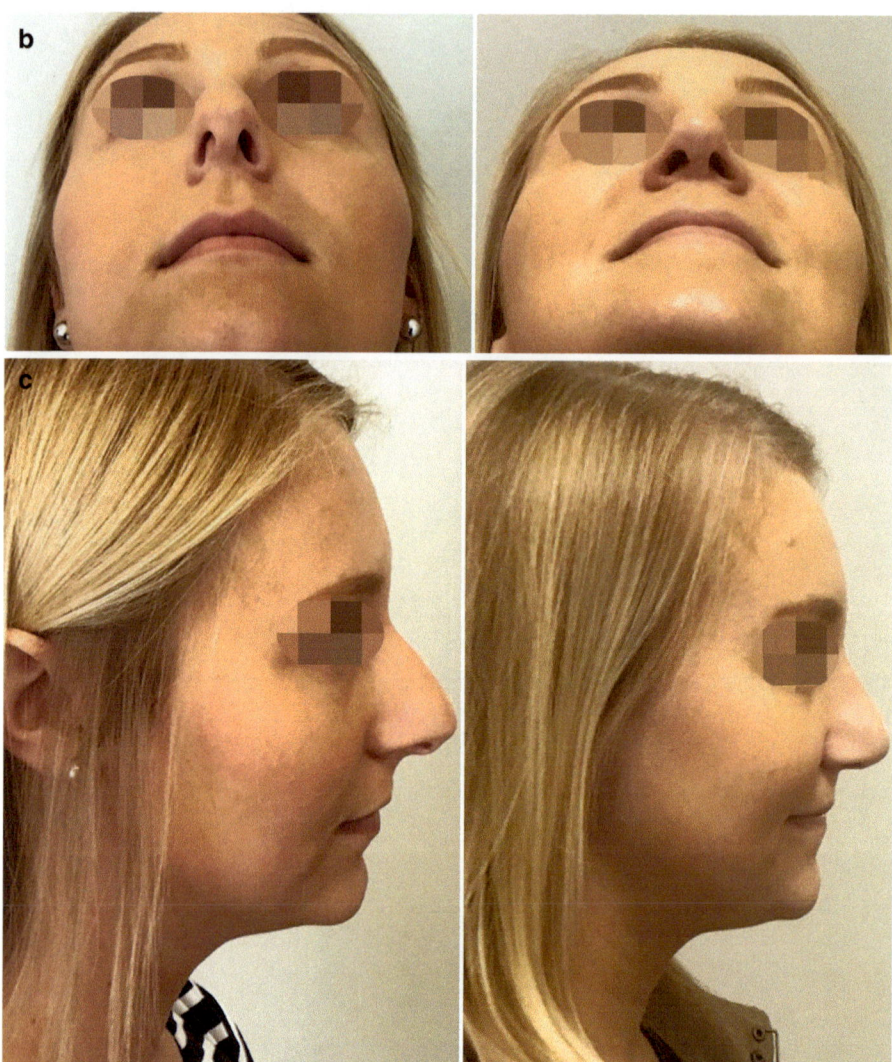

Fig. 7.35 (continued)

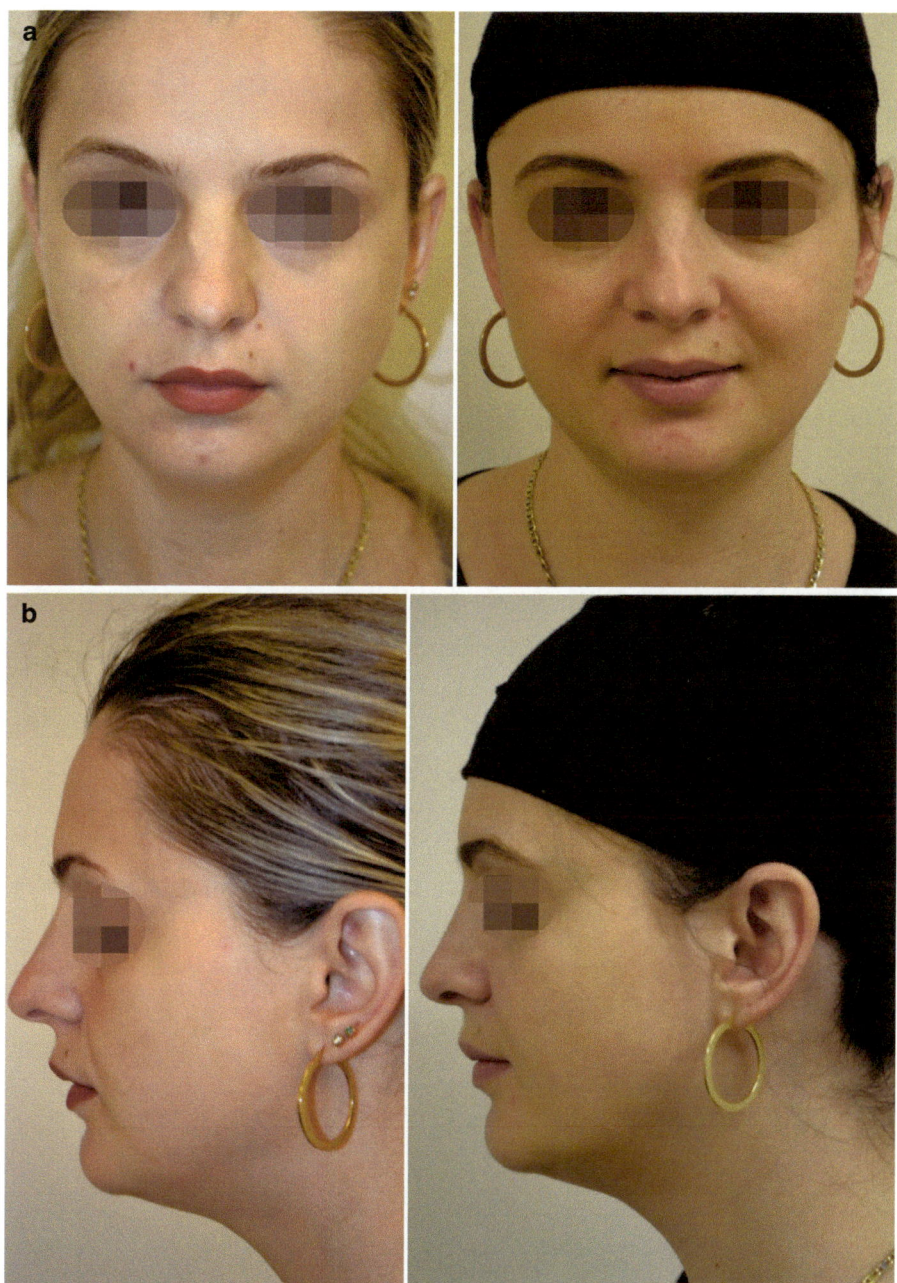

Fig. 7.36 Pre- (right side) and post-operative (left side) photographs of an AP+ SI+ (antero-posterior and superior excess patient). (**a**) shows the frontal view, (**b**) shows the left lateral view, and (**c**) shows the base view. Notice the framework size reduction, and the size increase of the nasal inlet or nostril. Rapid Eye Movement (stage) (REM) Apnea Hypopnea Index (AHI) improved from 34 to 9, while overall AHI improved from 9 to 2, with NOSE scores improving from 100 to 15. (Photographs courtesy of Wolters-Kluwer). Shuaib et al. [9]

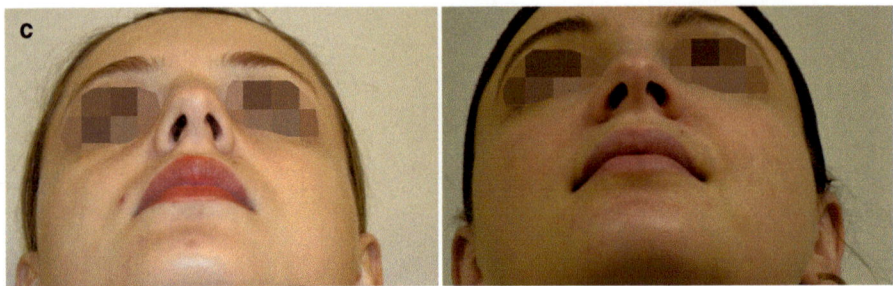

Fig. 7.36 (continued)

References

1. Ho Y, Deeb R, Westreich R, Lawson W. Effect of depressor septi resection in rhinoplasty on upper lip length. JAMA Facial Plast Surg. 2014;16(4):272–6.
2. Kridel RW, Scott BA, Foda HM. The tongue-in-groove technique in septorhinoplasty. A 10-year experience. Arch Facial Plast Surg. 1999;1(4):246–56; discussion 257.
3. Wilson MA, Mobley SR. Extracorporeal septoplasty: complications and new techniques. Arch Facial Plast Surg. 2011;13(2):85–90.
4. Orwell, G. Nineteen eighty-four. London: Harvill Secker; 1949.
5. Wong BJF, Friedman O, Hamilton GS 3rd. Grafting techniques in primary and revision rhinoplasty. Facial Plast Surg Clin North Am. 2018;26(2):205–23.
6. Toriumi DM, Rosenberger E. Rhinoplasty of the aging nose. Facial Plast Surg. 2016;32(1):59–69.
7. Stupak HD, Johnson CM Jr. Rhinoplasty for the aging nose. Ear Nose Throat J. 2006;85(3):154–5.
8. Quatela VC, Pearson JM. Management of the aging nose. Facial Plast Surg. 2009;25(4):215–21.
9. Shuaib SW, Undavia S, Lin J, Johnson CM Jr, Stupak HD. Can functional septorhinoplasty independently treat obstructive sleep apnea? Plast Reconstr Surg. 2015;135(6):1554–65.
10. Stupak HD, Weinstock M. Bony/cartilaginous mismatch: a radiologic investigation into the etiology of tension nose deformity. Plast Reconstr Surg. 2018;141(2):312–21.
11. Hyman AJ, Fastenberg JH, Stupak HD. Orientation of the premaxilla in the origin of septal deviation. Eur Arch Otorhinolaryngol. 2019;276(11):3147–51.

Chapter 8
Complementary Procedures to the Framework Strategy (The Canopy Layer)

For many events, roughly 80% of the effects come from 20% of the causes, [and the remaining 20% of effects come from the lower 80% of causes.]—Vilfredo Pareto

As in the classic 80-20 rule coined by Pareto (see above), I would very roughly estimate that 80% of the reason for seeking rhinoplasty is generally due to septal framework causes. This fits the concept, as perhaps this structure is only one of five major components of the nose with the nasal bones, upper lateral cartilages, lower lateral cartilages, and skin. Conversely, from my perspective, despite the widespread popularity of surgery of the tripod, in my opinion, the structure only accounts for 20% of structural problems because we mistakenly see indirect effects of the septal framework upon the tripod as being primarily due to the tripod itself. This, however, does not mean that the canopy layer is irrelevant, but just a little less so than commonly advertised. In the next section, we discuss how an understanding of this framework/tripod interaction can complement strategies utilized in the previous chapter.

Goal of Canopy Surgery

Re-sizing and repositioning the nasal framework is critical to achieving any efficacy in the rhinoplasty procedure. We have discussed treatment of the foundation and framework at length, including the root cause of the problem, and how to appropriately address the problem. But, what about surgery for the overlying canopy layer, which includes the skin and soft-tissue envelope and alar cartilages using the Dynamic Triangular Prism Model (DTPM)? As discussed in the previous chapter, MOST of the changes to the canopy are INDIRECT, with framework changes yielding changes in tension to the canopy layer (skin and alar cartilages). Indirect treatment is superior to direct treatment of this layer, as adding grafts or removing structure at this layer can create a much more unnatural appearance with forces of

© Springer Nature Switzerland AG 2020
H. D. Stupak, *Rethinking Rhinoplasty and Facial Surgery*,
https://doi.org/10.1007/978-3-030-44674-1_8

contracture in this layer having an oversized effect. Worse, attempting to overcome framework problems by adding structures (grafts) or sutures to the canopy is akin to modifying the roof of a residential structure while ignoring frame deficiencies. For this reason, cartilage "memory" and "warping" are cited as a frequent cause of failure in the open rhinoplasty "camouflage" procedures, where the real problem is the wrong layer was approached and treated. This chapter is thus not meant as an ALTERNATIVE to the framework procedure of the prior chapter (as come have previously conceived), but as a COMPLEMENT to framework improvements, which must be considered primary. In fact, it should be an uncommon occurrence to undertake rhinoplasty surgery simply for canopy layer modification. Problems in the canopy layer are almost always due to underlying structural framework problems, and the rare times that they are not, the surgery can be unwise to perform because canopy layer-only surgery can be less predictable, and the patients seeking this surgery may be overly self-critical.

Thus, the vastly most important and common reason to operate on the canopy layer is AFTER extensive re-sizing, to match the alar cartilages and skin and soft-tissue envelope to the newly re-sized nose. While the septum appeared over-size to the facial skeleton in the AP+ and SI+ configurations giving a long and prominent nose, after shortening and set-back, the entire nose is substantially smaller. The skin contracts to fit the new framework, and the elasticity of the alar cartilage will allow the tip to mobilize to a more superior and posterior position (DTPM figure). However, when there is a deficiency of elasticity of the skin, or alar cartilages, due either to age or an abundance of excess skin from a severe reduction, there is a tendency toward incomplete mobilization of the skin and tip. This can manifest as a persistently ptotic tip, a broad tip, or a wide nose due to excess skin and soft-tissue. This excess skin can recede and contract over time, and this can require a massive amount of patience to wait the shrinkage of the soft-tissue envelope to the new framework. In addition, in the severe AP+ or SI+ models, especially in older patients whose tissues have lost some elasticity, the lateral aspect of the lateral crura of the alar cartilage can stretch its ligamentous attachments to the spring-like scroll. Not only does this cause ptosis when the medial scroll is damaged, but loss of the central part of the scroll-spring can exacerbate a bulbous or broad tip, because the lateral crura essentially "roll up" from this loss of supportive tensioning much like the popular kid's "slap bracelet" in its curved configuration (Fig. 8.1).

The lateral crura furl like these spring bracelets when their natural scroll-spring tensing is lost. The crura in their ideal state are adhered to the upper lateral cartilage via the scroll, the lateral aspect to a fibrous connection to the pyriform aperture, and medially to the septum, and posteriorly to the vestibular mucosa. Loss of enough of specifically the lateral attachments will cause the flat crural cartilage to curl-up like a spring-loaded snap bracelet, while the medial domes remain in position. This can be readily seen if one has done enough cephalic trim via the open rhinoplasty approach. The careful observer will see that when performing the aggressive "cephalic trim," the cartilage will paradoxically curl more, making an even more "bulbous" or broad tip MORE broad. When both the medial and lateral portion of the scroll suspension spring are destroyed, tip ptosis can occur as well.

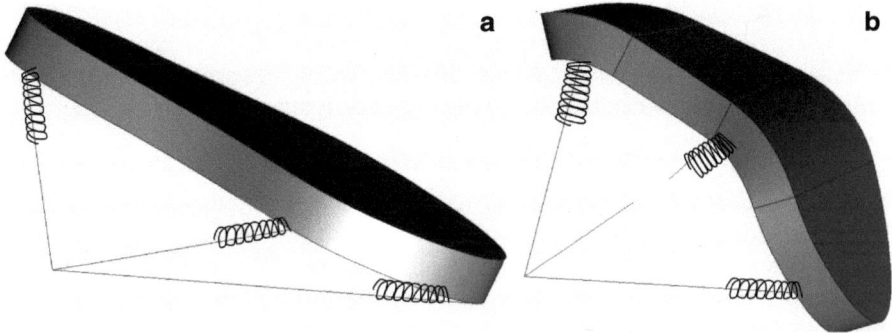

Fig. 8.1 Diagram of detail in (**a**) the spring (scroll) supported lateral crus retains its shape, (**b**) but if part of the scroll/spring is damaged, the lateral crus can curl-up or furl, creating the appearance of bulbosity to the nasal tip

The take-home message here is that after septal re-sizing and repositioning, there can be a size or positional nasal tip or alar cartilage disparity with the new framework structure. Is this a disaster that REQUIRES fixing? No, it does not. It is generally a subtle aesthetic disparity that can be ignored or even dealt with later. Actually, for surgeons just beginning to use the rhinoplasty compass and performing nasal re-sizing and repositioning, I advise against dealing with the (canopy layer) tip and skin directly and focus instead primarily on the framework. This way, you will not risk making the same mistake as many current surgeons to focus on various tactics in the canopy layer while missing the major flaw that must be addressed in the framework layer. Keeping the procedure as simple as possible while you are in a developmental phase will permit you to learn as much as possible about the simplicity of treating the framework and will you will not be confused by confounding factors.

The decision to approach the tip should not be taken lightly. The nasal re-framing surgery can be achieved almost exclusively through limited endonasal incisions. Re-sizing, repositioning, or re-supporting the tip cartilages also require an approach to first release the tensions that caused these problems.

If after successful framework surgery I anticipate a persistently ptotic, asymmetric, or broad tip, I initiate an open approach ONLY to skeletonize the alar cartilages. The open approach has been described at length in many texts and articles, so we will not waste your time with a lengthy discussion of it here. Essentially, using multiple point counter-traction, the alar domes and lateral crura are dissected in a subperichondrial plane after a columellar incision.

Once exposed, the cartilages can be seen and felt to be overly prominent relative to the framework, either in an inferior direction (ptosis), or bulging anteriorly or with excess lateral bowing. In theory, one could address all of these problems by identifying lateral crura and after extensive release, adjust the relationship or overlap with this structure with the scroll and upper lateral cartilage using an intercartilaginous incision (See re-tensioning procedures in Chap. 6).

My preference, however, is to completely re-size the entire canopy layer and alar cartilage to match the newly re-sized framework. The medial and lateral crura can be reduced with mucosal-sparing dome division. The domes are divided symmetrically from cephalic to caudal, preserving the underlying mucosal layer. The crura can be then separated sharply from medial to lateral, and once completely released from its deep attachments, the crura will overlap each other and must be trimmed by a few millimeters at the dome incision in order to reduce the redundancy and ptosis. If removed adequately, the medial and lateral crura will practically re-approximate of their own accord, creating a less-projecting, less bowed, and less ptotic tripod. Of course, to reinforce this, once the tension has been released, several sutures are placed to reinstate the domal architecture. Finally, to re-tense the lateral crura and prevent further reduce lateral bowing, the cephalic portion of the lateral crura are sutured together creating an "inter-crural" suture that over-rides the dorsal septum (Fig. 8.2).

In general, this is how simplified my approach to the tip is, in the relatively unusual circumstances that I do address this region. Even this limited approach causes collateral damage. Unfortunately, reducing the framework size, and then re-sizing the alar cartilages, despite the aesthetic and functional benefits does create an additional problem: Excess skin that early in the healing process can manifest as an imbalanced columellar scar especially in the early period despite a good result (Fig. 8.3a–d).

In general, the skin layer of the canopy will contract to match the new framework over a period of time. Unfortunately, it is hard to know how long this period is, and it can be very frustrating for patients and the surgeon to await its change. Frequently, it is a matter of weeks, sometimes months, and in some cases longer. The excess

Fig. 8.2 Diagram of (**a**) paired overly furled lateral crus of the alar cartilages with yellow mark indicating incision location for dome division. (**b**) After dome division and re-approximation of the alar cartilages with inter-crural re-approximation restores the tension that had been lost with an inadequately functioning scroll/spring

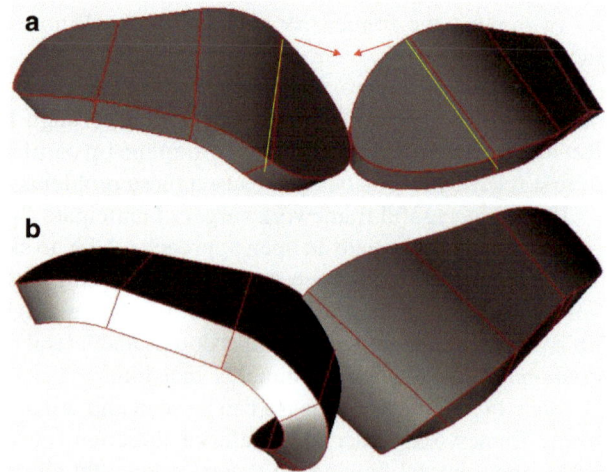

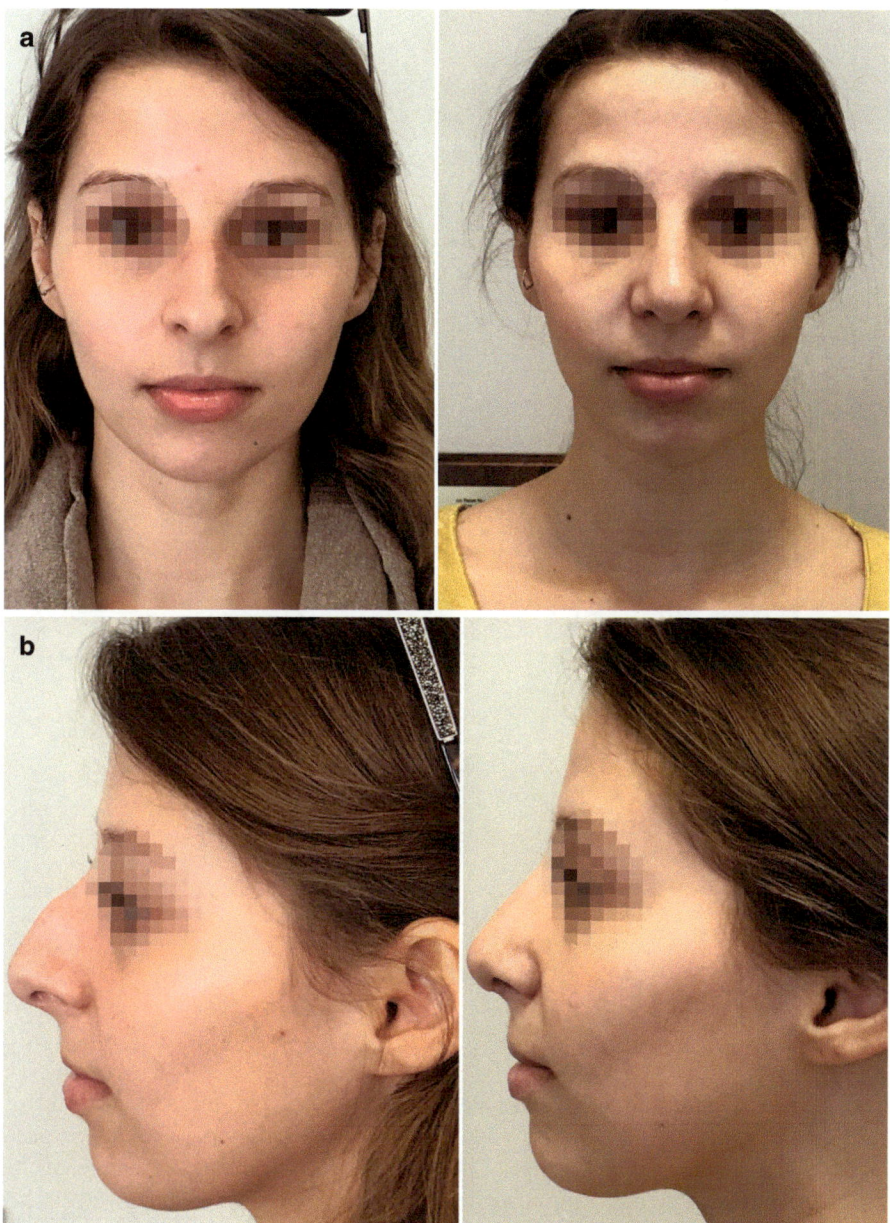

Fig. 8.3 Pre- (right side) and post-operative (left side) photographs of an AP+ SI 0 (antero-posterior excess supero-inferior neutral patient). (**a**) Frontal view, (**b**) left lateral view, (**c**) Right oblique view, and (**d**) base view

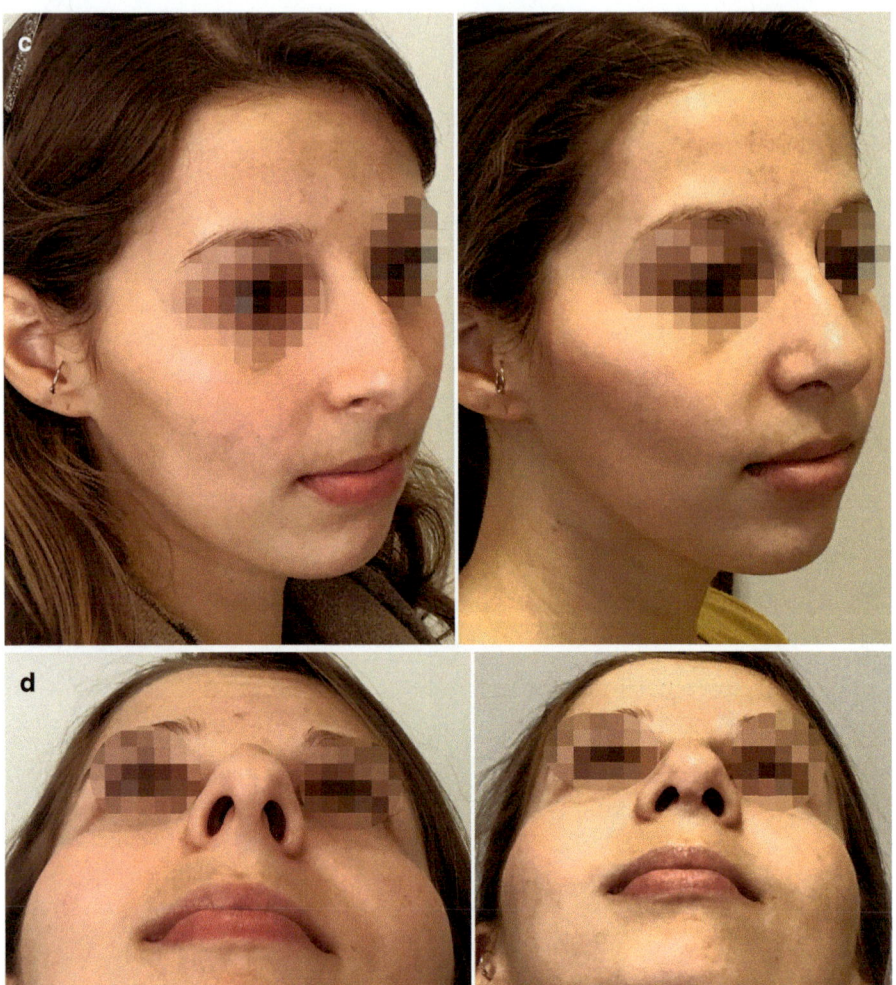

Fig. 8.3 (continued)

skin manifests almost exclusively in the nasal tip region, and in cases where the re-sizing was substantial, the tip can appear larger than its pre-operative appearance. This can be best managed with pre-operative counseling about the nature of this problem, and I frequently remind patients that the over-defined narrowed tip has almost completely gone out of style, and perhaps was never too attractive or functional. Steroid injections in the peri-operative period to the tip subdermis may be of use as well, but this is not clear, and I think this should be done conservatively to avoid discoloration of the skin.

While these conservative treatments take some patience, I have recently begun using a possibly more direct technique: skin excision at the columellar incision. In the severe re-sizing cases AP+/SI+ to AP 0/SI 0, where open rhinoplasty has been performed to re-size the tip and alar cartilages to match the framework layer, I began to notice that the tip-side of the columellar incision from the reduction in framework was so redundant that it literally overlapped the lip-side of the incision, in some cases by several millimeters. In some cases, despite vigilant attempts to close this incision in a level fashion, the mismatch of the two sides became quite apparent in very unfavorable scars that required multiple steroid injections and even consideration of scar revision much later. My mentor, Calvin Johnson, anticipated these problems, and his solution was to re-project the tip substantially using grafts, thus drawing the excess skin away from the incision. Others recommended excising skin from the dorsum [1–3].

Learning from the problem my own way, however, I began to excise a few millimeters of excess, much like in a rhytidectomy procedure, from the tip-side of the columellar incision (Fig. 8.4). The excised skin would have to match the W-shaped incision pattern of the other end of the incision, so this was not easy at first on the loose skin and was anxiety-provoking for me. Gradually, however the merits of matching the skin portion of the canopy layer to the alar cartilages and the underlying framework proved rewarding, albeit an imperfect solution. While the incision is flatter, the excision creates a slightly different texture pattern to the other end of the incision when viewed from the base. This being said, however, the improvement to the tip via removal of the excessive skin can be highly rewarding. Figure 8.5a shows overly enlarged tip cartilages right before surgery and after exposure. Figure 8.5b is the tip skin at the end of the procedure after reduction and reduction of the cartilage size as discussed above.

In other cases, complete endonasal release and repair of the scroll-spring combined with open lateral crural cartilage re-sizing can be useful with extreme tip ptosis or bulbosity to match the canopy to the re-sized framework. This combination of procedures must be done with great caution, as over-rotation can easily occur, and in general, I prefer using either one or the other.

Fig. 8.4 Diagram of broad nasal sill from front view, with orange ellipse demarcating area excised during sill reduction, with orange line indicating optional extension for additional dissection and mobilization. Green indicates the direction of mobilization

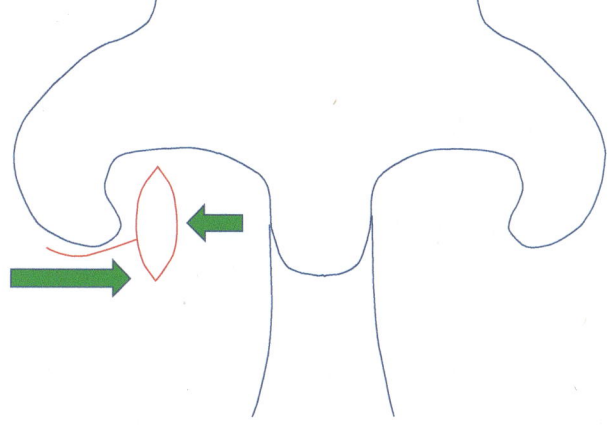

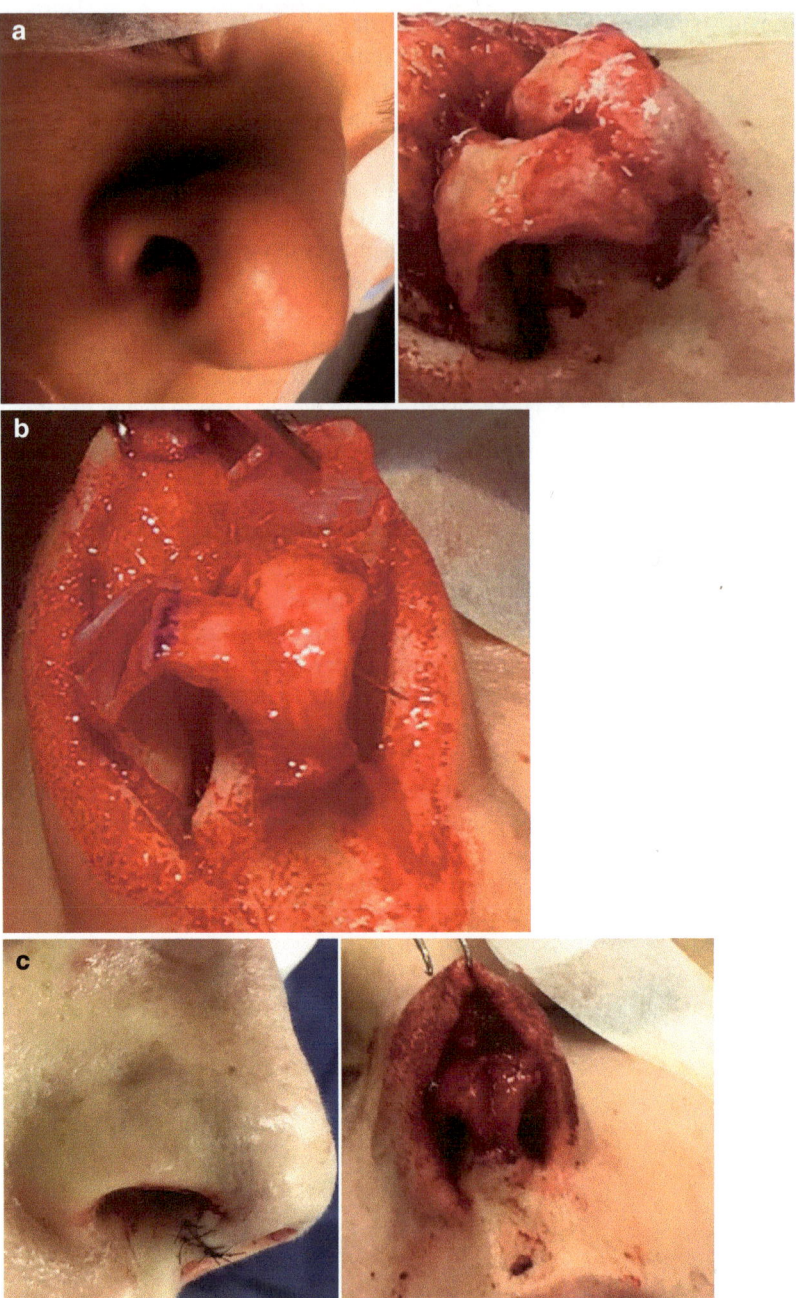

Fig. 8.5 Intra-operative view of "bulbous" lateral crura that are overly curled, after the completion of the intra-nasal framework re-sizing. (**a**) Left side shows bulbous tip before open approach. Right side shows the skeletonized bulbous over-sized crura. (**b**) After dome division and mucosal preservation (**c**) Left side shows skin after re-draping and re-sizing and tensioning of lateral crura, right side shows after domal re-approximation and re-sizing

Broad Nostrils and the Alar Base

In another canopy problem, particularly in the AP–/SI– case, the nose can appear overly flat and broad to the observer, sometimes with excessively wide nostrils. In these cases, the canopy/skin layer of the nasal sill or floor of the nostril can be effectively reduced. This is similar to the concept of the alar rim reductions of the lateral nostril [4, 5], except that effort is concentrated at the nasal sill. After an effort is made to change the framework from AP– to AP 0, thus narrowing the bridge and tip, including a septal repositioning and lateral osteotomy, an elliptical excision of nasal sill is made (Fig. 8.5), from mucosal to upper lip skin. Then, release is performed via sub-dermal undermining of the columella and alar side of the sill as much as possible to permit repositioning of the alar rims toward the midline. A relaxing incision can be created and eventually repaired along the inferior alar rim (Fig. 8.5). This sill excision and alar rim medial advancement can also create more bulk in the region over the diminutive nasal spine (pre-maxillary deficiency), giving the illusion of further improvement of the AP–/SI nose.

A final note on the canopy layer: Defocus both yours and the patient's attention away from the structures of the canopy layer (skin and tip). This can be accomplished by zeroing-in your efforts on the framework layer both in surgery and in consultation. This can be achieved by explaining how the canopy layer is simply a superficial layer that should be de-emphasized, regardless of what they read on the web or analyzed themselves. You will have less control over this layer than of the framework, so do not overstate expectations in an area where you might not deliver. Every time we make promises to patients that we cannot keep, we discredit ourselves and our profession.

Patient Selection

The strategy of release, re-size, and reposition of the nasal framework has broad application in rhinoplasty. However, as this is a strategy (e.g., problems occur because septum is oversized, so we can improve via septal re-sizing) and not a simple tactic (e.g., let's try spreader grafts to open the airway), the concept ONLY works if the septum is not of neutral size pre-operatively. Thus, patients who have undergone prior rhinoplasty with excessive lateral crural removal or reduction and have subsequently collapsed sidewalls and nostrils will not in any way benefit from septal re-sizing surgery if their septum is of neutral size AP and SI. Similarly, if excessive intra-nasal or external scarring and contracture has damaged the skin layer, or has caused nostril stenosis because of soft-tissue damage, no amount of nasal-re-sizing will fix this problem, and the patient will continue to have poor aesthetic and functional outcomes. So, my advice is to completely avoid the normal "tactical" thinking of "let's try that new nasal re-sizing procedure" in any cases where there is any doubt as to what the rhinoplasty compass diagnosis is, they are

AP/SI neutral, OR, when there is too much soft-tissue damage that even successful re-sizing or repositioning will be irrelevant because the tissue is already so damaged. This is not to say, however, that this strategy should not be employed in revision rhinoplasty. On the contrary, it is an excellent strategy for a "completion" version of a revision rhinoplasty where the otherwise decent nose remains over- or under-sized on the AP/SI compass, and simple maneuvers can neutralize this septum. In other words, if you have made a diagnosis using the rhinoplasty compass, and a patient reasonably agrees with this and has an adequate soft-tissue or canopy layer, there is no reason, if well-executed why you should not achieve surgical success.

References

1. Caterson SA, Singh M, Kueckelhaus M, Caterson EJ, Eriksson E. Skin excision as an adjunctive technique to rhinoplasty in middle-aged and elderly patients. Plast Reconstr Surg Glob Open. 2015;3(10):e532.
2. Quatela VC, Sherris DA, Johnson CM Jr. Skin excision revision rhinoplasty. Arch Otolaryngol Head Neck Surg. 1993;119(5):542–6; discussion 547.
3. Kabaker SS. An adjunctive technique to rhinoplasty of the aging nose. Head Neck Surg. 1980;2(4):276–81.
4. Ohba N, Ohba M. Preservation of nostril morphology in nasal base reduction. Aesthet Plast Surg. 2016;40(5):680–4.
5. Kridel RW, Castellano RD. A simplified approach to alar base reduction: a review of 124 patients over 20 years. Arch Facial Plast Surg. 2005;7(2):81–93. PubMed PMID: 15781717.

Chapter 9
Strategies for Addressing Mouth-Breathing Treatment with an "Adequate" Nose

Tis of little use ... for any to strive to get out of their elements, since it's natur' to stay in 'em, and natur' will have its way.—James Fenimore Cooper in Deerslayer

We have spent the past few chapters carefully explaining the difference between true nasal *obstruction* and the more common nasal *underuse*. We discussed how the symptomatology can be similar, and even experienced physicians can be confused between findings of actual blockage (cartilage or bone in non-ideal position), and reactive tissue enlargement due to chronic mouth-breathing (i.e., turbinate or adenoid hypertrophy). Once this concept was developed and we discussed strategy to differentiate the two opposing conditions, we spent Chaps. 7 and 8 describing a strategy to address, classify, and treat the *truly* obstructed nose. The goal of this chapter, in contrast, assumes that a patient has been confirmed to have an adequately functioning nose. *Adequate* function can be the result either after surgical framework repair, if they used a variety of nasal dilators that adequately restored the airway at night, or most commonly if they were fortunate enough to have a good enough nasal architecture to have a baseline adequately structured nose. If *these* patients are mouth-breathing, it is NOT due to nasal obstruction, but to nasal underuse related to tone and jaw/facial structure (see Chap. 5). To summarize, this underuse creates a buildup of negative pressure in the nasal cavities and sinuses, and the patient develop symptoms that mirror true nasal obstruction.

In this chapter, unlike the past two, we will employ strategy in this chapter to consider complementary treatments to prevent or treat nasal *underuse* (coined as disuse by Guilleminault and colleagues) [1], and not obstruction simply by utilizing tactics to achieve mouth-closure at night.

I will not pretend to know any one best way to achieve night-time jaw closure. Despite what most experts say, there probably is not one perfect one-size-fits-all solution. In lieu of an ideal solution, I will discuss alternatives to reverse jaw-relaxation mouth-breathing by breaking the concept into two main categories: I. The temporary, yet effective wearable or insertable mouth-closure device that can be very effective, but uncomfortable, and II. The long-term mouth-closure or

© Springer Nature Switzerland AG 2020
H. D. Stupak, *Rethinking Rhinoplasty and Facial Surgery*,
https://doi.org/10.1007/978-3-030-44674-1_9

musculoskeletal modification that can have nebulous outcomes but can be permanent and ideal if success is achieved.

Short-term (Temporary) Mouth-closure devices

1. Jaw-closure wearable devices (Garments/straps/tape)
2. Intra-oral appliances to support the jaws

   Long-term Mouth-closure solutions

3. Muscle re-training exercises (Myofunctional therapy)
4. Jaw expansion appliances
5. Jaw expansion surgery

Being an individual with a generally adequate nose but suffering from night-time jaw-relaxation, I myself am prone to night-time mouth-breathing, and thus when left untreated, like the rest of my fellow *Homo sapiens*, can experience the varied symptoms of nasal underuse (disuse). Because of this, I have through years of self-experimentation and practice found semi-successful solutions for my own problem. Also, as my father and one of my sons bear great resemblance to me, and face a similar problem of nightly jaw-relaxation, I have also been able to seek solutions for an older and younger variation of myself, and I will discuss these findings as well. These solutions are neither perfect nor the ideal solution, and I of course have not tested all of the possible variations, but I will begin with the answers that have brought me some personal success and also present what the evidence from the medical literature has to say about these solutions

Temporary Mouth-Closure Devices

Jaw closure wearable devices (Garments, straps, and tape)

As is obvious by the name, this class of therapeutic strategy involves the use of external devices, or even sleep position to keep the jaw closed during sleep where low tone stages cause relaxation of the muscles that support the jaw and lips, or worse, where counterproductive musculature actually causes jaw opening due to habitual mouth-breathing. I have found this class to be superior in achieving immediate results (and rest) compared to other classes, because if the device successfully keeps the jaw locked closed, the tongue will remain locked between the upper and lower jaws and thus cannot collapse into the airway. This strategy permits the adequately functioning nose to do its "job" humidifying the inspired air and maintaining a retro-lingual and retro-palatal column of air. Unfortunately, applying enough stable pressure to the undersurface of the jaw in the correct vector of lift can be both uncomfortable for the user (due to compressive pressure on the skin) and have a lack of stability if the patient is a restless sleeper. So, if an external jaw support device is too uncomfortable for the user, or too unstable during deep sleep, or does not provide enough force to counteract the forces of jaw opening, it will be useless. If the nasal airway is inadequate to independently provide respiration, the device is also not helpful, but as long as the lips are not taped shut (see below), mouth-breathing is still possible if the device was used inadvertently by someone with too much nasal obstruction, or who has developed acute nasal obstruction. Finally, recommending these devices to patients will frequently cause them to look at you like you have lost your mind. But, be persistent if you think it is warranted. They will thank you later.

A study from Taiwan testing a rudimentary silicone device that the authors called a POP (porous oral patch) used objective measures of efficacy of a mouth-closure device [2]. The study has one of the best explanations of how mouth-breathing, nasal obstruction, snoring, and sleep apnea are related. Although from my gathering, this brilliant paper is largely ignored by the surgical community.

The authors begin by introducing their project, "In patients with OSA, the mouth is opened during sleep and is associated with inferior movement of the mandible that decreases the pharyngeal diameter. Mouth opening during sleep is also accompanied by a reduction in the length of upper airway dilator muscles that lie between the mandible and the hyoid bone, which exacerbates snoring and OSA. Relief from severe nasal obstruction during sleep is related to a significant normalization of mouth breathing, enhancement of the sleep-stage architecture, and a modest reduction in the severity of OSA. However, many snoring individuals and patients with OSA are accustomed to opening their mouths during sleep in spite of the patent nasal pathway. In these patients, the symptoms of snoring and OSA may persist despite undergoing nasal or oropharyngeal surgery. Therefore, close-mouth-breathing must be maintained during sleep to reduce snoring and OSA for these patients. Conventional dental appliances may stabilize the upper airway by preventing the mouth from falling open during sleep. However, the dental appliance may cause excessive salivation, temporomandibular joint discomfort, and changes in occlusive alignment. This study used a porous oral patch (POP) to treat patients with mild OSA and OMB during sleep. The subjective and objective outcomes were evaluated" [2].

They went on to describe their study as a "prospective study conducted on patients who complained of snoring and habitual mouth opening during sleep, as observed by the bed partner. Each patient underwent a complete workup, including a thorough medical history review, physical examination, overnight polysomnography, and fiberoptic nasopharyngolaryngoscopy with the Mueller maneuver." They enrolled patients with mild obstructive sleep apnea (OSA) by polysomnogram, and excluded patients with severe pathology like very large tonsils or severely obstructed septal deviation after institutional review board approval. The patches worn by the patients, called the Porous Oral Patch (POP), consisted of a silicone sheet, and polyurethane foam and film, and is placed over the mouth during sleep, sealing the oral opening. They tested this over three nights and measured subjective and objective polysomnographic and cephalometric outcomes, compared using statistical measures. In this 30 patient study, "Every individual was able to sleep while wearing a POP and did not appear to have removed it … The median Apnea hypopnea index (AHI) score was significantly decreased by using a POP from 12.0 per hour before treatment to 7.8 per hour during treatment ($P < 0.01$ Wilcoxon Rank Test)." The

POP also radically improved symptoms of snoring, dry mouth, and drooling as well as cephalometric airway measures [2].

The research team wisely evaluated *"only patients without nasal obstructions,"* revealing their insight into the cause of the mouth-breathing (not the nose, but tone!). The flaw of the study besides its relatively small number of patients is possibly that the design of the device could be improved. Specifically, if you look at the figure, the device only closes the lips. However, while they discuss chin straps, I have found from personal experience that support of the jaw in a closed position is critical to mouth-closure efficacy and simply closing the lips is not enough [2].

While one study one showed no objective improvement in AHI [3], when looking at the chin strap utilized by the researchers, it is obvious that this device is neither stable nor lifting of the chin, but quite flimsy with the incorrect vector of lift. If the device fails to close the jaw comfortably during the night, the device is automatically a failure. However, failure of a single device does not mean that mouth-closure does not prevent apnea. This is an error in logic. It is my opinion that with complete mouth-closure, apneas will cease. However, because no treatment studied adequately achieves *complete* mouth-closure, we are led to believe that mouth-closure is only a footnote in the management of sleep apnea, especially when we are motivated to find a surgical option. In reality, it is likely that the efficacy of the treatment is proportional to the degree of the mouth-closure. However, the better the device achieves mouth-closure during sleep (which requires substantial force), the less comfortable the device will feel.

Personal Experience and Thoughts on Temporary Mouth-Closure Devices

At some point several years ago, around age 42, I became aware that I was snoring, (my wife let me know) and mouth-breathing (I awoke with a dry mouth), particularly when supine, or after a very long day that left me exhausted. Initially, I assumed that this was the inevitable manifestation of age and paid it little attention. At around this same period, I was working with a device company in the development of a nasal valve device to treat obstruction. During this time, a particularly astute executive with the company named Joel Granier told me that he was puzzled how the nose was involved with sleep apnea. Initially, I responded that by most accounts the literature reported only a slight symptomatic association between the two, and that largely nasal surgery could only be performed to "improve CPAP compliance," as was the mantra of the time. But, the question got me thinking, and after some investigation, and even some clinical studies I became convinced that the nose was intimately related to OSA, and that the primary culprit was obstruction of the nasal valve. So, applying the concept to myself, I began to self-experiment with Breatheright™ strips of many varieties, even doing home sleep studies on myself to test efficacy. However, this was to almost no avail as the strips at best marginally improved my symptoms, despite diminishing any nasal blockage. How, I wondered, could mouth-breathing be the problem, when improving nasal airflow did nothing to alleviate my OSA symptoms or AHI?

Unexpectedly, a cleaning by a dental hygienist turned-up the solution in ways I never could have imagined. My hygienist at the time, who eventually attended dental school noticed excess plaque on the lingual surface of my lower incisors, and he told me that this meant that my mouth-breathing at night was quite severe. I of course informed him that I was aware of this and had been studying the problem for years and self-treating. He patiently listened to my explanation, and then suggested that I tape my mouth closed at night, as he had heard of this concept from an expert in California on YouTube™. After I was done laughing and ridiculing the foolishness of his suggestion, I looked up the videos he suggested that night. But, as foolish as it sounded, I couldn't resist trying it that very night. Amazingly, my wife informed me that I had less snoring that night, and I experienced less dry throat sensation on waking up and had more energy the next day. The lip taping was a huge step in the right direction toward the basic understanding that mouth-breathing was independent from nasal obstruction. In other words, I previously thought, as counter-intuitive as this sounds that nasal obstruction was THE cause of mouth-breathing, as I suspect many of my fellow clinicians do. As I was learning, though, mouth-breathing is actually related jaw-relaxation, NOT blockage of the nose (see Chap. 5). So, I finally switched my goal of attempting to solely dilate the nasal valve of myself and OSA patients, and re-focused the goal on maintaining an ADEQUATE nasal airway with nasal dilators or valve/septal surgery but more importantly supporting jaw, lip, and mouth-closure during sleep. Over time, the simple mouth tape evolved into peri-oral taping, and very strong jaw support tape that was adequate to keep the mouth entirely closed at night even with some loosening with salivation or stretching. I tested the jaw/mouth-closure taping on myself combined with nasal dilator tape using a Watermark home sleep study test system all night in the supine position with three nights with, and three nights without the device (unpublished data—Fig. 9.1). As you can see, my supine AHI decreased from the mid-teens to the low single digits, as in the POP study. Multiple family members use similar systems, from diving hoods cut to support the chin, to commercially available anti-snore devices. For all of us, jaw support devices, regardless of the style, material or type has been life-changing, and has the possibility to improve the lives of millions of people who have symptoms of nasal underuse/nasal disuse or mouth-breathing, many of which are currently treated in a compartmentalized fashion by many types of providers, and includes, headache, facial pressure, negative ear pressure (popping and hearing loss), sore throat, upper respiratory infection (URI), and the many variations of chronic fatigue (actually sleep apnea). Currently, we are in the early stages of obtaining Institutional Review of a clinical study that tests split-night sleep studies using jaw support devices in adult and pediatric patients in patients with an adequate functioning nose. As mentioned, the "Catch-22" of jaw support devices that keep the mouth closed is that efficacy is inversely proportional to comfort. In other words, there is a substantial amount of force required to reverse the pull of gravity to maintain a stable jaw closure for the

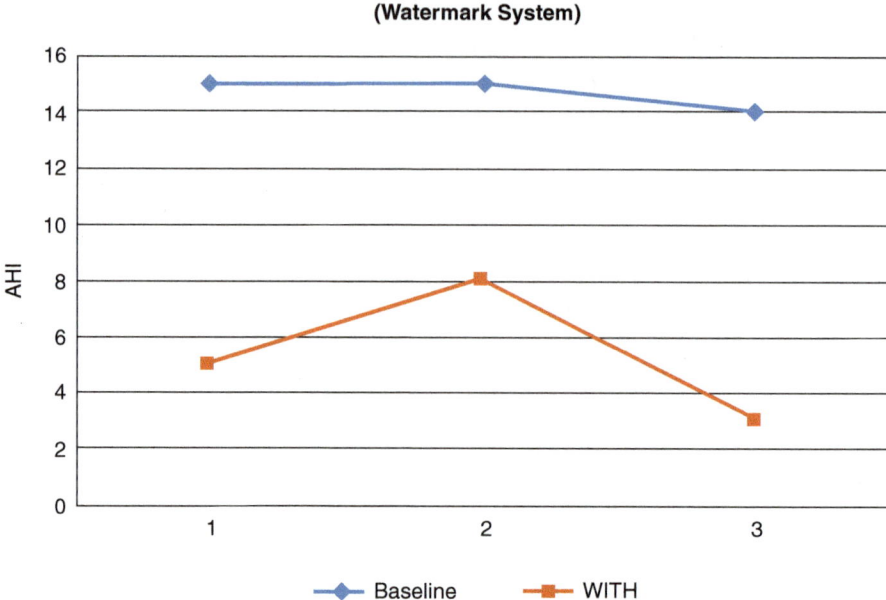

Fig. 9.1 Supine AHI (*Y*-axis) of author in 2015 over three nights (*x*-axis), both with (blue) and without (orange) the jaw closure device (three nights each for a total of six nights) using the Watermark home sleep study system

duration of the night. This force can feel quite uncomfortable on top of the head or as tape pulling on the cheekbones. The device is ineffective if it is too uncomfortable to wear, and ineffective if it fails to completely lift the jaw to a closed position. A common error is to use a jaw closure device like a chin strap that either uses the incorrect vector, or is so "comfortable" and slim that it fails to close the mouth. This "comfortable" jaw strap stays on possibly, but fails to do its job, and the wearer instead of trying a more effective but less comfortable version assumes that the jaw-closure concept is ineffective, so abandons it completely. The ideal device worn externally could be a web of jaw supporting tape, anchored to the zygomatic arch skin under some tension or could be a tight "diving hood" type device that has a broad vector of vertical lift below the chin, and diffuses the pinpoint tension of a typical narrow chin strap over the surface of the scalp. Finally, it will be resistant to sweat and saliva, as well as resistant to dislodgement during restless sleep. Can this ideal device be found? Probably, but may end up as different solutions for different individuals, instead of a perfect solution for all. Even in my own family, I use Durapore™ tape from 3 M, one of my children uses a modified latex diving hood with ear-holes cut, while a parent uses a continuous positive airway pressure (CPAP) device. All with generally the same problem to various degrees, but with multiple solutions due to personal comforts and preferences.

Oral Appliances

There is a tremendous amount of information about oral appliances and sleep apnea in the literature and on the web. I have no problem with the use of oral appliances for OSA as long as they keep the mouth closed and do not cause chronic change to occlusion or function of the temporomandibular joint (both real possibilities). To paraphrase Douglas Adams in his fictional two-word entry of the description of the planet earth in "The hitchhikers guide to the galaxy," all I can say about these devices in general is that to me, they appear generally benign [4].

The jaw advancement devices that take mouth-closure to a new level (beyond normal occlusive closure) sound particularly uncomfortable to me, and I have no desire to test these devices, nor do I have an interest in exploring the temporomandibular joint discomfort that I would imagine goes along with these devices. The literature seems to consider the effects of the mandibular advancement devices (MAD) as controversial on its effects on the bite or Temperomandibular joint (TMJ) condyle [6, 7].

A final note on temporary mouth-closure devices: Mouth or jaw closure devices should only be used with an adequate nasal airway. This means being able to breathe comfortably for several minutes in the office with the mouth closed and not any occasional mouth-breaths. In an ideal world, for physicians to recommend these devices, a physical exam that determines that the nasal airway is adequate, a NOSE score below 30 [5], or use of a device like the thermal imaging device that has a ΔT value above the threshold considered as an adequately functioning nose would be assessed before recommending or dispensing one of these devices (see Chap. 5). The combination of these assessments could be stored in a document similar to the audiogram and could be called a "thermo-nasogram."

Most importantly, after functional rhinoplasty, where the main goal may be to convert one from a mouth-breathing individual to a nasal-breathing individual, once the adequate nasal airway has been established, jaw support or mouth-closure devices may make an excellent adjunctive treatment modality.

Long-Term Strategies to Prevent Mouth-Breathing via Musculoskeletal Improvement

The long-term, but less direct approach to prevention of mouth-breathing is to attempt to enhance the musculoskeletal function and structure to encourage nocturnal closure of the jaw. There is much written about this online, and in the medical literature, and there are many approaches employed in this process. However, because it is by definition an *indirect* treatment, instead of the direct mouth-closure techniques from the previous section, there is really no way to know for certain that these long-term techniques truly work. Clinical studies are helpful, as we can see shortly, but because there are so many confounding variables, like continued growth in children and people who concurrently use multiple techniques, I find that even good clinical data from very reliable sources cannot be completely reliable. From a reasoning perspective, I recommend using short-term mouth-closure devices or positioning (avoiding the supine position during sleep as this is most apnea and mouth-breathing prone) [8] while concurrently pursuing long-term solutions. I do this both for myself, my family, and I recommend this to my patients too.

Myofunctional Therapy

First, I will discuss an entity known as "myofunctional therapy," which is essentially a version of physical therapy designed to strengthen the tongue and jaw muscles to encourage nightly jaw closure. This therapy is typically coached by someone from the dental profession, frequently an individual trained along the dental hygiene pathway with extensive knowledge of non-procedural care of the oral cavity. Myofunctional therapy consists of isometric and isotonic exercise that target the function of the lip as well as the structures of the pharynx. Despite a heterogeneity of exercises, a systematic review and meta-analysis by Camacho et al. showed a consistent improvement (approximately 50% AHI reduction) in objective sleep measures by polysomnography in all age groups [9]. While the exercises were variable, the effects were consistent, raising into question how exactly the therapy improves sleep function. Is it overall muscle tone increases, a reduction in fatty deposits, or just awareness by the individual to maintain mouth-closure?

Another study compared myofunctional therapy and something called "passive" myofunctional therapy which consisted of a beaded device contained in the mouth during the night. They noted a major problem with compliance and myofunctional therapy, and that even objective results could be distorted due to high drop-out rates in studies. Their study preferred the "passive" device, but in reality, this is really an oral appliance (see prior section) and faces the same consideration of results on TMJ function and occlusion and does not really involve exercises besides the patient being instructed to "roll" the intra-oral bead at night [10].

My son and I are participating in a myofunctional therapy program for the past 6 months with a very engaging, thoughtful, and intelligent therapist named Sarah Hornsby RD, of Seattle, Washington. The excercises are varied and seem useful for strengthening the muscles of the lips and tongue. My favorite one involves lip strengthening by holding a weighted popsicle stick between the lips for 10 minute intervals. I feel like I had a lip "workout" with all of the usual soreness of classic weight-lifting but just on the lips. Another really positive one was to hold a plastic disk on the roof of the mouth while maintaining lip closure. With this as well, once could feel "the burn" on the lips. Finally, putting small rubber tubes under the upper and lower lips while maintaining closure for 5–10 minutes was also a very positive experience.

While my son's sleep seems subjectively fine now with almost no snoring and adequate rest, he also uses a supportive garment to keep his jaw closed at night, making for a very confounding variable. During the day, even with the exercises he still seems to favor keeping his jaw open despite reminders, but not as much as before. We also are not super-compliant with the exercises. To me, the overall goal is to assist an individual in attaining the awareness and muscle strength to keep the jaw closed at all times or at least most of the time. It does not seem that despite tone improvement with myofunctional therapy, it is not necessarily a complete cure for mouth-breathing in the presence of an adequately breathing nose, but it seems very helpful! My overall view of myofunctional therapy after 6 months of treatment is that while it seems very helpful, it is very difficult to maintain compliance in a child. In a motivated adult, this is different, and results may be much better. The true benefit from myofunctional therapy appears to me to be the *awareness* and reflection upon the importance of converting one's self from a mouth-breathing to a nasal-breathing individual. It is this newfound awareness that needs to be near-constant that may be most critical for an individual to be more driven to maintain a closed mouth both by day and by night. Myofunctional therapy, with or without a mouth-closure device may be a useful complement to functional rhinoplasty in maintaining the nasal airway.

Facial Bone Expansion Strategies

As we had discussed in Chap. 4, as it seems likely that the root cause of obstructive sleep apnea and sleep disordered breathing is the progressive diminishment of the human maxilla and mandible, it stands to reason that strategies that focus on expanding the maxilla or mandible would reverse sleep apnea. While this is theoretically true, the answer in actual practice is not necessarily the case. As we have discussed, the airway causing sleep apnea is not simple airway narrowing, but instead may be more related to mouth-breathing related to nocturnal jaw slackening with subsequent unleashing of the relaxed tongue into the pharynx. Thus, even successful re-expansion of the maxilla and mandible does not necessarily translate into cessation of mouth-breathing and related sleep disorders.

   That being said, there is abundantly clear evidence in the literature that variations of the maxillomandibular advancement procedure is highly effective in reducing the objective parameters of sleep-breathing disorders. A 2016 meta-analysis from Stanford University, in a group including the famed Guilleminault, Riley, and Powell analyzed 45 studies with individual data from 518 unique patients/interventions. The study showed: "Among patients for whom data were available, 197 of 268 (73.5%) had undergone prior surgery for OSA. Mean postoperative changes in the AHI and Respiratory Disturbance Index (RDI) after MMA were −47.8 (25.0) and −44.4 (33.0), respectively; mean (SE) reductions of AHI and RDI outcomes were 80.1% (1.8%) and 64.6% (4.0%), respectively; and 512 of 518 patients (98.8%) showed improvement. Significant improvements were also seen in the mean (SD) postoperative oxygen saturation nadir (70.1% [15.6%] to 87.0% [5.2%]; $P < .001$) and Epworth Sleepiness Scale score (13.5 [5.2] to 3.2 [3.2]; $P < .001$). Rates of surgical success and cure were 389 (85.5%) and 175 (38.5%), respectively, among

455 patients with AHI data and 44 (64.7%) and 13 (19.1%), respectively, among 68 patients with RDI data" [11].

Despite the efficacy of the procedure, it remains an unattractive option to most patients including myself. The invasiveness of any variation of the procedure involving osteotomies of the maxilla and mandible with permanent hardware fixation, airway support requirements including possible tracheotomy and maxilla-mandibular fixation (MMF) requirements, not even including the risk of actual surgical complications are almost all deal-breakers for most patients. In a study of 28 patients who had undergone maxilla-mandibular advancement, there was a total of 108 complications, 15 of which were major (requiring re-operation or admission). Interestingly, the authors listed the major complication rate at 13.9%, using major complications as the numerator and total complications as the denominator. Fifteen major complications in 28 patients is a 53.5% major complication rate, most of which were infections per the authors [12].

In this study, the authors also minimized the total complication rates by comparing the OSA MMA complications with a cohort of patients who had maxillo-mandibular advancement for non-OSA reasons, and tested statistical significance only *between the groups*, thus not mentioning the total complication rates that I re-calculated above.

As a rhinoplasty surgeon, one will also note an additional complication that is rarely discussed by even many maxilla-mandibular advancement surgeons: Secondary nasal/septal deviation. The etiology of this problem is not dissimilar to the common form of septal deviation as discussed in the previous chapters. In this case however, the septum remains in its original position, while the lower maxilla is advanced after LeFort osteotomy anteriorly. The upward sloping maxillary crest now exists in the midline spot that is currently occupied by the quadrangular cartilage. This causes the quadrangular septal cartilage to be displaced and buckle at its caudal end, even if released! (Fig. 9.2). As I said, this is not dissimilar to the bony/cartilaginous mismatch in developmental cases. In the Stanford University experience, this complication must be recognized, and expected to occur in 18.7% of cases, as they demonstrated in a retrospective study of 379 patients [13]. They did find a high level of surgical success (76.3% based on RDI criteria), and 71 patients underwent nasal surgery, including aesthetic nasal surgery. The authors provided excellent insight that patients must be counseled in advance about this problem's likelihood (subclinical cases may have a much higher incidence of postoperative septal deviation and valve compromise). Another excellent paper from a team in South Korea recommended a solution to this problem [14]. They advised that at the conclusion of the MMA, the septum be evaluated for deviation as well as the nasal valve. If abnormality is identified, the authors recommend resection of the caudal-most portion of the L-strut and including refinement of the nasal spine via an intra-oral upper lip vestibular approach. I do not disagree with this approach, but it can also be achieved via a transfixion incision as described in previous chapters. Either way, the problem should be addressed pro-actively as these authors recommend, and not after the patient develops nasal obstructive complaints, or develops worsened mouth-breathing or deviation-related aesthetics. I have seen several instances

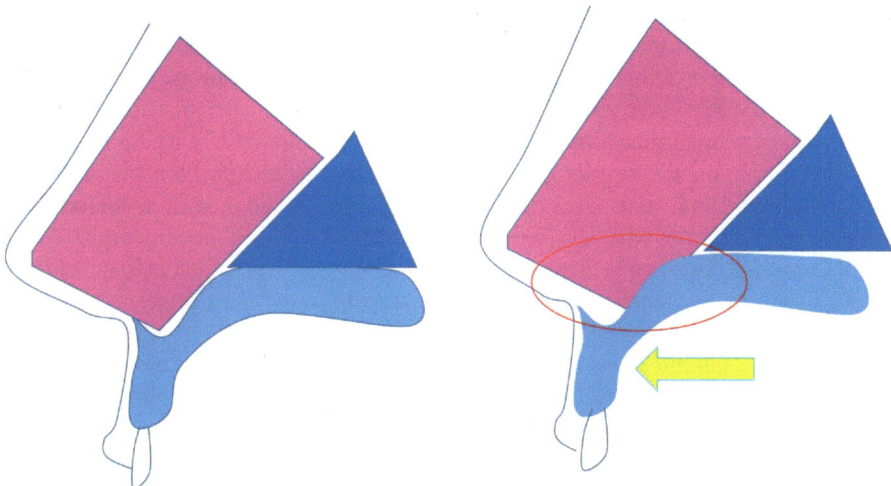

Fig. 9.2 Schematic of sagittal view of the nasal septum (pink) at its intersection with the maxilla (light blue) and with the vomer (dark blue). With LeFort I osteotomy and advancement of the maxillary segment (yellow arrow), even WITH complete release of the septum from the maxillary crest, will compete for space in the midline at the point encircled, and will create septal buckling with subsequent nasal breathing and discomfort. Do not confuse this for sinusitis

of patients who were not only surprised about their new nasal obstruction and deviation after MMA, but were told repeatedly that they simply had developed and were treated for "sinusitis." Of course the patients had evidence of inflammation of the maxillary sinuses, having them divided literally in half by the maxillary osteotomy, but the symptoms of nasal obstruction, pressure, congestion, and discharge is related to the newly deviated septum or perhaps a local reaction to hardware and osteotomy and is obviously not classic "sinusitis." This is not, unfortunately an isolated scenario but can be common where this procedure is performed commonly, and is almost always confused for sinusitis by the treating team, who frequently will refer for surgical treatment of this disorder. On a similar note, a similar line of thinking exists for infected dental implants, that providers can blame "sinusitis" instead of the obvious foreign implant that is triggering inflammation.

> Encouraging bony growth naturally: Reversal of "gracilization."
> Cryin' won't help you, prayin' won't do you no goodNow cryin' won't help you, prayin' won't do you no good
> Kansas Joe McCoy and Memphis Minnie in 1929, from "When the levee breaks"

As clinicians, we are generally taught to keep our patients happy and find solutions that sound palatable to them. After all, they are the client even if the insurance company may be the one actually paying you. So, we typically have some treatment options like a medication, or surgery that may have some upsides and downsides to offer, or maybe offer some unpleasant advice, but in general, we tend to avoid making life-altering pronouncements like in the quote above from a song popularized by Led Zeppelin. In the lyrics, the narrator is cautioning that the two easy options (crying or praying) will not do the listener much good. Instead, only the option of moving remains. This is not dissimilar to the problem of the patient who expects the surgeon to fix their chronic problems with a simple procedure or the physician with a medication. Especially when these problems are chronic nasal disuse and mouth-breathing, neither surgical options nor medical options do too much help in the long run. In my opinion, the best long-term option to reverse these problems is to encourage musculoskeletal tone via extensive exercise and avoidance of sedentarism, a generally healthy diet without excessive consumption of food, and high quality and sufficient sleep. This can be applicable to all age groups, from toddlers to the elderly.

As we discussed in a previous chapter how perhaps the most important cause of human facial diminishment is the process of "gracilization." Gracilization is the reduction of bone thickness and muscle tone over the course of human history, as technological advances has resulted in less requirements for extensive physical exertion to gather and prepare food. These advances include the development of fire for processing food for easier digestion, agriculture for easier gathering, and even blenders, which make food easier for chewing. Chirchir (2015) studied "peripheral quantitative CT and microtomography to measure trabecular bone of limb epiphyses (long bone articular ends) in modern humans and chimpanzees and in fossil hominins attributed to *Australopithecus africanus*, *Paranthropus robustus*/early *Homo* from Swartkrans, *Homo neanderthalensis*, and early Homo sapiens." They found that evidence that "the low trabecular density of the recent modern human skeleton evolved late in our evolutionary history, potentially resulting from increased sedentarism and reliance on technological and cultural innovations" [15].

Further, Ryan and Shaw showed in another comparative anatomy study that this gracilization or weakening of the skeleton is due to decreased biomechanical loading. Their study sampled femur Computed Tomography (CT) scans of 229 individuals from multiple primate species, and 59 individuals from distinct archaeological human populations. They showed that foraging human populations had bone thickness more similar in structure to wild non-human primates of similar size [16]. Other authors have confirmed that our recent and distant ancestors had more robust skeletons due to increased physical activity requirements [17].

While these studies focus upon long bones, the facial bones could follow a similar trajectory and can be related to masticatory loading or even an overall activity level. A comparative study of chimp masseter muscles disclosed that "Powerful masticatory muscles are found in most primates; contrarily, in both modern and fossil member Homo, these muscles are considerably smaller. The evolving hominid masticatory apparatus shifted towards a pattern of gracilization nearly simultaneously with accelerated encephalization in early *Homo sapiens*" [18].

So, what is the unpleasant answer to the patient asking for the easy solution? The gracilization process must be reversed, from birth to death. That means seriously increased exercise requirements and severe reductions in sedentarism and poor diet. Through near-constant physical activity, the thinning of our bones, possibly including our diminished maxilla and mandible bones can be reversed, possibly including a diet of less processed foods. This is hard, particularly in the modern world of cubicles, constant WIFI connectivity, and fast food. It is much easier to sit and watch Netflix or catchup on Facebook or Instagram. But as Memphis Minnie and Kansas Joe McCoy remind us, crying or praying isn't going to be of much help here. Many of the problems described in the previous chapters can be reversed simply through intense exercise and a healthy diet.

Studies have shown that "exercise regimes combining resistance and impact training should provide larger bone response than either one of them alone in growing children" [19]. Further, "mechanical loading is a major regulator of bone mass and geometry. The osteocytes network is considered the main sensor of loads, through the shear stress generated by strain induced fluid flow in the lacuno-canalicular system. Intracellular transduction implies several kinases and phosphorylation of the estrogen receptor. Several extra-cellular mediators, among which NO and prostaglandins are transducing the signal to the effector cells. Disuse results in osteocytes apoptosis and rapid imbalanced bone resorption, leading to severe osteoporosis. Exercising during growth increases peak bone mass and could be beneficial with regards to osteoporosis later in life, but the gain could be lost if training is abandoned [20].

Finally, a study showed that increases in bone density and strength followed increases in muscle mass during the pubertal growth spurt. They described the "mechanostat" theory, that these increases in bone strength are specifically due to increased loads "imposed" by muscle forces. Gain in lean body mass (a surrogate for muscle bulk) preceded bone mineral content increases by over half a year in males and females. While the authors acknowledged that this muscle growth preceding bony growth could be genetically determined, they felt it was more likely that the bone strength increases were resultant to the increase in muscle loading [21].

While this may not have perfect translation to the maxilla and mandible, and these bones may be just as much effected by occlusal loading as systemic exercise loading, one cannot help but observe that the most active and athletic individuals also frequently have associated adequate facial structure [22].

Perhaps the exercise causes the facial growth, or the good sleep quality permits more and higher quality exercise, or perhaps there is a feedback loop that has not been discovered. Either way, my own pre-pubertal children are encouraged to have as extensive high impact exercise as possible. This is achieved through participation in contact sports, (where my personal belief is that the benefits outweigh the risks, in contrast to conventional modern wisdom), hiking, swimming, and anything else we can think of. Of course, the outcome is not able to prove anything one way or another, but I feel it is my personal duty to push as much exercise at this stage and beyond as possible while they are in my care. As Nicholas Taleb's "anti-fragile" concept extolls, physical stressors like heavy exercise has the potential to be protective against actual hazards, unlike an over-protective strategy to avoid and stress or conflict for one's offspring that may have resulted in modern "gracilization" [23]. How well this strategy will work still remains to be seen. On a strenuous hike up Mount Mansfield in Vermont, all three of my children informed me that they hate me and that I am a horrible person. Fortunately, by lunchtime, they seemed to have forgotten this animosity, and I continue to hope that the fresh air and physical stress of the hike will yield health benefits.

Why does this not translate much into patient care? The answer may be found in game theory's "prisoner's dilemma" model, according to a brilliant 2004 study: Essentially, in this scenario, the patient and clinician are opponents in a simple game, where a patient with poor lifestyle choices that has resulted in medical problems now visits a physician in consultation. The physician can choose to offer the "easy" answer to their problem (pills or surgery), which can improve symptoms temporarily, but will not address the root cause, or permit a permanent solution, or the "hard" solution of changing lifestyle completely with a long discussion and counseling. The health-care model rewards the physician for taking the easy route financially for procedures and a short visit. The patient, likewise, can choose to seek the easy or hard solution, the easy one being more favorable to the patient who has had a lifetime of poor health choices. Only when the physician and patient cooperate to choose the "hard" solution, going against their own internal short-term reward pathways, can the patient truly recover [24]. Essentially, only the shared goal of becoming better people will motivate both parties to purposely seek the hard answer. In the current culture of our western world, this is not common. While this may be too late for my generation and its predecessors, perhaps the future generations will seek this type of enlightenment not found in most medical clinics today. In the current Covid-19 era, this game theory failure by both parties may be at least partially responsible for the severity experienced by the least healthy patients (see Chap. 10 and appendix).

Functional appliances for jaw expansion:

Q: What do I think of the efficacy of functional intra-oral appliances?

A: I remain both optimistic and skeptical about the utility of these devices and do not have enough practical information to decide.

References

1. Lee SY, Guilleminault C, Chiu HY, Sullivan SS. Mouth breathing, "nasal disuse," and pediatric sleep-disordered breathing. Sleep Breath. 2015;19(4):1257–64.
2. Huang TW, Young TH. Novel porous oral patches for patients with mild obstructive sleep apnea an mouth breathing: a pilot study. Otolaryngol Head Neck Surg. 2015;152(2):369–73.
3. Bhat S, et al. The efficacy of a chinstrap in treating sleep disordered breathing and snoring. J Clin Sleep Med. 2014;10(8):887–92. Published online 2014 Aug.
4. Adams D. The hitchhikers guide to the galaxy. London: Pan Books; 1979.
5. Lipen MJ, Most SM. Development of a severity classification system for subjective nasal obstruction. JAMA FPRS. 2013;15(5):358–61.
6. Knappe SW, Bakke M, Svanholt P, Petersson A, Sonnesen L. Long-term side effects on the temporomandibular joints and oro-facial function in patients with obstructive sleep apnoea treated with a mandibular advancement device. J Oral Rehabil. 2017;44(5):354–62.
7. Heidsieck DSP, Koolstra JH, de Ruiter MHT, Hoekema A, de Lange J. Biomechanical effects of a mandibular advancement device on the temporomandibular joint. J Craniomaxillofac Surg. 2018;46(2):288–92.
8. Omoboni O, Quan SF. Positional therapy in the management of positional obstructive sleep apnea – a review of the current literature. Sleep Breath. 2018;22(2):297–304.

9. Camacho M, et al. Myofunctional therapy to treat obstructive sleep apnea: a systematic review and meta-analysis. Sleep. 2015;38(5):669–75.
10. Huang YS, Hsu SC, Guilleminault CG, Chuang LC. Myofunctional therapy: role in pediatric osa. Sleep Med Clin. 2019;14:135–42.
11. Zaghi S, Holty JE, Certal V, Abdullatif J, Guilleminault C, Powell NB, Riley RW, Camacho M. Maxillomandibular advancement for treatment of obstructive sleep apnea: a meta-analysis. JAMA Otolaryngol Head Neck Surg. 2016;142(1):58–66.
12. Passeri LA, Choi JG, Kaban LB, Lahey ET 3rd. Morbidity and mortality rates after maxillo-mandibular advancement (MMA) for treatment of obstructive sleep apnea. J Oral Maxillofac Surg. 2016;74(10):2033–43.
13. Liu SY, Lee PJ, Awad M, Riley RW, Zaghi S. Corrective nasal surgery after maxillomandibular advancement for obstructive sleep apnea: experience from 379 cases. Otolaryngol Head Neck Surg. 2017;157(1):156–9.
14. Shin YM, Lee ST, Kwon TG. Surgical correction of septal deviation after Le Fort I osteotomy. Maxillofac Plast Reconstr Surg. 2016;38(1):21.
15. Chirchir H, Kivell TL, Ruff CB, Hublin J-J, Carlson KJ, Zipfel B, Brian G. Richmond recent origin of low trabecular bone density. PNAS. 2015;112(2):366–71.
16. Ryan TM, Shaw CN. Skeletal gracility in modern humans. PNAS. 2015;112(2):372–7.
17. Stock JT, Pfeiffer SK, Chazan M, Janetski J. F-81 skeleton from Wadi Mataha, Jordan, and its bearing on human variability in the Epipaleolithic of the Levant. Am J Phys Anthropol. 2005;128(2):453–65.
18. Favaloro A, Speranza G, Rezza S, Gatta V, Vaccarino G, Stuppia L, Festa F, Anastasi G. Muscle-specific integrins in masseter muscle fibers of chimpanzees: an immunohistochemical study. Folia Histochem Cytobiol. 2009;47(4):551–8.
19. Wang Q, Alén M, Nicholson P, Suominen H, Koistinen A, Kröger H, Cheng S. Weight-bearing, muscle loading and bone mineral accrual in pubertal girls–a 2-year longitudinal study. Bone. 2007;40(5):1196–202.
20. Bergmann P, Body JJ, Boonen S, Boutsen Y, Devogelaer JP, Goemaere S, Kaufman J, Reginster JY, Rozenberg S. Loading and skeletal development and maintenance. J Osteoporos. 2010;2011:786752.
21. Rauch F, Bailey DA, Baxter-Jones A, Mirwald R, Faulkner R. The 'muscle-bone unit' during the pubertal growth spurt. Bone. 2004;34(5):771–5.
22. Hichijo N, Tanaka E, Kawai N, van Ruijven LJ, Langenbach GEJ. Effects of decreased occlusal loading during growth on the mandibular bone characteristics. PLoS One. 2015;10(6):e0129290.
23. Taleb NN. Anti-fragile. London: Random House; 2012.
24. Tarrant C, Stokes T, Colman AM. Models of the medical consultation: opportunities and limitations of a game theory perspective. Qual Saf Health Care. 2004;13:461–6.

Chapter 10
Breaking the Barriers Between Specialties: Toward a Universal Understanding of Anatomy and Function

What we wish, we readily believe, and what we ourselves think, we imagine others think also.—Julius Caesar

Sometimes, we are not even aware of what we don't know. When we stick to practicing narrowly within our specialty closely following guidelines, this concept seems to be generally irrelevant, and we can happily continue to perform procedures, etc. without a deep understanding of causation. Unfortunately, while this has become the norm in our society, it does not mean it is the correct pathway. In the physical world, there are universal truths that must be acknowledged regardless of one's background and training. This is no different in surgery, where despite what we have been trained, there *must be* universal concepts of anatomy, pathology, and function of the facial structure, airway, and aesthetics interaction that defy our simplified attempt to artificially divide disease management by specialty. This compartmentalization, as described in Chap. 1 may be the root of why we tend to fail to see a bigger picture beyond current treatment standards of care. I know that I have personally learned most from stepping outside of my limited world, into the perspectives farthest from my own, often initially against my will. (As you have seen throughout this book, in addition to my traditional mentors and colleagues, I have learned amazing things from dental hygienists, medical students, device executives, zoo-keepers, anthropologists, aeronautical engineers, ornithologists, dentists, orthodontists, and oral surgeons, and even a lot from a few of my children's lacrosse and football coaches.) While I will not claim to know the universal truths in understanding this physiology, I do think we must work as a culture to disrupt economic driven turf battles, and the specialties must interact, with specific aspects of disease or health management criticized or praised by honest assessment from impartial individuals, combining reason with evidence. It is not acceptable to even inadvertently mislead the public by simply working to increase procedure rates or indications. Instead, we can strive toward a universal-type specialty of the face and airway, not necessarily where all perform the same function, but where common goals of treating cause is recognized as primary over symptomatic-based treatment.

© Springer Nature Switzerland AG 2020
H. D. Stupak, *Rethinking Rhinoplasty and Facial Surgery*,
https://doi.org/10.1007/978-3-030-44674-1_10

Throughout this book, we have repeated the theme that the shrinking maxilla and mandible in *Homo sapiens* over the course of time has resulted in a series of problems. Most obviously, this results in aesthetic problems from a receded chin, to flattening of the cheekbones and zygoma. This can result in a mismatch of skin and soft-tissue to musculoskeletal support, creating the appearance of excess tissue and pre-mature aging of the face or at least less facial "definition." These diminished facial bones can be more susceptible to fracture (although routine violence and contact has been reduced over time as well fortunately) and exhibit crowding of the teeth due to insufficient space. This also includes nasal deformity from a mismatch between the conserved nasal septal size resulting in extrusion and deviation. It also includes a predisposition to mouth-breathing and nasal disuse or "underuse" because of musculoskeletal tone. This combination of nasal obstruction and nasal disuse goes well beyond the expected clinical symptoms of simple dry mouth and nasal stuffiness, in that during sleep, a combination of negative pressure build-up from tongue collapse and desiccation from mouth-breathing can wreak havoc to the entire upper airway from the sinuses and turbinates, through the pharynx and larynx to the trachea and beyond [1].

In this final chapter, we will move beyond discussing simple strategies to correct the functional and aesthetic structures alone, and discuss how to avoid the specialist "compartmentalization" tactical high-tech algorithm oriented thinking that we are so accustomed to, and shift to more global strategies that minimize risk, over-operation, excessive technology to achieve better long-term outcomes beyond short-term "satisfaction." To complete this discussion using the unified principle of pervasive facial diminishment, we will divide the facial skeleton into (1) external facial skeleton (esthetics/trauma) and (2) internal facial skeleton (upper airway). We will specifically *exclude* digestive function, neurologic and inner ear function, and treatment of head and neck cancer, as these clinical conditions lie well outside the present discussion and my expertise.

By understanding that the face (external skeleton) and airway (internal facial skeleton) are essentially one unified structure, we can begin to see beyond the classic specialty compartmentalization that has resulted in many ineffective and overly simplified treatments. In each section below, we will predict how the surgeon/clinician "of the future" may recommend strategic treatment, in contrast to the prevailing "futurist" view of how only hot concepts like Artificial Intelligence (AI), "personalized medicine," and gene manipulation hold the key to the future. In other words, it will be a re-discovery of rationality and strategy that will be the antidote to the mediocre results that are already becoming evident in the world of constantly "improving" technology. Increasingly, young physicians and other clinicians are entering the work-force believing that if their scopes were just a little more high-definition (HD), and their guidance systems were just a little more high-tech and accurate, that they would have better outcomes and fewer complications. I have encountered this attitude more than once, that high complication rates are due only to a lack of the highest technology equipment, and not much all related to patient selection or strategic thinking. Dan Pedersen, who was the founder of the Navy's Topgun School for combat aviators described an almost identical situation in his book Topgun: An American Story (2019) where beginning with the Vietnam conflict, skill, and thoughtfulness gained via experience was mistakenly substituted with high-tech systems, resulting in near-disastrous results. The foundation of the Topgun training program helped avert catastrophe where thoughtful leaders re-imagined air combat and disseminated their conceptual strategies [2].

External Facial Skeleton (Aesthetics/Trauma)

Facial Skin/Soft-Tissue

As physicians, we tend to think of specific aesthetic "deformities," more than analyzing the components of attractiveness that are universal to our species. Nowhere is this concept more applicable than in the skin and soft-tissue of the face. With a United States cosmeceutical industry estimated to be $15 billion and growing rapidly (Source: statista.com), attention to everything from skin blemishes to wrinkles is ever-present in our culture. There is increasing pressure on individuals to address these "flaws" from the media, celebrities, YouTube channels, dermatologists, and of course even from physicians in our field.

From my perspective, however, this focus on "fixing" these specific flaws is simply incorrect. I am not against facial improvement, but I do believe that we are going about it almost completely backwards, by focusing on fixing the details like "wrinkle removal" or "lip enhancement." In essence, as the old English expression goes, we can't see the forest for the trees. These concepts are overly simple "tactics" or maneuvers that in the big picture make little aesthetic sense in the thoughtful enhancement of attractiveness. Individuals with wrinkles removed or filled, or lips that are "plumped" beyond normal anatomy look in no way more attractive or youthful than their peers. In fact, removing or filling wrinkles, as is commonly recommended results in odd, alien appearances that even in small doses is very obvious to the expert and gives observers the impression that the person who has undergone the treatments is attention-seeking and "trying too hard." Even when done with subtlety, the treatment fails to achieve any objective beyond simple "smoothing." Further, poor regulation of the individual non-pharmacologic treatments from lasers, to creams results in frequent side-effects, ineffective but expensive treatments that are simply the result of effective misleading marketing campaigns. The public, fed on these "wrinkle removal, facial enhancement" strategies by pseudo-experts, (from television hosts to celebrities peddling products to clinicians) who usually have an undisclosed conflict of interest frequently remains completely confused. The average person then performs "research" that is so inaccurate that they end up disappointed by false promises, or else they completely withdraws from the market choosing "to age naturally," not realizing that safe and effective strategies do exist.

The solution to this pervasive problem is, of course, strategic thinking (and possibly better marketing transparency). First, instead of focusing on wrinkles, lip fullness, and skin blemishes, that are typically thought of by conventional skin-treating providers, a re-analysis of facial attractiveness and aging reveals a much different perspective. Just as diminishment of the facial structure has caused the nasal aesthetic and functional airway problems described in previous chapters, again the musculoskeletal structure of the face plays a major role. In general, with age, a mismatch between the soft-tissue structures of the face and the underlying petite facial structural framework creates a laxity of soft-tissue that tends to sag in upright position. This is more or less pronounced in various parts of the face, and we will address each region independently.

Starting from the top, we will begin with the forehead and brow position. That the brow descends over the course of an individual's life is not debated and is even common knowledge. It is believed commonly that the brow descends due to ligamental laxity over the superior orbital rim. This aging brow is known to be associated with various "wrinkles," the glabellar vertical furrows (11's), the horizontal forehead rhytids, and the "crow's feet" fan-shaped lines at the lateral portion of the orbit. With the best of intentions, the conventional treatments promote the flattening of these "line" groups with agents like botulinum toxin, some with filling them from the base, and others flattening with abrasive agents like lasers, mechanical irritants (dermabrasion), or with chemicals (skin care or peels.). Finally, brow position can be corrected with a browlift to replace its position, all while smoothing the skin of the forehead and removing the corrugator muscle!

The improved smoothness of the skin can be impressive, but does not necessarily result in improved attractiveness or youth. In contrast, it creates a very distinct "botoxed" look of a shiny forehead that has strange and limited mobility, with the brow frequently at an odd angle. While the surgical browlift achieves lift, and corrugator reduction, it can be unpredictable and is quite invasive.

Rather than viewing the brow and forehead region as a series of wrinkles that must be smoothed, or a brow that must be physically moved to a new position, one can re-imagine that the brow position is essentially located at the equilibrium point between the brow-lifting muscles (frontalis), and downward and medial-pulling muscles (orbicularis oculi and corrugators). Over the course of an individual's lifetime, this equilibrium evolves causing the brow to be in a more favorable position during youth, and a more descended position later in life. In those who exhibit more squinting or brow furrowing expressiveness, the downward pull can be excessive, making the equilibrium shift inferiorly prematurely. In mature males, a descended brow may not appear unattractive, in contrast, can be an appealing feature of masculinity. In females, however, a depressed and medialized brow is universally interpreted as aged, tired, or a sign of experiencing emotional distress [3].

With an understanding of this musculoskeletal equilibrium, and with a knowledge of the male/female brow aesthetic, we can now find a strategic reversal to the depressed brow equilibrium aesthetic problem. The simple answer is to completely de-activate the down-pulling muscles (corrugator, procerus, and upper

Fig. 10.1 Early brow ptosis caused by excessive depressor muscle activity (top), with blue Xs representing injection sites for 2.5 U of botulinum toxin A. At the bottom, a few weeks later, the brow position is improved at rest

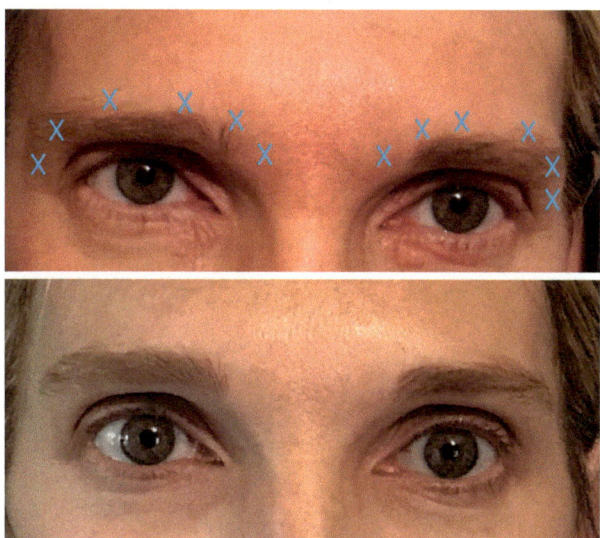

orbicularis) and completely PRESERVE the upward-pulling muscles (Frontalis). This can be completely and successfully accomplished using injection of botulinum toxin into the complete down-pulling muscle groups, and by explaining to patients why the frontalis should never be injected, despite popular opinion to the contrary. This is a strategic modification of the "chemical browlift" described 20 years ago [4, 5], and where botulinum toxin can be safely injected into the depressors of the central part of the brow, despite the reported risk for eyelid ptosis, but of course this would be an off-label usage of this product (Fig. 10.1). In my belief, the reported eyelid ptosis that is so feared is not due to migration of the botox to the levator palpebrae muscle as believed, but may be due simply to confounding from a weakened frontalis muscle due to injection and is actually brow descent.

Cheeks and Jawline

Again, while the mainstream approach for the lower part of the face consists of wrinkle elimination to many, in reality this may not the only solution. Instead, we can analyze *why* the cheeks, jowls, and jawline age, or appear less than aesthetically appealing. As with the brow, the wrinkles/lines may be just "fellow-travelers" with facial aging and are not the root cause of the aesthetic problem, even though conventional wisdom dictates otherwise. It all goes back to our understanding that the facial skeleton has been diminishing over generations and is of course more pronounced in some individuals than others. So, just as in the origin of the over-sized nose and nasal deformity, the petite midface/maxillary/zygomatic structure is small relative to a larger skin- and soft-tissue layer [6].

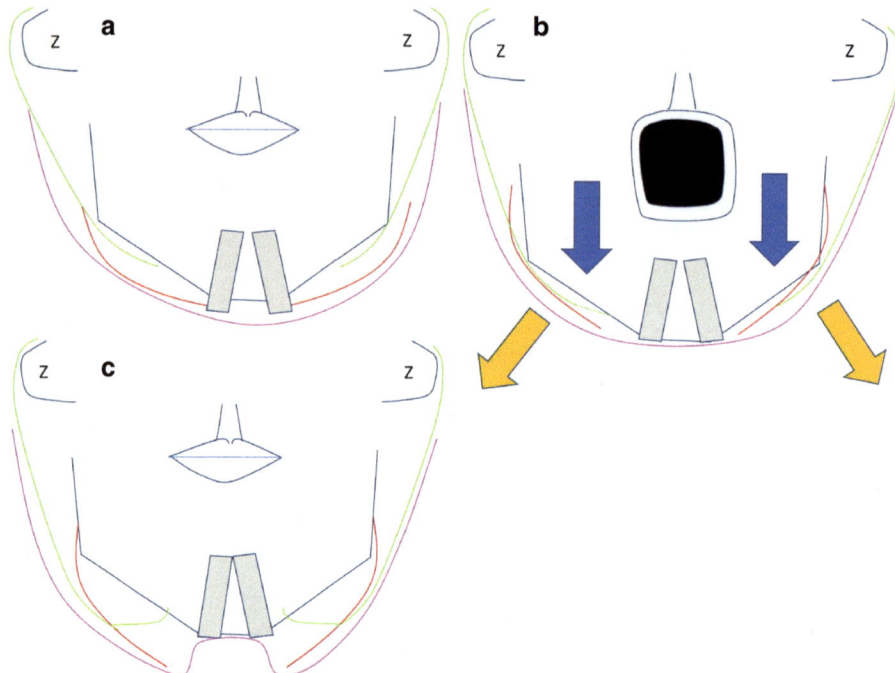

Fig. 10.2 Schematic diagram of the effect of mouth-breathing on soft-tissue laxity of the neck and jowl. (**a**) Mandible in closed-mouth position, with neck/jowl soft-tissue in youthful taut state. (**b**) Mandible in open-mouthed position, as repeated nightly over the course of a lifetime. As the mandible proceeds inferiorly, it deflects and stretches the platysma, skin, and jowl infero-laterally, while in the midline there is little stretching, aided by the sub-labial musculature. (**c**) Mandible in closed-mouth position, but after many years of nocturnal open-mouthed stretch as in 2B. Note how the midline remains little stretched, while the platysmal bands have formed, and the jowl has substantially stretched, creating folds of excess tissue. *Key*: Z—zygoma, platysma—red line, sublabial musculature—grey trapezoid, jowl—green line, neck skin—pink line

As one will note, however, this process accelerates as the facial bones, particularly tooth-bearing areas diminish with time. This can appear to be ligamental laxity [7], but is also due to loss of bony contour and fat in the cheek areas *relative* to the facial structure. Further, it is my view that chronic nocturnal mouth-breathing as discussed throughout this book stretches the facial skin and soft-tissue envelope in an inferior direction over time creating the classic aged neck and jawline. This is not dissimilar to the concept of "creep" or non-recoverable elongation of soft-tissues that is discussed in the tissue-expander reconstruction literature. As seen in Fig. 10.2, chronic nocturnal mouth-breathing or opening over many years can also explain why jowls and platysmal bands form lateral to the midline structure in many patients due to the limited midline stretching of tissues aided by the sub-labial muscles, while laterally, there is limited muscular attachment to the mandible at the jowl.

In essence, then as the facial soft-tissue is stretched relative to a shrinking facial structure, creating an unfavorable soft-tissue to framework ratio or relationship, and the result is droopy tissue, stretched ligaments, deflated malar eminences, and a sagging neck and jawline. This laxity secondarily creates folds of overlap like the melolabial folds, and an unfavorable positioning of the medial platysma into an unfavorable infero-lateral location. When one observes patients with pronounced melo-labial folds and platysmal sagging with a purposeful mouth-open position, the excess folds disappear, supporting the concept that this stretched-skin position is a possible cause of the laxity. In contrast, because we see the patients in our office during daytime, the nocturnal mouth-breathing is of course not evident, so we do not consider this in an aesthetics practice.

So, in addition to just camouflage for these varied problems, the key to appropriate and natural appearing results is to restore the normal soft-tissue to skeletal frame work relationship, not only from filling folds that are actually secondary to the root cause. This includes restoring the height of the malar eminence through any means (I prefer the use of long-term hyaluronic acid fillers as these can be both firm enough to actually project and soft enough to feel natural, and can have more added slowly over time to titrate desired amount until a steady-state or equilibrium is reached.) This skeletal enhancement can be complemented with a lower neck and jawline deep plane facelift in select cases to further improve the soft-tissue to skeletal ration. In almost all cases, the neck and jawline facelift should be combined with restoration of the malar eminence over the long-term. I tend to avoid chin and cheek alloplastic implants as these can appear unnatural or asymmetric after long-term contracture and cannot be enhanced as easily as progressive filling can be. Using only fixed procedures like implants or isolated facelifts can be problematic in the long run, as these fixed one-time procedures do not permit evolution of treatment in the individual patient. Improving the *lateral* aspect of the zygoma and malar eminence is most important, and should not be confused with filling the depressions of the cheek area anteriorly, or as midface injections. The filler goes directly above the bone to give the "high cheekbone look." This is done more like sculpting the lateral-most zygomatic/malar arch by diffusing the material than by placing filler into depressed areas below the arch. In contrast, with this technique, depressions can be *increased*, and are at least ignored, but overall aesthetics looks much more natural and attractive, not just filled [8]. Figures 10.3 and 10.4 show the pre- and post-rhinoplasty photos of a young woman with ideal lateral cheek bones and brow position (all natural) that are accentuated by the subtle re-sizing of the nose.

External Facial Skeleton: Trauma

Along the same theme of this book, as expected, with more delicate and petite facial bones, more minor trauma may be more likely to induce clinically significant facial fractures. As violence rates decline, a higher percentage of facial fractures occur in elderly patients, in some cases on the extreme end of the "gracilization" picture, with bones considered to be atrophic by physicians, and even exhibiting pathologic fractures, where limited force was involved, as in a fall from standing.

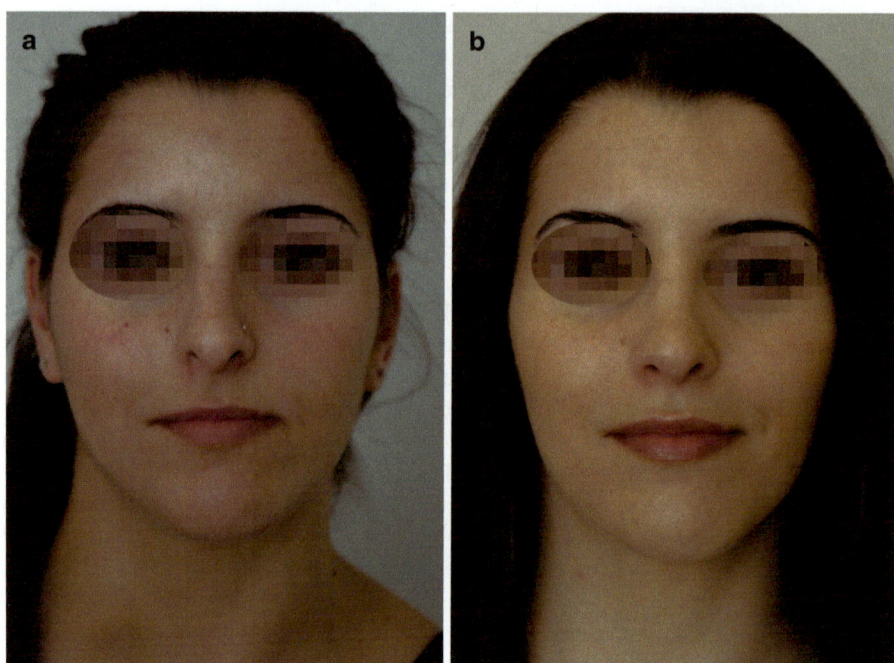

Fig. 10.3 (**a**) Pre- and (**b**) post-rhinoplasty frontal photographs of patient with excellent lateral cheek bone projection. Note how with subtle nasal shortening the cheek bones seem even more improved relatively and without direct treatment

These pathologic fractures, specifically of the mandible, are considered to be among the most difficult to treat. I attended several educational trauma meetings as a resident and remember being surprised that the recommended treatment for these challenging fractures was to place the largest reconstruction plate possible through an open approach, the most aggressive of approaches. The goal of surgery for these patients is in many cases just to permit usage of dentures. But the theme of the courses I attended was to paraphrase, "bigger and more plates are better." The risk/benefit ratio did not completely add up to me at the time, but who was I to question the distinguished and seasoned faculty.

So, as I entered practice, despite my course experience, I felt some instinctual aversion to do maximally big procedures to achieve little things, particularly in older patients, especially having seen how debilitating such procedures were to the patients despite the excellent radiologic results. I also noted over time that other clinicians at the time (early 2000s) also felt that more surgery, plates, and exposure in facial fractures was always better than less, with the goal of achieving better stability. For example, in several conferences I regularly attended, a general theme was that any fracture or bony crack must be "explored" or "stabilized." This is counter to reason, where we know that most bones do heal, and that the only thing the surgeon can really control is ensuring alignment of displaced bones! So, strategic

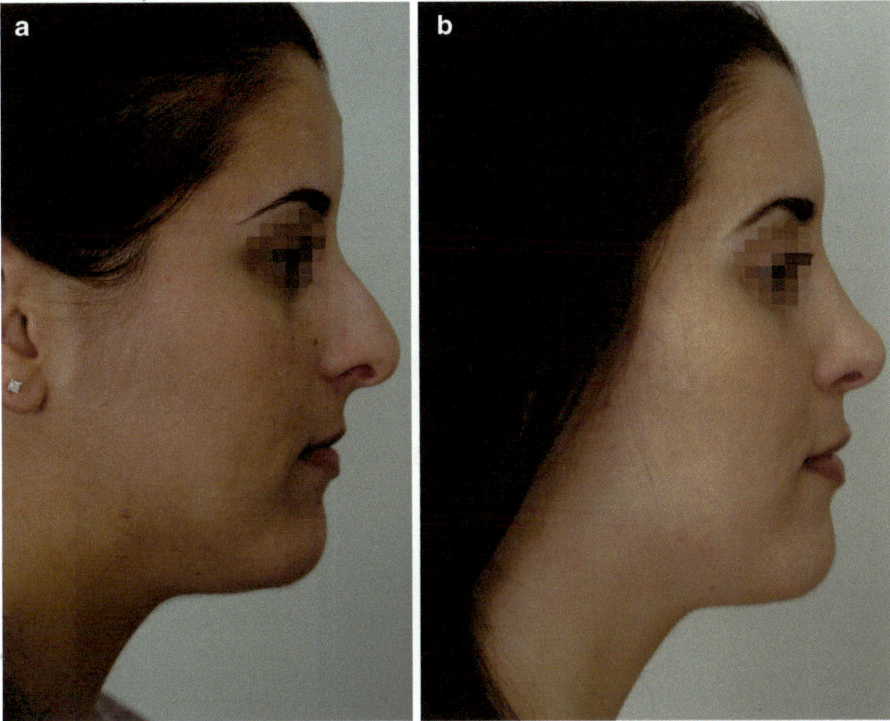

Fig. 10.4 (a) Pre- and (b) post-rhinoplasty lateral photographs of patient with excellent lateral cheek bone projection. Note how with subtle nasal shortening the cheek bones seem even more improved relatively and without direct treatment

thinking dictates that only bones that are out of position causing clinically significant sequelae should be repositioned using the most minimal approaches to avoid harm to the patient with the most minimal reinforcement required with the shortest surgery and hospital stay as possible. Any extra approaches or hardware placed, despite the intention of the clinician, is an extra risk of problems. As we discussed in the rhinoplasty chapters, of the stages of approach, reduction, and reposition, and reinforcement (plating and suturing), only reduction and repositioning of the bone is therapeutic to the patient. From a logic perspective, of course the least amount of re-inforcement (plating) in order to stabilize the reduction is ideal, and any extra implant bulk only increases the risk of future problems, and any additional approach only creates more soft-tissue damage, despite how "pretty" computed tomography (CT) images of extensively plated fractures plated may appear. The indication/contra-indication list-type thinking we are taught in texts is a contributor to this flawed thinking as is the confusing "favorable versus unfavorable fractures" and "load-sharing and load-bearing plates" concepts in the field of craniofacial trauma.

I also learned more about the device industry and was surprised to find out that some device plating manufacturers had complex relationships with non-profit educational organizations (Source SEC telephone call) [9].

Interestingly, Cochrane database reviews of both atrophic mandible fractures [10] and interventions for all mandible fractures [11] show that there is no real evidence of one particular approach over another on analysis of the greater literature. Thus, with essentially complete lack of evidence for one approach over another, reason-based strategy (goal to restore bone position with the least intervention and collateral damage) can be useful.

In one of the most intuitive and useful articles I have read, Ellis explains how the most important factor in failure in the surgical management of mandible fractures is actually rotational torsion of one segment of bone relative to the other, as is most evident in cases of double fractures [12].

Before I read and re-read this article, I unfortunately had a two-dimensional view of mandible fractures. After exposing the fracture, I imagined that the plates prevented distraction of the segments in two-dimension, as one would conceive by looking at a two-dimensional x-ray of a fracture like a plain film or panorex (Fig. 10.5). My mind was changed when I read the article and finally began to visualize two segments of the mandible rotating relative to the other (Fig. 10.6).

This three-dimensional rotational torsional view of mandible fracture treatment failure was one of the most interesting insights I have ever read in a single article. It helped everything make more sense to me. It explained why the mucosal incisions break down so frequently after surgery, especially double fractures due to the literal

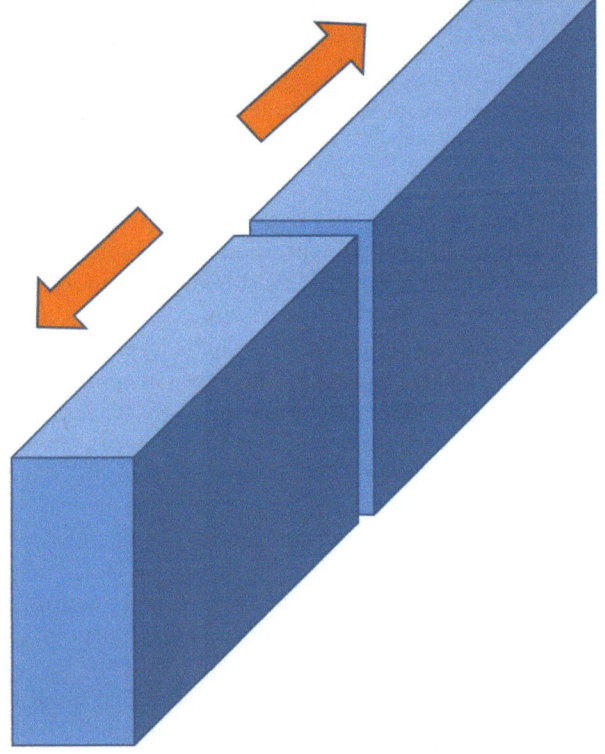

Fig. 10.5 Schematic of two-dimensional conception of mandible fracture failure, with the blue bars representing the segments of the mandible on either side of the fracture being distracted in the direction of the orange arrows

Fig. 10.6 Schematic of three-dimensional conception of mandible fracture failure, with the blue bars representing the segments of the mandible on either side of the fracture. In this diagram, the orange arrow represents the segments rotating with reference to each other as described by Ellis

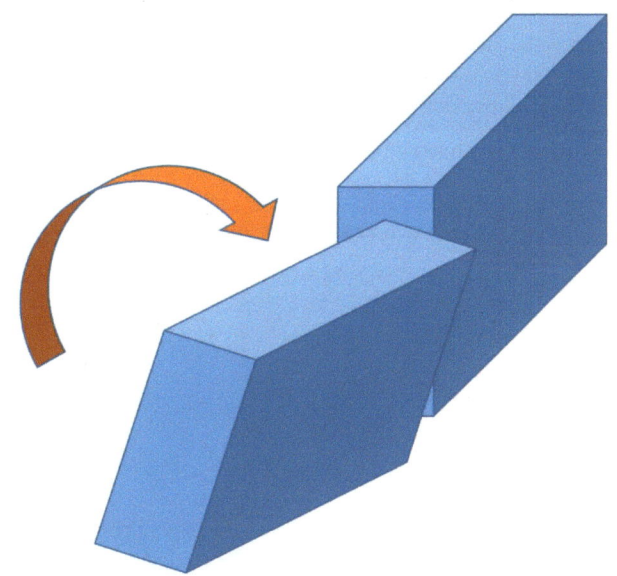

stretching of the wound. The torsional rotational forces of the two segments rotate away from each other, distracting the mucosal wound edges, and preventing healing. The same force also can prevent bone healing completely in patients in poor health (non-union), and malocclusion (mal-union) in patients with adequate bone healing, because the teeth are shifted in axis to the occlusal plane.

Only by making the plate larger, and more rigid, argues Ellis can these torsional forces be minimized and prevented [12, 13]. While this is probably true, biomechanical testing shows that there is a more efficient way to prevent torsion at the occlusal surface of the jaw. Instead of increasing the amount of rigidity at the inferior border of the mandible with larger, thicker (and more expensive) plates, (Fig. 10.7) increasing the number of points of vertical fixation can be more efficient (Fig. 10.8). A vastly smaller dissection area is required, and substantially less hardware is utilized. Using a torque wrench, we compared in a synthetic mandible whether vertical points of fixation compared to horizontal rigid fixation prevented torsional failure of repair. We found that "the vertical box plate provided greater stability and 150% of the resistance against torsional forces when compared with traditional linear plating" [14]. In an analogy using door hinges, one can see a similar progression from horizontal hinges from the colonial era and before, and the vertically fixed hinges that take up less room. As expected, the vertical plate requires much less dissection in a horizontal plane, and thus has less soft-tissue side-effects and time of surgery to complete. A clinical study of 84 patients comparing vertical fixation plating using box plates with traditional plating "showed vertical plating was associated with a lower incidence of postoperative neurosensory disturbance (25 [38%] patients treated with vertical plating vs 0 patients treated with box plating; $P = .002$) and a lower risk of any complication (41 [62%] vs 6 [33%],

Fig. 10.7 Schematic of conception of mandible fracture repair, with the blue bars representing the segments of the mandible on either side of the fracture and green bars representing conventional horizontal plates to counter the segmental rotational forces

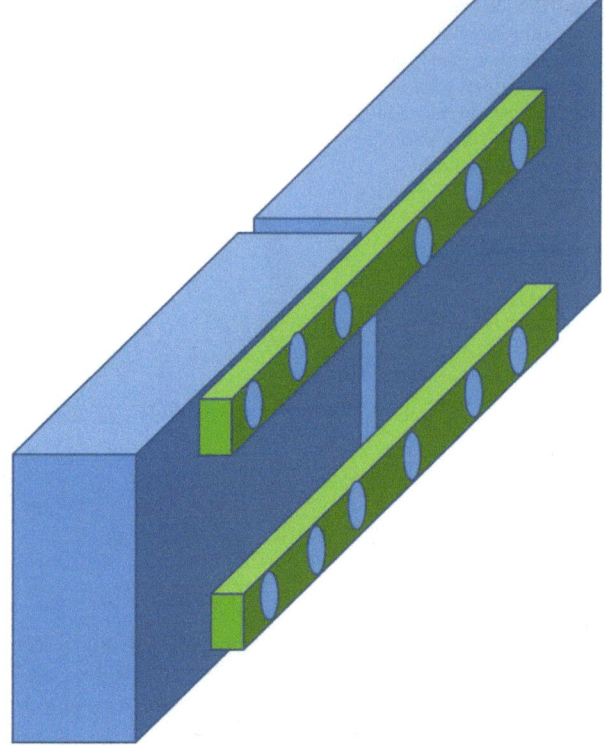

Fig. 10.8 Schematic of conception of mandible fracture repair, with the blue bars representing the segments of the mandible on either side of the fracture and the green bar representing a vertical plate to counter the segmental rotational forces. Notice what a narrower field of dissection is required to approach when compared to the broad horizontal area and vertical area of Fig. 10.6

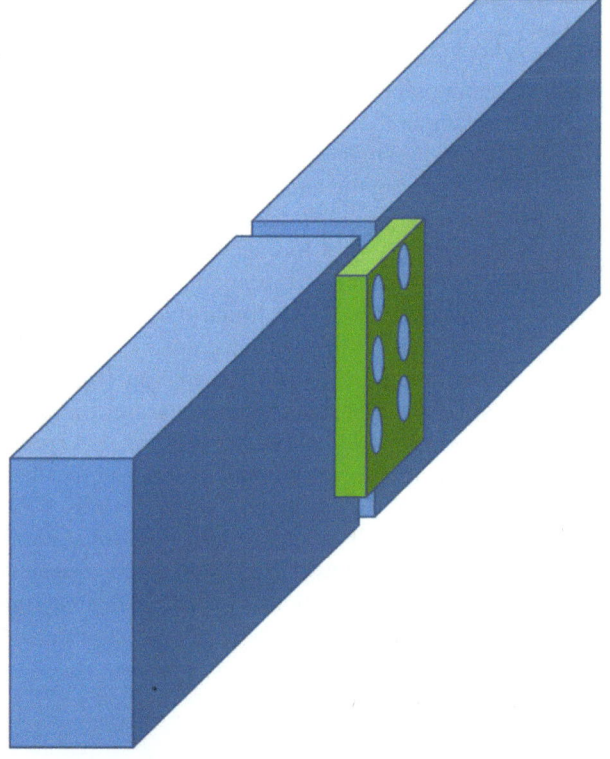

respectively; relative risk, 0.54; 95% CI, 0.27–1.06; P = .03). Vertical plating was associated with reduced operative time (134 minutes vs 70 minutes, respectively; P < .001)" [14]. In a well-written and thoughtful commentary about the concept, Humphrey and Kriet said, "Although the 3-D vertical box or strut plate is still not considered a load-bearing repair, these newer plates demonstrate a resistance to torsional forces during bone healing similar to reconstruction plates. Perhaps 3-D vertical box or strut plates can 'build in the compliance' without the considerable challenges of properly implanting a larger reconstruction plate. The load-sharing vs load-bearing distinction is still important for educating the novice surgeon. But, an experienced facial trauma surgeon often views load-bearing to load-sharing as a continuum, rather than as distinct categories. Along this continuum, the 3-D vertical box or strut plate feels much closer to a load-bearing repair compared with single or even multiple miniplates" [15].

In a similar but earlier study, we confirmed the findings of Champy, who much earlier showed that his three-dimensional angle plate, twisted to prevent torsional rotation along the oblique ridge of the mandible similarly was much lower cost with many fewer complications [16].

These concepts can be universalized, that in general, minimizing extent of approach, focus on three-dimensionally adequate reduction, then stabilization with as little plating as possible can cause the least collateral damage to the patient, regardless of how comprehensive the traditional "more is better" plating system appears on a radiologic exam.

Internal Facial Skeleton (Airway)

I am tremendously fortunate to have the privilege to practice within the field of Otolaryngology/Head and Neck Surgery, at its intersection with Facial Plastic and Reconstructive Surgery. The overlap and connection between the two fields has expanded so much in my personal experience, that the boundaries between them has blurred, despite what I believed at the end of training. I have enjoyed participating and practicing in this field since the day I was introduced to the anatomy of the airway during medical school, and I could not ask for a better group of colleagues and teachers: Sophisticated, polite, diverse, well-spoken, and well-mannered, dedicated to education and research, and overall enjoyable to be around. I could not think of practicing in another specialty.

I also have been at times concerned for the long-term health of my specialty, not because of the individual physicians, but because of the direction taken by some. So, in this last section of the last chapter of this book, I intend to discuss how the newer knowledge of the facial structure, as described during the course of this text may be critical to having a broader view of the diseases of the airway that are commonly treated by otolaryngologists and others. Unfortunately, as you will see, this understanding may not mesh well with the conventional clinical model, so I do anticipate some resistance to this concept.

A recent trade journal explained how researchers can seek increasing roles for FESS (functional endoscopic sinus surgery), while *protecting* the growth of the use of this procedure. While I am not opposed to optimism about a procedure by an academic organization, I do anticipate that a hope to expand procedural indications and "protecting" growth may not be as helpful to public health as a genuine search for most efficient and least cost treatment plans. This is not unique to this organization of course, but has become endemic to specialty medicine on the whole, and may be beginning to erode the trust of our patients, as they begin to notice that it is not only for their interests for which we strive.

While some with a faith in technology could insist that procedural expansion goals are for the good of all, I unfortunately cannot help but feel that this is more likely due to concept described by Julius Caesar from the beginning of this chapter: "What we wish, we readily believe, and what we ourselves think, we imagine others think also." To maintain persistent growth in our field, our leaders of course would wish that our research, medical knowledge, and our carefully codified standards of care all would coincide together like a synchronized swimming team, summing up the American Academy of Otolaryngology's motto, "We are One." This is what worries me about the future: At the expense of free-discussion, open-mindedness, and exploration of deeper understanding of the origins of disease, we must instead choose *conformity* as our mission. It seems that some would prefer that we simply partner with industry to find more higher-definition scopes, more aggressive drugs to complement more surgeries, and more indications for more billable treatments to maintain our growing businesses, instead of using thoughtfulness and reason to provide real value to patients while being maximally efficient.

I have found that the most aggressively marketed and pushed products and practices also tend to provide the least true value to the patient and the public. A massive practice near me is known for a physician incentive system that rewards the excess use of testing, (audiograms and fiberoptic endoscopy for all patients, etc.) of course forced upon patients (and their insurance companies) under the guise of pre-emptive treatments, but of course to maximize corporate profit. In another example, several companies of nasal breathing devices provided large payments to many physician leaders (source Centers for Medicare and Medicaid Services [CMS] Sunshine act website: https://openpaymentsdata.cms.gov/search/companies) upon their launch to help popularize devices that have favorable billing profiles for physicians, but whose therapeutic targets actually make no practical/anatomic sense (imagine small scale Theranos-style companies – see Home Box Office (HBO) film's "The Inventor: Out for Blood in Silicon Valley"). By the way, you can look me up too on the CMS Sunshine Act website, to see that I am compensated for the intellectual property for a device that I have licensed (see disclosures in Chap. 6). However, from my perspective, there is a substantial difference between receiving royalties for device sales when obtaining intellectual property than for compensating many "experts" with payments for "consultation" to essentially promote a product.

Despite these few outliers, however, the vast majority of practitioners do have the patient's best interests in mind and most do the right thing. Unfortunately, the failure rate of many offered "standard of care" treatments and procedures are high, and sometimes this lack of widespread treatment success is not efficiently communicated to the public in the manner of the risk/benefit ratio, but more as physician recommendations. I believe this is partially due to the rigid algorithm-based training of specialists that always recommends a "next step" bigger procedure after the previous less invasive step fails regardless of how much reason is lacking. In other cases, high failure rates are just accepted as the norm.

For example, there are high but poorly acknowledged failure rates in sinus surgery, adeno-tonsillectomy for sleep apnea, and turbinate reduction and classic steroid treatments that are the mainstays of practice, so we portray the disorders themselves as vague and difficult to treat, and use outcome measures that are equally as vague. We typically minimize the failures as well by referring to failures as "refractory patients," as though the treatment was fine, but there was some resistance in the patient.

While the typical answer is to "double down" on more expensive and high-tech versions of these treatment algorithms (like better scopes, anti-inflammatory agents, and hemostasis devices), the better answer may be to obtain a better understanding of the disease process that causes our current treatments to fail so frequently, even if difficult to discuss and generating unpleasantly less revenue and growth.

Reality for best patient care unfortunately may not completely fit current practice models of more testing, procedures as better. As we have discussed in the previous chapters, the progressively shrinking facial skeleton, particularly since modern times has created a deficiency in airway support that has resulted in a tendency toward mouth-breathing in lieu of consistent nasal breathing. This oral airway path, particularly during sleep, creates airway exposure desiccation, particularly in the low humidity winters. Worse, during sleep, the palate and tongue during this relaxation induced mouth-opening can collapse and generate pockets of airway negative pressure (as described in Chap. 4) [1]. This synergistic airway desiccation and airway negative pressure buildup create focal areas of mucosal barrier disruption (MBD). It is this resultant MBD and the sensation of the desiccation and negative pressure airway barotrauma that may be the origin of most upper airway diseases, both acute and chronic variations of the "upper respiratory infection," causing resultant inflammation that we are aware of from the turbinates at the top of the airway, to the bronchioles at the other end.

Of course, this MBD can manifest in any part of the airway, particularly in the fixed internal chambers of the skull of the middle ear, nasal cavity, sinuses, and pharynx. Of course, we name the variations of MBD not by the forces that cause the problem, but by the resultant downstream inflammatory response to the initial problem (otitis, rhinitis, sinusitis, pharyngitis, and tonsillitis), assuming that the event is initiated solely by a pathogen, or the body's own immune system.

The location of peak negative pressure can determine the location of MBD and the resultant inflammatory process. To illustrate this, we will use the example of a hose connected to a vacuum source. Imagine a soft tube connected to a vacuum that simulates inspiratory pressure generated by the expansion of the chest cavity. If one occludes or plugs the other end of the tube, the tube will narrow just distally (closer to the vacuum). This narrowing marks the area of peak negative pressure and

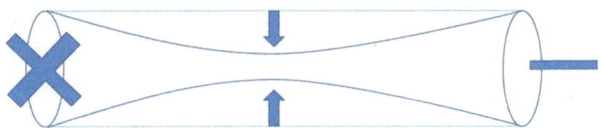

Fig. 10.9 Diagram representing a soft-walled tube, with negative pressure applied on one end (minus sign), and obstructed on the other end (X). The walls will be drawn inward as illustrated here. This is translatable to the entire upper airway

mucosal stretching. In the airway, the intra-luminally stretched mucosa is just distal to the site of obstruction. Thus, if the nasal valve is obstructed, maximal mucosal in-stretching can occur at the turbinates and sinuses, giving the appearance of enlarged turbinates or thickened sinus mucosa, adenoid thickening or even "allergy." When the palate collapses, the mucosa around the tonsil area stretches and is damaged especially with dehydration from mouth-breathing in a lower humidity environment. Similarly, when the tongue-base is the source of obstruction in patients with a more severe loss of tone, the resultant MBD occurs distally from the epiglottis to the larynx (Fig. 10.9). The mucosal stretching of course damages the submucosa and is compounded by desiccation. This mucosal trauma results in a submucosal inflammatory process that to the observer, becomes the hallmark of the disease, as rarely is the nocturnal obstruction or desiccation (see Appendix).

Because we focus our diagnosis, pathologic examination and research primarily on the inflammatory process and the micro-organisms associated with this process, our treatments nearly exclusively focus on treating primarily the inflammatory process as well, both in acute and chronic MBD. Thus, the root cause of airway disease (the invisible nocturnal barotrauma and desiccation forces) is largely ignored by most clinicians in favor of the more traditional surgical (remove inflammatory tissue, i.e., FESS and tonsillectomy, turbinate reduction) or medical (prevent secondary inflammation, i.e., steroids, or secondary microbial invasion, i.e., antibiotics). This is the equivalent of having a persistently leaky pipe in the ceiling, but only repeatedly cleaning the floor of water as a means to fix the problem, while ignoring the root cause. Even from a reasoning perspective, removing diseased, damaged, and inflamed tissue cannot possibly address the root cause and permanently correct the disorder, as something had to cause the tissue damage in the first place, and no one will pretend that surgery removes only the offending organisms, in an airway covered with organisms.

So, the bottom line is that while tradition and our practice model calls for us to follow a tactical algorithm that chiefly identifies the location and extent of airway disease though history, examination, radiographic analysis, and fiberoptic endoscopy, in reality we may be failing to routinely recognize the invisible forces that are the root cause of airway disease. Further, our treatment of airway disease, from sinusitis to sleep apnea to otitis media addresses only the inflammation and secondary infection through medication and surgery.

Let me clarify and summarize this concept, as this is really the theme of this book: Essentially, a subclinical skeletal deficiency that is usually manifest as simply a "less-attractive" phenotype (weaker chin, over-bite, etc.) predisposes to

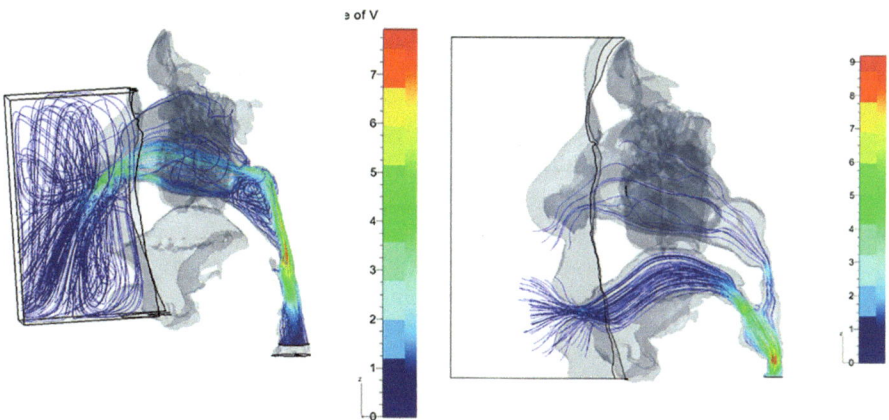

Fig. 10.10 Computational Flow Dynamics of nasal (*left*) versus oral (*right*) breathing routes. (Courtesy: Suzuki and Tanuma [1]. Permission: Copyright: © 2020 Suzuki, Tanuma. This is an open access article distributed under the terms of the Creative Commons Attribution License, which permits unrestricted use, distribution, and reproduction in any medium, provided the original author and source are credited)

mouth-breathing because this unfavorable skeletal structure creates increased work required to close the jaw during low tone states like sleep. This tone and work are affected by BMI, age, and sedation/arousal levels. Mouth-breathing in turn causes tongue collapse and build-up of negative pressure in the pharynx/airway (Fig. 10.10). This vacuum effect, especially when combined with mucosal dehydrating states can cause disruption of the upper airway anatomy, creating a spectrum of symptoms from ear discomfort and pressure when transmitted through the Eustachian tubes, to acute epiglottitis when occurring acutely in a lower part of the airway, the disrupted site determined by the peak negative pressure point and acuity. Essentially, what I am implying is that nearly all otolaryngologic complaints seen in our clinics (excluding sensorineural hearing loss and head and neck oncology/ smoking related disorders) are essentially explained by this process, and should be reversed or treated not by tissue removal alone, but by reversal of the chain of events in the root cause IN ADDITION to conventional treatments.

In an ideal world what could be done differently? First, we can change our mindset. While rigid one-size-fits-all tactical algorithmic thinking can prevent disasters much like aviation checklists, and standardize our business models, we also can re-invigorate our practices by re-incorporating strategic thinking. In an ideal world, we can limit specialty "compartmentalization," where the artificial borders between specialties that are procedure-driven can be limited. In the ideal world, the "universal specialist" would have a strong grasp of the internal and external facial skeleton and would be able to recognize the invisible forces, from human evolution to mouth-breathing to negative pressure that are the root causes of disease. Instead of treating simple symptoms like sinus headaches, we would take a broader view and treat the underlying cause.

First, we need strategies to help people develop adequate facial bone structure. How? I don't know, but we discussed possibilities in previous chapters, from expansion surgery to resistance exercise, or even using pediatric endocrinology treatments like growth hormone to enlarge bone. Two, we need to help people reduce mouth-breathing, possibly with devices, exercises, or even surgery—this is the ultimate goal as Guilleminault pointed out in one of his final papers [17]. Third, we need to be able to help people achieve adequate nasal airways through surgery only when there is primary obstruction, and not just mucosal compensation to obstruction. We can continue to use our classic tactical treatments as complementary procedures, from sinus surgery to tonsillectomy to turbinate reduction, but we must have the understanding that these do not address cause, and are just adjunct procedures to "clean-up" already hopelessly diseased or damaged tissue. And finally, we must be able to communicate this concept to patients effectively, and to our family and friends so that care can be delivered efficiently, without wasted excess, or poorly conceived treatments that are all too common.

A focus on achieving a higher level of success due to a better understanding of anatomic cause and effect, even with a smaller numbers of cases may be more beneficial in the long run than the ever-popular attempt to increase surgical volume at all cost. As Margaret Thatcher once said, "Don't follow the crowd. Let the crowd follow you." Evidence-based medicine (EBM) and the algorithms established by experts of course remain critical in many aspects of our field. However, individual clinicians can balance the use of these with careful reasoning, logic, and deeper thought about cause and effect relationships. In the end, only the individual operator is responsible for the structural changes that will affect the outcome, not the algorithm they followed.

Let this simple rethinking of rhinoplasty and facial surgery text be simply a springboard to your own ideas and development of real-world anatomic knowledge. Instead of the instinct to add more high-tech equipment or algorithms to solve problems, spend more time considering the ways of nature. This is not just to help you relax or prevent "burnout," but to guide you in the ways of the universal laws of physics that more accurately reflects how our anatomic structures function beyond what a textbook can teach. In the end, as it was for our pre-industrial ancestors, these forces may be our best instructor of the nature of structure, esthetics, and function. Technology combined with evidence-based medicine has shown us where the dots are on the page ... but now, the job falls upon human *reason* to connect the dots and make sense of the patterns.

The hostile attitude of conquering nature ignores the basic interdependence of all things and events. —Alan Watts (courtesy of Alan Watts Association)
After a certain high level of technical skill is attained, science and art tend to coalesce in aesthetics, plasticity, and form. The greatest scientists are always artists as well.—Albert Einstein
With permission: As recalled by Mathematician, Archibald Henderson (from an article, *Henderson Recalls Shaw, Einstein Association*, in **Durham Morning Herald**,) August 21, 1955—AEA 33-257.

References

1. Suzuki M, Tadashi T, Lee P-L. The effect of nasal and oral breathing on airway collapsibility in patients with obstructive sleep apnea: Computational fluid dynamics analyses. PLOS ONE. 2020;15(4):e0231262. https://doi.org/10.1371/journal.pone.0231262
2. Pedersen D. Topgun: an American story. New York: Hachette; 2019.
3. Johnson CM Jr, Alsarraf R. The aging face: a systematic approach. Philadelphia: W.B. Saunders; 2002.
4. Stupak HD, Maas CS. New procedures in facial plastic surgery using botulinum toxin A. Facial Plast Surg Clin North Am. 2003;11(4):515–20.
5. Frankel AS, Kamer FM. Chemical browlift. Arch Otolaryngol Head Neck Surg. 1998;124(3):321–3.
6. Wong CH, Mendelson B. Newer understanding of specific anatomic targets in the aging face as applied to injectables: aging changes in the craniofacial skeleton and facial ligaments. Plast Reconstr Surg. 2015;136(5 Suppl):44S–8S.
7. Kang MS, Kang HG, Nam YS, Kim IB. Detailed anatomy of the retaining ligaments of the mandible for facial rejuvenation. Craniomaxillofac Surg. 2016;44(9):1126–30. https://doi.org/10.1016/j.jcms.2016.06.018. Epub 2016 Jun 23.
8. Li D, Wang X, Wu Y, Sun J, Li Q, Guo S, Jia Y, Murphy DK. A randomized, controlled, multicenter study of Juvéderm Voluma for enhancement of malar volume in Chinese subjects. Plast Reconstr Surg. 2017;139(6):1250e–9e.
9. https://www.sec.gov/Archives/edgar/data/200406/000095015711000267/form425.htm.
10. Nasser M, Fedorowicz Z, Ebadifar A. Management of the fractured edentulous atrophic mandible. Cochrane Database Syst Rev. 2007;(1):CD006087. Review. Update in: Cochrane Database Syst Rev. 2013.
11. Nasser M, Pandis N, Fleming PS, Fedorowicz Z, Ellis E, Ali K. Interventions for the management of mandibular fractures. Cochrane Database Syst Rev. 2013;(7):CD006087.
12. Ellis E 3rd. Open reduction and internal fixation of combined angle and body/symphysis fractures of the mandible: how much fixation is enough? J Oral Maxillofac Surg. 2013;71(4):726–33.
13. Ellis E III, Miles BA. Fractures of the mandible: a technical perspective. Plast Reconstr Surg. 2007;120(7):76S–89S.
14. Demesh D, Leonard JA, Schechter CB, Dhillon P, Hsueh W, Stupak H. Evaluation of a vertical box plating technique for mandibular body fractures and retrospective analysis of patient outcomes. JAMA Facial Plast Surg. 2019;21(4):271–6.
15. Humphrey CD, Kriet JD. Simplifying mandible fracture repair. JAMA Facial Plast Surg. 2019;21(4):276–7.
16. Hsueh WD, Schechter CB, Tien Shaw I, Stupak HD. Comparison of intraoral and extraoral approaches to mandibular angle fracture repair with cost implications. Laryngoscope. 2016;126(3):591–5.
17. Torre C, Guilleminault C. Establishment of nasal breathing should be the ultimate goal to secure adequate craniofacial and airway development in children. J Pediatr. 2018;94(2):101–3.

Appendix: Notes on Severity of the Upper Respiratory Infection in the Covid-19 Era (Interplay of Ambient Humidity and Mouth-Breathing)

Highlights Ambient humidity and mouth-breathing may be synergistic in the genesis of the upper respiratory infection (URI) after eposure.

- Mucosal barrier disruption (MBD) may be the inciting cause of the URI.
- Chronic airway inflammation and related clinical conditions from sinusitis to tonsillitis may be related to MBD.

In the development of the upper respiratory infection (URI), the the prediction of severity of disease is not only based on the degree of exposure to a pathogen (e.g Covid-19), but also on host factors beyond the status of the general immune system. In the period just prior to the pandemic, several landmark experimental reports permit a better understanding of the physical factors that may be also important in cause and effect in URI severity.

First, in 2018, Christian Guilleminault and colleagues showed in a study of nearly 7000 patients that rhinosinusitus, otitis, and antibiotic usage were highly associated with sleep-related reported mouth-breathing [1]. Second, in early 2019, a team at Yale University using experiments in a mouse model explained the link between the seasonality of URI (influenza in this case) and their tendency to be associated with cold, dry (low ambient humidity) periods: disruption of the upper respiratory mucous membrane barrier and mucociliary transport system [2].

Instead of the URI simply representing the invasion of host airway tissue by pathogens, URI may be *initially* incited by a mucosal barrier disruption (MBD) caused by the desiccation of the airway mucous membranes from a potential synergistic combination of environmental dryness (decreased relative humidity) and exposure (nocturnal mouth-breathing). This is even further supported by a study that contradicts the prevailing belief that the reason for influenza's increased prevalence in low humidity environments is due to increased viral aerosol stabilization. In the third landmark study also from 2018, a research team demonstrated that "viruses remain highly stable and infectious in aerosols across a wide range of relative humidities" [3].

© Springer Nature Switzerland AG 2020
H. D. Stupak, *Rethinking Rhinoplasty and Facial Surgery*,
https://doi.org/10.1007/978-3-030-44674-1

Acceptance of the conventional concept may be incomplete, especially that beyond "presence of comorbidities", little explanation is usually given for why some patients develop severe respiratory infection while others remain completely asymptomatic. One cannot help but question the comprehensiveness of this paradigm when we consider that there is so much variability in the development of disease in individuals, especially those who fail to develop disease when "exposed" and in response to treatment.

In other words, in the spectrum from the "common cold" to deaths from influenza or Covid-19, the physical breach of the airway mucosal barrier may be as important as host immune factors and pathogen load and aggressiveness in the determination of URI disease and outcome.

This alternative paradigm rests on the concept that instead of the pathogen itself being the root cause of the URI, physical/environmental forces acting on the host airway cause the mucosal barrier disruption. Then, pathogen invasion is permitted, with eventual pathogen proliferation and onset of classic disease. By deepening our understanding of the nature of these MBD forces, in addition to knowledge of pathogens and their treatment, we can consider low-cost/low-risk barrier protecting interventions.

Airway MBD may be initiated primarily by the synergistic forces of ambient humidity and exposure-induced dehydration or mechanical barometric disruption of the mucosa. Thus, the risk of URI and its outcome will be related to mucosal hydration status combined with the extent of mechanical disruption.

The hydration status of the airway mucosal barrier and its function "depends strongly on the humidity and heat in the inhaled air, the exposure time, and the health of the individual" [4]. The extent of exposure is determined by the route of breathing (nasal versus oral). Pure mouth-breathing will expose the wet mucosa to drier environmental air when compared to pure nasal breathing (more mucosal humidification) [5]. Thus, the hydration status of the mucosa may be determined primarily by the ambient/environmental humidity and the tendency for an individual to utilize primarily oral breathing. This could explain why most URIs, including influenza,and possibly Covid-19 are most apparent in the low humidity winter months where indoor heating systems dehydrate the room air. In contrast, in overly high humidity seasons/regions, barrier disruption can be due to *excess* pharyngeal water vapor, as in tropical climates, influenza peaks during high humidity [6]. In regions of very high humidity, fungal infections are endemic, not because of the prevalence of the fungus, but because essentially of the presence of excess moisture present in the airways.

Further, mechanical disruption of the mucosal barrier can be due to high levels of negative pharyngeal pressure, which builds up in the airway due to inspiration with partial upper airway obstruction. Typically, this occurs intermittently during low-tone sleep stages where due to relaxation of jaw and tongue musculature (that normally counter the effects of gravitational forces) the mouth opens, releasing the tongue into the airway and causing obstruction (aka sleep disordered breathing

[SDB] or obstructive sleep apnea [OSA]) and generating negative pressure build-up in the airway [7]. This negative pressure stretches the mucosa intra-luminally, creating focal micro-traumas upon the mucosa and resulting in the typical inflammatory response found in tonsillar, adenoid, and uvular specimen [8]. In addition, exacerbation of the disease in the upper airways can cause a build-up of negative pressure in the lower airways and alveoli, causing alveolar "stress" with eventual alveolar collapse and clinical scenario of severe acute respiratory distress. These focal areas of negative pressure–induced inflammation, if also undergoing desiccation from low ambient humidity, can become the breach-point for MBD [9].

Temporally, after pathogen exposure, the acute onset of any of these conditions (i.e., winter humidity or temporary predisposition to mouth-breathing) could induce an acute URI, while chronic exacerbations of these conditions (i.e., long-term diminished tone in the setting of elevated BMI resulting in increased OSA/SDB severity with long-term mouth-breathing) can result in chronic, or severe symptoms. An acute flu-like systemic illness could result if the barrier-breach lacks a regionally built-up immune response (like Waldeyer's ring) while systemic illness can be limited by the build-up of chronic regional immune response from chronic exposure.

Anatomic location of the MBD can be predicted as well using the "tube law" of collapsible pipes. Negative pressure build-up in the airway maximally exerts its effects on collapsing the soft mucosal sidewalls in an inward fashion at a location *just distal* from the *inspiratory* obstruction. Thus, with septal deviation or nostril narrowing, sinus mucosal in-drawing will manifest, while with nocturnal palatal collapse, the mucosal in-stretching will occur in the pharynx. More downstream obstruction, with tongue collapse in more severe sleep apnea patients (i.e, with elevated BMI), will mount excess negative pressure in the lower airways, making this area prone to MBD.

In summary, MBD may be due to the interplay of humidity-induced mucosal dehydration and mechanical damage due to negative pressure build-up in the airway during sleep from mouth-breathing/OSA/SDB. The anatomic location and temporality of URI may depend on the acuity of onset of these forces and location of maximal airway collapse, respectively.

In addition to exposure reduction strategies like social distancing, etc, patients can be redirected to attempt mucosal barrier restoration using manipulation of environmental humidity (e.g., check and adjust room humidity to 40–60%) as well as encouraging mechanical techniques to reduce mouth-breathing via mouth-closure combined with nasal dilation and OSA treatment, but more evidence is required to confirm these findings. Putting these concepts together, a severity index for respiratory infections, where the probability of severe disease is calculated for individuals or populations could be roughly equivalent to: Severity Index = Exposure (number of human contacts) × Airway Tone (Age × BMI) × Inhaled toxin exposure (pack years)/outdoor temperature as a surrogate for indoor humidity.

References

1. Kukwa W, Guilleminault C, Tomaszewska M, Kukwa A, Krzeski A, Migacz E. Prevalence of upper respiratory tract infections in habitually snoring and mouth breathing children. Int J Pediatr Otorhinolaryngol. 2018;107:37–41.
2. Kudo E, Song E, Yockey LJ, Rakib T, Wong PW, Homer RJ, Iwasaki A. Low ambient humidity impairs barrier function and innate resistance against influenzainfection. Proc Natl Acad Sci U S A. 2019;116(22):10905–10.
3. Kormuth KA, Lin K, Prussin AJ, Vejerano EP, Tiwari AJ, Cox SS, Myerburg MM, Lakdawala SS, Marr LC. Influenza virus infectivity is retained in aerosols and droplets independent of relative humidity. J Infect Dis. 2018;218(5):739–47.
4. Williams R, Rankin N, Smith T, Galler D, Seakins P. Relationship between the humidity and temperature of inspired gas and the function of the airway mucosa. Crit Care Med. 1996;24(11):1920–7.
5. Tamerius JD, Shaman J, Alonso WH, et al. Environmental predictors of seasonal influenza epidemics across temperate and tropical climates. PLoS Pathog. 2013;9(3):e1003194.
6. Naclerio RM, Pinto J, Assanasen P, Baroody FM. Observations on the ability of the nose to warm and humidify inspired air. Rhinology. 2007;45(2):102–11.
7. Zang HR, Li LF, Zhou B, Li YC, Wang T, Han DM. Pharyngeal aerodynamic characteristics of obstructive sleep apnea/hypopnea syndrome patients. Chin Med J. 2012;125(17):3039.
8. Almendros I, Carreras A, Ramírez J, Montserrat JM, Navajas D, Farré R. Upper airway collapse and reopening induce inflammation in a sleep apnoea model. Eur Respir J. 2008;32(2):399–404.
9. Ference RS, Leonard JA, Stupak HD. Physiologic model for seasonal patterns in flu transmission. Laryngoscope. 2020;130(2):309–13.

Index

© Springer Nature Switzerland AG 2020
H. D. Stupak, *Rethinking Rhinoplasty and Facial Surgery*,
https://doi.org/10.1007/978-3-030-44674-1